1992
YEAR BOOK OF
VASCULAR SURGERY®

The 1992 Year Book® Series

Year Book of Anesthesia and Pain Management: Drs. Miller, Kirby, Ostheimer, Roizen, and Stoelting

Year Book of Cardiology®: Drs. Schlant, Collins, Engle, Frye, Kaplan, and O'Rourke

Year Book of Critical Care Medicine®: Drs. Rogers and Parrillo

Year Book of Dentistry®: Drs. Meskin, Currier, Kennedy, Leinfelder, Matukas, and Rovin

Year Book of Dermatologic Surgery: Drs. Swanson, Salasche, and Glogau

Year Book of Dermatology®: Drs. Sober and Fitzpatrick

Year Book of Diagnostic Radiology®: Drs. Federle, Clark, Gross, Madewell, Maynard, Sackett, and Young

Year Book of Digestive Diseases®: Drs. Greenberger and Moody

Year Book of Drug Therapy®: Drs. Lasagna and Weintraub

Year Book of Emergency Medicine®: Drs. Wagner, Burdick, Davidson, Roberts, and Spivey

Year Book of Endocrinology®: Drs. Bagdade, Braverman, Horton, Kannan, Landsberg, Molitch, Morley, Odell, Rogol, Ryan, and Sherwin

Year Book of Family Practice®: Drs. Berg, Bowman, Davidson, Dietrich, and Scherger

Year Book of Geriatrics and Gerontology®: Drs. Beck, Abrass, Burton, Cummings, Makinodan, and Small

Year Book of Hand Surgery®: Drs. Amadio and Hentz

Year Book of Health Care Management: Drs. Heyssel, Brock, King, and Steinberg, Ms. Avakian, and Messrs. Berman, Kues, and Rosenberg

Year Book of Hematology®: Drs. Spivak, Bell, Ness, Quesenberry, and Wiernik

Year Book of Infectious Diseases®: Drs. Wolff, Barza, Keusch, Klempner, and Snydman

Year Book of Infertility: Drs. Mishell, Paulsen, and Lobo

Year Book of Medicine®: Drs. Rogers, Bone, Cline, Braunwald, Greenberger, Utiger, Epstein, and Malawista

Year Book of Neonatal and Perinatal Medicine: Drs. Klaus and Fanaroff

Year Book of Nephrology®: Drs. Coe, Favus, Henderson, Kashgarian, Luke, Myers, and Strom

Year Book of Neurology and Neurosurgery®: Drs. Currier and Crowell

Year Book of Neuroradiology: Drs. Osborn, Harnsberger, Halbach, and Grossman

Year Book of Nuclear Medicine®: Drs. Hoffer, Gore, Gottschalk, Sostman, Zaret, and Zubal

Year Book of Obstetrics and Gynecology®: Drs. Mishell, Kirschbaum, and Morrow

Year Book of Occupational and Environmental Medicine: Drs. Emmett, Brooks, Harris, and Schenker

Year Book of Oncology: Drs. Young, Longo, Ozols, Simone, Steele, and Weichselbaum

Year Book of Ophthalmology®: Drs. Laibson, Adams, Augsberger, Benson, Cohen, Eagle, Flanagan, Nelson, Reinecke, Sergott, and Wilson

Year Book of Orthopedics®: Drs. Sledge, Poss, Cofield, Frymoyer, Griffin, Hansen, Johnson, Simmons, and Springfield

Year Book of Otolaryngology–Head and Neck Surgery®: Drs. Bailey and Paparella

Year Book of Pathology and Clinical Pathology®: Drs. Gardner, Bennett, Cousar, Garvin, and Worsham

Year Book of Pediatrics®: Dr. Stockman

Year Book of Plastic, Reconstructive, and Aesthetic Surgery: Drs. Miller, Cohen, McKinney, Robson, Ruberg, and Whitaker

Year Book of Podiatric Medicine and Surgery®: Dr. La Porta

Year Book of Psychiatry and Applied Mental Health®: Drs. Talbott, Frances, Freedman, Meltzer, Perry, Schowalter, and Yudofsky

Year Book of Pulmonary Disease®: Drs. Bone and Petty

Year Book of Speech, Language, and Hearing: Drs. Bernthal, Hall, and Tomblin

Year Book of Sports Medicine®: Drs. Shephard, Eichner, Sutton, and Torg, Col. Anderson, and Mr. George

Year Book of Surgery®: Drs. Schwartz, Jonasson, Robson, Shires, Spencer, and Thompson

Year Book of Transplantation: Drs. Ascher, Hansen, and Strom

Year Book of Ultrasound: Drs. Merritt, Mittelstaedt, Carroll, and Nyberg

Year Book of Urology®: Drs. Gillenwater and Howards

Year Book of Vascular Surgery®: Dr. Bergan

Roundsmanship '92–'93: A Year Book® Guide to Clinical Medicine: Drs. Dan, Feigin, Quilligan, Schrock, Stein, and Talbott

1992

The Year Book of VASCULAR SURGERY®

Editor

John J. Bergan, M.D., F.A.C.S., Hon. F.R.C.S. (Eng)
Clinical Professor of Surgery, University of California, San Diego; Clinical Professor of Surgery, Uniformed Services, University of Health Sciences, Washington, D.C.; Professor of Surgery, Emeritus, Northwestern University Medical School, Chicago

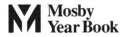

Mosby Year Book

St. Louis   Baltimore   Boston   Chicago   London   Philadelphia   Sydney   Toronto

Editor-in-Chief, Year Book Publishing: Kenneth H. Killion
Sponsoring Editor: Linda Steiner
Manager, Literature Services: Edith M. Podrazik
Senior Information Specialist: Terri Santo
Senior Medical Writer: David A. Cramer, M.D.
Assistant Director, Manuscript Services: Frances M. Perveiler
Associate Managing Editor, Year Book Editing Services: Elizabeth Fitch
Editorial Assistant: Tamara L. Smith
Production Coordinator: Max F. Perez
Proofroom Manager: Barbara M. Kelly

Copyright © April 1992 by Mosby–Year Book, Inc.
A Year Book Medical Publishers imprint of Mosby–Year Book, Inc.

Mosby–Year Book, Inc.
11830 Westline Industrial Drive
St. Louis, MO 63146

Editorial Office:
Mosby–Year Book, Inc.
200 North LaSalle St.
Chicago, IL 60601

International Standard Serial Number: 0749-4041
International Standard Book Number: 0-8151-0681-5

Contributing Editors

Alexander W. Clowes, M.D.
Professor of Surgery, University of Washington, Seattle
Ralph G. DePalma, M.D.
Professor and Chairman, Department of Surgery, George Washington University Medical Center, Washington, D.C.
Lazar J. Greenfield, M.D.
Professor and Chairman, Department of Surgery, University of Michigan Medical School, Ann Arbor, Michigan
Roger M. Greenhalgh, M.A., M.D., MChir, F.A.C.S.
Charing-Cross and Westminster Medical School, London
Kaj Johanssen, M.D.
Professor of Surgery, University of Washington, Seattle
Steven L. Moulton, M.D.
Surgical Resident, Department of Surgery, University of California
Charles S. O'Mara, M.D.
Clinical Assistant, Professor of Surgery, University of Mississippi School of Medicine; Chief of Surgery, Mississippi Baptist Medical Center, Jackson
Shirley M. Otis, M.D.
Head, Division of Neurology, Scripps Clinic and Research Foundation, La Jolla, California
David Rosenthal, M.D.
Clinical Professor of Surgery, Medical College of Georgia, Atlanta

Table of Contents

The material covered in this volume represents literature reviewed through June 1991.

Journals Represented

Mosby–Year Book subscribes to and surveys nearly 900 U.S. and foreign medical and allied health journals. From these journals, the Editors select the articles to be abstracted. Journals represented in this YEAR BOOK are listed below.

Acta Chirurgica Scandinavica
Acta Obstetricia et Gynecologica Scandinavica
American Heart Journal
American Journal of Cardiology
American Journal of Diseases of Children
American Journal of Emergency Medicine
American Journal of Gastroenterology
American Journal of Human Genetics
American Journal of Medicine
American Journal of Neuroradiology
American Journal of Pathology
American Journal of Roentgenology
American Journal of Surgery
American Surgeon
Angiology
Annales de Radiologie
Annals of Emergency Medicine
Annals of Internal Medicine
Annals of Surgery
Annals of Thoracic Surgery
Annals of Vascular Surgery
Annals of the Royal College of Surgeons of England
Archives of Dermatology
Archives of Internal Medicine
Archives of Neurology
Archives of Otolaryngology–Head and Neck Surgery
Archives of Physical Medicine and Rehabilitation
Archives of Surgery
Arteriosclerosis and Thrombosis
Artificial Organs
Atherosclerosis
British Journal of Radiology
British Journal of Surgery
British Medical Journal
Canadian Journal of Surgery
Cancer
Cardiology
Catheterization and Cardiovascular Diagnosis
Chest
Chirurg
Circulation
Circulation Research
Clinical Imaging
Clinical Orthopaedics and Related Research
Clinical Radiology
Complications in Surgery
Critical Care Medicine
European Journal of Obstetrics, Gynecology, and Reproductive Biology

European Journal of Surgery
European Journal of Vascular Surgery
Gastroenterology
Head and Neck
Histopathology
Human Pathology
Infections in Surgery
International Angiology
Israel Journal of Medical Sciences
Journal de Chirurgie
Journal de Radiologie
Journal of Biomechanics
Journal of Bone and Joint Surgery (American Volume)
Journal of Cardiovascular Surgery
Journal of Clinical Investigation
Journal of Dermatologic Surgery and Oncology
Journal of Hand Surgery (American)
Journal of Interventional Radiology
Journal of Neurology
Journal of Thoracic Imaging
Journal of Thoracic and Cardiovascular Surgery
Journal of Trauma
Journal of Urology
Journal of Vascular Surgery
Journal of the American Academy of Dermatology
Journal of the American College of Cardiology
Journal of the American Geriatrics Society
Journal of the American Medical Association
Journal of the Neurological Sciences
Journal of the Royal College of Surgeons of Edinburgh
Laboratory Investigation
Magnetic Resonance Imaging
Mayo Clinic Proceedings
Metabolism
Neurology
Neurosurgery
New England Journal of Medicine
New York State Journal of Medicine
Plastic and Reconstructive Surgery
Postgraduate Medical Journal
Presse Medicale
Proceedings of the National Academy of Sciences
Quarterly Journal of Medicine
ROFO: Fortschritte Auf Dem Gebiete Der Rontgenstrahlen Und Der
Nuklearmedizin
Radiology
Revue Neurologique
S.A.M.J./S.A.M.T.—South African Medical Journal
Scandinavian Journal of Clinical and Laboratory Investigation
Scandinavian Journal of Rehabilitation Medicine
Semaine des Hopitaux
Southern Medical Journal

Stroke
Surgery
Surgery, Gynecology and Obstetrics
Surgical Research Communications
Thorax
Ultrasound in Medicine and Biology
VASA: Zeitschrift fur Gefasskrankheiten
Virchows Archiv A: Pathological Anatomy and Histopathology
Western Journal of Medicine

STANDARD ABBREVIATIONS

The following terms are abbreviated in this edition: acquired immunodeficiency syndrome (AIDS), central nervous system (CNS), cerebrospinal fluid (CSF), computed tomography (CT), electrocardiography (ECG), human immunodeficiency virus (HIV), and magnetic resonance (MR) imaging (MRI).

Publisher's Preface

Publication of this volume of the YEAR BOOK OF VASCULAR SURGERY marks the end of an outstanding era of editorship by John J. Bergan, M.D., who co-edited this publication since its inception in 1986 with James S. T. Yao, M.D., Ph.D., through the 1991 edition, and served as solo editor for the 1992 edition.

During their term as editors, Drs. Bergan and Yao provided YEAR BOOK readers with discerning and informative literature selections and editorial commentary of the highest caliber. We, on our part, have been treated to a most enjoyable association. We extend our sincere thanks to them and to their Board of Contributing Editors for the service they have provided and for their ever-present commitment to the YEAR BOOK.

Beginning with the 1993 YEAR BOOK OF VASCULAR SURGERY, John M. Porter, M.D., Professor of Surgery, Oregon Health Sciences University, will edit this publication. We welcome Dr. Porter, while we extend our heartfelt thanks and appreciation to Drs. Bergan and Yao and their colleagues for their many years of excellent service.

As publishers, we feel challenged to seek ways of presenting complex information in a clear and readable manner. To this end, the 1992 YEAR BOOK OF VASCULAR SURGERY now provides structured abstracts in which the various components of a study can easily be identified through headings. These headings are not the same in all abstracts but, rather, are those that most accurately designate the content of each particular journal article. We are confident that our readers will find the information contained in our abstracts to be more accessible than ever before. We welcome your comments.

Introduction

Medical science, including vascular surgery, exhibits progress according to the laws of wave theory. First, there is an accumulation of observed facts. This is followed by a tumultuous cresting as new developments based on new observations are presented. Then there is a smooth decline of progress to a placid interval in which a consolidation of activity occurs. This interval precedes the next swell of observations. Frequently, during accumulation of new facts, the old ideas are revisited and recycled. Some of these even masquerade as new thoughts. In contrast, new technology frequently brings truly legitimate and authentically new observations to light. The 1992 YEAR BOOK OF VASCULAR SURGERY demonstrates all of these phenomena.

The first 2 years of this past decade of the 20th century could be characterized as a time of consolidation of ideas in vascular surgery. The flurry of new observations that surrounded the introduction of endovascular techniques in the 1980s was replaced by a period of watchful waiting in the '90s. During the furious application of laser technology and the distal extension of balloon angioplasty and atherectomy activity that followed, the old specter of myointimal hyperplasia as a response to arterial wall injury surfaced once again. It first appeared as a shadow on the horizon and then rapidly enlarged to obscure the entire frontier and bring to a sharp halt the progress in endovascular techniques.

Previous editions of the YEAR BOOK stands in contrast. Instead, the chapter titled Basic Considerations introduces the new observations that we hope, will lead to control of myointimal hyperplasia. This, in turn, would lead to a reopening of the field of minimal interventional surgery and allow treatment of the minimal symptoms of arterial occlusive disease.

In contrast to the shutting down of the field of endovascular surgery, the arena of vascular imaging has become heavily populated. Many imaging techniques compete for the attention of the clinical vascular surgeon. Which of these techniques will emerge to become definitive is uncertain. However, it will probably be the technique that is totally noninvasive and causes no side effects, yet produces clear, sharp-edged, high-contrast visualizations of the arterial wall and vascular abnormalities. Increasingly, it appears that the competition will be between MRI and ultrasound imaging. If this is true, then cost considerations will favor the application of ultrasound.

The vineyard of arterial reconstruction is where vascular surgeons till the soil. Here there is a distinct consolidation of activity. Carotid surgery has returned to the operating theater, and indications for its use have become increasingly clarified. Although basic scientific research in aortic aneurysm development has not reduced the need for surgical correction of this entity, it has produced a heightened interest. Furthermore, experience with the management of ruptured abdominal aortic aneurysms has delivered the uncomfortable truth that a hasty transport to the operating room and swift surgery by an experienced team does not reduce the mortality rate. Instead, a higher figure is produced, reflecting the larger number of premorbid patients who undergo surgery. The inescapable conclusion to be derived from this is that aneurysm screening must develop. Individuals at risk must have their aortic aneurysms detected and treated before symptoms occur.

Perhaps the most significant contribution of modern vascular surgery is the prevention of amputation and its disability. To accomplish this, vascular surgery has proceeded more distally—even onto the plantar vessels themselves. On the treatment team, including a plastic surgeon, with his knowledge of free tissue transfer techniques and microscopic anastomoses, is of further help in the prevention of amputation. This is true especially in the management of diabetic patients with infectious tissue necrosis as well as ischemic necrosis.

During this time of consolidation in vascular surgery, this founding editor of the YEAR BOOK OF VASCULAR SURGERY is taking advantage of the relative placidity of the trough between cresting waves and is passing the baton to John Porter's competent hands. It was thrilling indeed in 1984 to receive the invitation from Year Book Medical Publishers, Inc. to produce the first YEAR BOOK OF VASCULAR SURGERY. Subsequently, the increasing acceptance of the YEAR BOOK as a source of information was most heartening. Comments made to me by friends, and even strangers, reinforced the idea that the YEAR BOOK was a resource of information that made good reading at bedtime or during cross-country travel, and even provided occasional amusement.

Now that the YEAR BOOK is totally accepted and has a stable base of subscribers, it can look forward to further growth in the next century. Therefore, it seems appropriate for me to step aside. This is done with the firm conviction that John Porter, M.D., the new editor, and his staff will carry the banner of the YEAR BOOK forward in exemplary fashion. May God speed their work and guide future developments in our chosen field of vascular surgery.

John J. Bergan, M.D.

1 Basic Considerations

Epidemiology of Some Peripheral Arterial Findings in Diabetic Men and Women: Experiences from the Framingham Study
Abbott RD, Brand FN, Kannel WB (Univ of Virginia; Boston Univ)
Am J Med 88:376–381, 1990   1–1

Introduction.—There is evidence from the Framingham Study that diabetes is an important risk factor of peripheral arterial disease in the lower extremities. However, the effect of diabetes on peripheral arterial disease at other locations has not been well documented. Therefore, a study was designed to investigate the relationship between diabetes and carotid bruits, femoral bruits, and nonpalpable pedal pulses. The study also assessed the cardiovascular prognosis associated with these 3 arterial findings.

Patients.—The study population consisted of 1,196 men and 1,582 women who had been followed for 20 years as part of the Framingham study. A total of 169 men and 175 women had diabetes; in 60 men and 55 women the disease was diagnosed after follow-up began. The average age at the start of follow-up was 61.8 years for men without diabetes, 64 years for men with diabetes, 65.2 years for women without diabetes, and 62.1 years for women with diabetes.

Results.—Among the men and women without diabetes, the incidence of carotid bruits and nonpalpable pedal pulses increased significantly with age, but without any apparent difference for gender. In contrast, the diabetic men and women had an increased risk of all 3 peripheral arterial conditions, regardless of age. Compared with women without diabetes, the women with diabetes had a nearly twofold excess of femoral bruits and a 50% excess of nonpalpable pedal pulses. Among the men, the presence of diabetes nearly doubled the risk of carotid bruits. Men and women with both diabetes and symptoms of peripheral arterial disease had an especially high risk of incident cardiovascular events. The nonpalpable pedal pulses were associated with more than a twofold excess of coronary heart disease and stroke in diabetic women and more than a twofold excess of coronary heart disease and cardiac failure in diabetic men. Femoral bruits in diabetic men doubled the risk of coronary heart disease.

Conclusion.—The increased risk of acute cardiovascular events in diabetic patients is further enhanced by the presence of peripheral arterial disease. Diabetic patients should therefore be carefully monitored for signs of peripheral arterial disease by examining the peripheral arterial pulses and checking for the presence of carotid and femoral bruits.

▶ It seems remarkable that the tremendous effort of the Framingham study has yielded so little information on peripheral arterial occlusive disease and its manifestations. Perhaps the input of knowledge from a clinical vascular surgeon would be of help to the researchers who continue to analyze the data obtained in that study.

Relationship of Atherosclerosis in Young Men to Serum Lipoprotein Cholesterol Concentrations and Smoking: A Preliminary Report From the Pathobiological Determinants of Atherosclerosis in Youth (PDAY) Research Group

Pathobiological Determinants of Atherosclerosis in Youth (PDAY) Research Group (Univ of Texas; San Antonio)
JAMA 264:3018–3024, 1990   1–2

Background.—Predictors of frank coronary heart disease such as serum lipid and lipoprotein levels are associated with aortic and coronary artery atherosclerosis in adults. This relationship has rarely been examined in young indivduals, despite the fact that atherosclerosis begins in these sites during childhood. A large-scale collaborative study (14 centers) examined the relationships of serum cholesterol and smoking to atherosclerosis in teens and young adults.

Methods.—The series included 390 young men (217 white, 173 black; age, 15–34 years) who had died of violent causes within 72 hours of injury. At autopsy, a longitudinal half of the aorta and the right coronary artery (RCA) were fixed for shipment to a central facility where they were analyzed visually. Pathologists estimated the expanse of intimal surface involved with fatty streaks and raised lesions. The raised lesions included fibrous plaques (greatest percentage), rare complicated lesions (plaques with hemorrhage, thrombosis, or ulceration), and calcified lesions. Frozen serum was analyzed centrally for thiocyanate level (a reliable indicator of smoking) and for cholesterol, high-density-lipoprotein cholesterol (HDL-C), and very-low-density-lipoprotein plus low-density-lipoprotein cholesterol (VLDL + LDL-C).

Results.—Young white males had significantly higher serum cholesterol levels than blacks. This was accounted for by significantly higher VLDL + LDL-C and lower HDL-C levels. The prevalence of smoking and the VLDL + LDL-C levels increased with age in both races. The percentages of intimal surface area involved in both total and raised lesions increased significantly with age for both groups in the abdominal aorta (AA) and RCA, and the surface area of raised lesions increased in the thoracic aorta (TA). The high VLDL + LDL-C levels were positively correlated with increasing lesion extent in the AA and RCA. Smoking predicted the prevalence of raised lesions in the AA and RCA. Except for total lesions in the TA, increasing age was the best predictor of lesion extent. Except for a greater prevalence of raised lesions in the RCA in whites, blacks had more lesions than whites.

Discussion.—This study provided the first evidence in individuals less than 25 years of age that smoking is associated with severe aortic atherosclerosis. The evident early relationship between high serum lipoprotein levels and lesion development in the aorta and coronary arteries sustains the argument that hyperlipidemia in the young will promote atherosclerosis. A greater prevalence of aortic lesions in young blacks compared with young whites confirms the results of previous studies. The racial relationship is reportedly reversed in older adults, and risk factors for coronary heart disease may be different in the 2 races.

▶ As indicated in this study, more research must be done on arterial occlusive disease in young adults. Although the vascular surgeon's interest has been confined to exploration of the causes of claudication in young individuals (especially young athletes), an enormously fertile field awaits cultivation in the study of atherosclerotic occlusive disease in the peripheral arteries of young individuals.

Lowering Cholesterol Concentrations and Mortality: A Quantitative Review of Primary Prevention Trials
Muldoon MF, Manuck SB, Matthews KA (Univ of Pittsburgh)
Br Med J 301:309–314, 1990   1–3

Objective.—Dietary or pharmacological reduction of serum cholesterol levels has been shown in several large clinical trials to diminish the frequency of coronary heart disease events—but only 1 study has demonstrated reduced mortality. Whether cholesterol reduction actually extends survival was determined by using the statistical technique of meta-analysis to combine the results of multiple randomized clinical primary prevention trials of serum cholesterol level reduction.

Methods.—Six studies that included 24,847 participants with a mean age of 47.5 years met the criteria for inclusion in the meta-analysis. All 6 studies were randomized clinical primary prevention trials that had found serum cholesterol levels to be significantly lower in a treatment group with dietary or pharmacological control of cholesterol, compared with a control group. Both total and cause-specific deaths were reported. Only data on males were included.

Results.—During the 119,000 person-years of follow-up, 1,147 mortalities occurred. There was no significant difference between cholesterol treatment and control groups in overall mortality. The tendency for lower mortality caused by coronary heart disease in men who received cholesterol-lowering treatment was borderline in significance; a highly significant, interesting finding was that the men in this group had double the mortality rate from causes not related to illness, that is, from accidents, suicide, or violence. The latter finding held in both individual studies and the meta-analysis. Lowering the serum cholesterol levels did not significantly increase the risk of death resulting from cancer.

Conclusions.—The results of this large-scale meta-analysis corroborate those of several individual studies—lowering serum cholesterol levels does not reduce overall mortality. Although there may be a modest reduction in the deaths caused by coronary heart disease in men with lowered serum cholesterol levels, this advantage is offset by a robust increase in the death rate resulting from other causes. The latter finding merits further investigation.

▶ The results of this large meta-analysis are disappointing. One could sense from previous information that, despite intensive intervention, regression of atherosclerotic lesions was difficult to prove. Now it seems that concentrating treatment on lowering the plasma lipids is relatively ineffective. This therapy should be categorized with the use of aspirin in the prevention of stroke.

Effect of Partial Ileal Bypass Surgery on Mortality and Morbidity From Coronary Heart Disease in Patients With Hypercholesterolemia: Report of the Program on the Surgical Control of the Hyperlipidemias (POSCH)
Buchwald H, Varco RL, Matts JP, Long JM, Fitch LL, Campbell GS, Pearce MB, Yellin AE, Edmiston WA, Smink RD Jr, Sawin HS Jr, Campos CT, Hansen BJ, Tuna N, Karnegis JN, Sanmarco ME, Amplatz K, Castaneda-Zuniga WR, Hunter DW, Bissett JK, Weber FJ, Stevenson JW, Leon AS, Chalmers TC and the POSCH Group (Univ of Minnesota; Univ of Arkansas; Univ of Southern California, Los Angeles; Lankenau Hosp and Research Ctr, Philadelphia; Univ of Nebraska; et al)
N Engl J Med 323:946–955, 1990   1–4

Objective.—The Program on the Surgical Control of the Hyperlipidemias (POSCH) is a randomized trial intended to demonstrate whether partial ileal bypass can lessen the overall morbidity and mortality from coronary heart disease by lowering the serum level of cholesterol. Surgery was performed in 421 of 838 patients who had survived a first myocardial infarction. Most of the group (90%) were men; the average age was 51 years. The patients were followed for a mean of nearly 10 years. Sur-

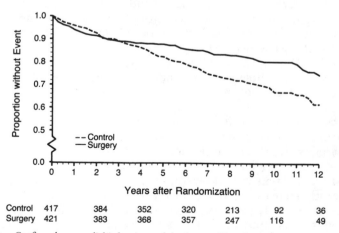

Control	417	384	352	320	213	92	36
Surgery	421	383	368	357	247	116	49

Fig 1–1.—Confirmed myocardial infarction and death caused by atherosclerotic coronary heart disease as a combined end point ("event") in the study groups. The difference between the groups was significant (*P* < .001). The numbers of patients at risk for an event are shown at 2-year intervals. (Courtesy of Buchwald H, Varco RL, Matts JP, et al: *N Engl J Med* 323:946–955, 1990.)

gery consisted of bypassing the distal 200 cm or the distal third of the small bowel, whichever was greater.

Findings.—Patients operated on had cholesterol levels that were 23% lower than those in control patients after 5 years. Their low-density-lipoprotein cholesterol was reduced by 38%, and their high-density-lipoprotein cholesterol level was 4% higher. The mortality from coronary heart disease was reduced, but not significantly, and the same was true for overall mortality. Nevertheless, death rates from coronary disease and nonfatal infarction were both reduced by 35% in the surgical group (Fig 1–1). Disease progression occurring up to 10 years after randomization was less marked in the surgical group. The ileal bypass caused no hospital deaths, and its chief side effect was diarrhea.

Conclusion.—Partial ileal bypass improves the blood lipids in patients who have had myocardial infarction and lowers the subsequent morbidity from coronary heart disease. The final role of this surgery remains uncertain, but the findings support the beneficial effects of lipid modification in countering the progression of atherosclerotic disease.

▶ As in Abstract 1–3, the relatively minor contribution of intensive lipid lowering to the survival of patients with established atherosclerotic occlusive disease is impressive. Although the procedure detailed in this report does reduce cardiac morbidity, the overall mortality and mortality caused by coronary heart disease were not significantly altered in the group as a whole compared with the control group.

Regression of Coronary Artery Disease as a Result of Intensive, Lipid-Lowering Therapy in Men With High Levels of Apolipoprotein B
Brown G, Albers JJ, Fisher LD, Schaefer SM, Lin J-T, Kaplan C, Zhao X-Q, Bisson BD, Fitzpatrick VF, Dodge HT (Univ of Washington)
N Engl J Med 323:1289–1298, 1990   1–5

Background.—With the advent of more effective therapies for hyperlipidemia, new arteriographic methods for assessing atherosclerosis, and new insights into atherogenesis, the question of whether progression of atherosclerosis can be retarded or reversed with treatment of hyperlipidemia can be addressed.

Study.—In a randomized, double-blind, placebo-controlled study, the effect of intensive lipid-lowering therapy on coronary atherosclerosis in men at high risk for cardiovascular events was assessed by quantitative arteriography. The series included 146 men, 62 years or younger, with elevated (>125 mg/dL) apolipoprotein B levels, documented coronary artery disease, and a family history of vascular disease, seen in a 2.5-year period.

Treatment.—The patients were given dietary counseling and assigned to 1 of 3 treatment groups: 20 mg of lovastatin twice a day and 10 mg of colestipol 3 times a day; 1 g of niacin 4 times a day and 10 g of colestipol 3 times a day; or conventional therapy with placebo [or colestipol if the low-density-lipoprotein cholesterol (LDL-C) level was elevated]. The primary end point was the average change between the initial and follow-up (after treatment) coronary arteriography in the percent stenosis of the worst lesion in each of 9 proximal segments.

Findings.—Among the 120 men who completed the study, the levels of LDL-C and high-density-lipoprotein cholesterol (HDL-C) changed only slightly in the conventional therapy group, but more substantially in the patients treated with levostatin and colestipol and in those treated with niacin and colestipol. Definite lesion progression as the only change occurred more frequently in conventionally treated patients (46%) than in those who received lovastatin and colestipol (21%) and niacin and colestipol (25%). Regression as the only change was uncommon in the conventionally treated patients (11%), whereas it was 3 times more common in the intensively treated patients (32% and 39%, respectively). Furthermore, intensive lipid-lowering therapy reduced the frequency of cardiovascular events such as death, myocardial infarction, or revascularization for worsening symptoms. Clinical events occurred in 3 of the 46 men treated with lovastatin and colestipol and in 2 of the 48 men who received niacin and colestipol, compared with 10 of the 52 men assigned to conventional therapy. Multivariate analysis showed that reduction in apolipoprotein B levels (or LDL-C) and systolic blood pressure, and increases in HDL-C correlated independently with regression of coronary lesions.

Conclusions.—Intensive lipid-lowering therapy in men with coronary artery disease who are at high risk for cardiovascular events appears to reduce the frequency of progression of coronary lesions, increase the frequency of regression, and reduce the incidence of cardiovascular events.

▶ This is another report confirming that intensive lipid-lowering therapy improves coronary arterial anatomy. A novel aspect of this study was the reduction of the apolipoprotein B levels. Although the study was not designed to assess the clinical outcomes, coronary events occurred in 10 of the 52 patients assigned to conventional therapy, compared with only 3 of the 46 assigned to receive lovastatin and colestipol and 2 of the 48 assigned to receive niacin and colestipol.

It is critical to note that substantial lipid changes were induced in the treatment groups, specifically −46% and −32% for LDL-C levels and +15% and +43% for HDL-C levels. These findings confirm the findings of previous reports, such as the CLAS Study (1), which showed statistically strong and consistent benefits to coronary anatomy after 2 years of lipid altering treatment. Similar results have been obtained by lowering LDL-C levels with the use of ileal bypass (2). These human results support previous long-term experimental observations in animals (3). The threshold reductions in the serum cholesterol level can affect anatomical changes in atherosclerotic plaques that result in less luminal intrusion. It now appears possible to achieve these effects on coronary plaques by diet and medical therapy in humans.—R. DePalma, M.D., Washington, D.C.

References

1. Blankenhorn DH, et al: *JAMA* 257:3233, 1987.
2. Buchwald H, et al: *N Engl J Med* 323:947, 1990.
3. DePalma RG, et al: *Surg Gynecol Obstet* 131:633, 1970.

n-3 Fatty Acids and Leukocyte Chemotaxis: Effects in Hyperlipidemia and Dose-Response Studies in Healthy Men

Schmidt EB, Pedersen JO, Varming K, Ernst E, Jersild C, Grunnet N, Dyerberg J (Aalborg Hosp, Denmark)
Arteriosclerosis Thrombosis 11:429–435, 1991   1–6

Background.—Dietary n-3 polyunsaturated fatty acids (n-3 PUFAs) may be valuable in the prevention of coronary artery disease (CAD). Dietary supplementation has been demonstrated to decrease the chemotactic response of monocytes and neutrophils in healthy men. The effect of dietary supplementation with n-3 PUFAs on monocytes and neutrophils was investigated in 17 patients with hyperlipidemia.

Technique.—The patients were administered 6 g of n-3 PUFAs daily for 6 weeks. Monocyte and neutrophil chemotaxis was analyzed before and after 6 weeks of supplementation, using the under-agarose assay, with autologous serum and N-formyl-methionyl-leucyl-phenylalanine as chemoattractions.

Results.—Patients with type IIa hyperlipidemia had increased monocyte chemotaxis before treatment. Dietary supplementation reduced chemotaxis in these patients but not in those with type IV hyperlipidemia.

Conclusion.—Dietary supplementation with low doses of n-3 PUFAs appears to have an effect on leukocyte chemotaxis. This may explain the observed antiatherosclerotic effect of low doses of n-3 PUFAs. The effect of dietary supplementation should be replicated in placebo-controlled studies.

▶ Increasingly, the role of leukocytes in atherogenesis and the progression of aneurysm disease has been recognized. Ross suggested this in his informative article in the *New England Journal of Medicine* in 1986, and his suggestion has led to fruitful research such as that done in this study (1). It is too early to tell where this research will lead us.

Reference

1. Ross R: *N Engl J Med* 314:488, 1986.

Immunohistochemical Characterization of Inflammatory Cells Associated With Advanced Atherosclerosis

Ramshaw AL, Parums DV (Univ of Oxford, England)
Histopathology 17:543–552, 1990   1–7

Background.—Chronic periaortitis (CPA), an infiltration of the aortic outer layer by immunoglobulin-secreting plasma cells and mononuclear cells that is associated with medial thinning, often attends advanced atherosclerosis. Although CPA may only be discerned histopathologically, severe CPA may produce clinical conditions described variously as "idio-

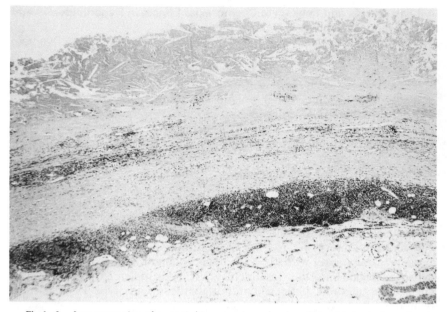

Fig 1–2.—Low-power view of an aortic biopsy specimen showing advanced intimal atherosclerosis, medial thinning, and a moderate aortic adventitial chronic inflammatory cell infiltrate consisting of lymphocytes, plasma cells, and macrophages, predominantly around the blood vessels. Hematoxylin-eosin. (Courtesy of Ramshaw AL, Parums DV: *Histopathology* 17:543–552, 1990.)

pathic retroperitoneal fibrosis," "inflammatory aneurysm," or "perianeurysmal retroperitoneal fibrosis." Atherosclerotic aneurysms may also show an underlying inflammatory process. Ceroid, which is composed of insoluble oxidized protein and lipid, is found in all progressed atherosclerotic plaques and is associated with IgG in plaques of patients with severe CPA. Antibodies to ceroid can always be found in the latter patients.

Methods.—Full-thickness biopsy specimens of the aortic wall were taken from 12 male patients during elective surgery to repair abdominal aortic aneurysms. Flash-frozen unfixed tissue was used for immunohistochemical studies and was labelled with monoclonal antibodies for leukocyte common antigen, B cells, and T cells. The presence of ceroid, varying degrees of aortic adventitial chronic inflammation, medial thinning, and the diagnosis of advanced intimal atherosclerosis were confirmed in fixed sections by standard histopathology (Fig 1–2).

Results.—Helper T cells and some T cytotoxic cells were found in both the aortic adventitia and in the atheromatous plaques. The helper T cells tended to surround the more dense, focal B cell accumulations; whereas the B cells, that constituted 60% of the total lymphocytes, were restricted to the outer layer of the aorta. An HLA-DR positive reaction was shown by all macrophages, most lymphocytes, and most vascular endothelial cells in the atheroma, media, and aortic adventitia. The proliferation of B cells and T cells was evidenced by Ki-67 staining. Sporadic activated lymphocytes were BerH2 positive.

Discussion.—The pattern of chronic inflammation described in these cases of CPA is consistent with an active, immunologically-mediated disease process. The lymphocytes in the adventitia stained with Ki-67 and BerH2 indicate that the inflammatory process is progressive. The presence of HLA-DR positive staining of the vascular smooth muscle cells suggests that these cells play a role in antigen presentation and may also aid in the attraction and targeting process of the lymphocytes. The B cells, that locally encounter antigens for which they have specific receptors, will be stimulated to remain, proliferate, and differentiate in the aortic adventitia and lymphoid follicles. This process may be further aided by locally-activated T-cells through the release of lymphokines, a possibility that is currently being investigated.

▶ As subsequent abstracts will show, an inflammatory cellular infiltrate is a characteristic of arterial wall damage that may lead to either stenotic disease or aneursymal degeneration. These studies reveal findings that are consistent with an active immunologically mediated disease process. This process may proceed in either direction (toward narrowing or dilation) and it is apparently dependent upon the interactions of proteolytic enzymes and the strength proteins in the arterial wall. An interesting concept has been introduced in this study: the severe forms of chronic periaortitis may present in patients with nondilated aortas and may be referred to as idiopathic, retroperitoneal fibrosis. In contrast, such a condition associated with dilation of the aortic wall will be referred to as an inflammatory aneurysm.

The Association of Elevated Plasma Homocyst(e)ine With Progression of Symptomatic Peripheral Arterial Disease
Taylor LM Jr, DeFrang RD, Harris EJ Jr, Porter JM (Oregon Health Sciences Univ)
J Vasc Surg 13:128–136, 1991   1–8

Background.—Several studies have suggested that elevated plasma levels of homocyst(e)ine (H[e]) are associated with an increased incidence of atherosclerotic disease, particularly in symptomatic patients. Therefore, the relationship of plasma levels of H(e) to the progression of symptomatic peripheral arterial disease was assessed.

Method.—Plasma levels of H(e) (defined as the sum of free and bound homocysteine, homocystine, and the mixed disulfide homocysteine-cysteine, expressed as homocysteine) were measured in 214 patients with symptomatic lower extremity arterial occlusive disease (LED) or symptomatic cerebral vascular disease (CVD), or both. They were also measured in 103 healthy controls. Progression of the disease was defined by clinical and vascular laboratory criteria.

Results.—The mean plasma level of H(e) was significantly higher in patients with peripheral arterial disease than in control subjects (mean, 14.37 nmol/mL versus 10.0 nmol/mL), with 38% of patients having plasma values of H(e) that were greater than 2 standard deviations above the control values. The incidence or level of risk factors for atherosclerosis (including age, male sex, diabetes, hypertension, smoking, renal failure, and plasma cholesterol) did not differ significantly between patients with increased plasma levels of H(e) and those with normal levels. The clinical progression of LED and coronary artery disease and the vascular laboratory progression of LED were significantly more likely to occur in patients with increased plasma levels of H(e). Furthermore, the rate of progression was significantly more rapid in patients with elevated plasma levels of H(e). This difference was not observed for CVD.

Summary.—This study confirms previous reports of the increased incidents of elevated plasma levels of H(e) in patients with symptomatic peripheral vascular disease, independent of other risk factors. In addition, patients with elevated plasma levels of H(e) have more rapid progression of disease. These data indicate that elevated plasma levels of H(e) are an independent risk factor for symptomatic atherosclerosis.

▶ The absolute establishment of an elevated level of plasma homocyst(e)ine with symptomatic arterial occlusive disease is another contribution of the University of Oregon vascular surgeons to the field of vascular surgery. These researchers are careful to point out that the relationship is true for symptomatic atherosclerosis. This is, after all, the condition that comes under treatment by vascular surgeons. As indicated in this abstract, the risk factors in symptomatic patients and asymptomatic controls were similar with regard to plasma, lipids, smoking, diabetes, hypertension, male sex, and age. This finding casts doubt on the idea that these factors may be as important as the level of hyperhomocyst(e)ine.

Hyperhomocysteinemia: An Independent Risk Factor for Vascular Disease
Clarke R, Daly L, Robinson K, Naughten E, Cahalane S, Fowler B, Graham I (Adelaide Hosp, Trinity College, Children's Hosp, University College, Dublin; Royal Manchester Children's Hosp, Manchester, England)
N Engl J Med 324:1149–1155, 1991   1–9

Background.—Although hyperhomocysteinemia caused by impaired methionine metabolism has been associated with premature cerebral, peripheral, and possibly coronary vascular disease, the strength of this association and its independence from other cardiovascular disease risk factors is not known. The extent to which the association could be explained by heterozygous cystathionine β-synthase deficiency was investigated.

Methods.—A diagnostic criterion for hyperhomocysteinemia was established by comparing the peak serum levels of homocysteine after a standard methionine-loading test was given to obligate heterozygotes and control subjects with respect to cystathionine β-synthase deficiency. Twenty-five heterozygotes whose children were homozygous for homocystinuria because of this enzyme defect and 27 unrelated age- and sex-matched normal persons were evaluated. A level of 24 μmol/L or more, that had a sensitivity of 92% and a specificity of 100%, was used in distinguishing the 2 groups. The peak serum homocysteine levels of the normal subjects wee then compared with those of 123 patients with vascular disease who were diagnosed before 55 years of age.

Results.—Hyperhomocysteinemia was diagnosed in 42% of the patients with cerebrovascular disease, 28% of those with peripheral vascular disease, and 30% of those with coronary vascular disease. None of the normal subjects had hyperhomocysteinemia. After conventional risk factors were controlled, the lower 95% confidence limit for the odds ratio of vascular diseases among patients with hyperhomocysteinemia compared with normal individuals was 3.2. The patients with vascular disease had a geometric-mean peak serum homocysteine level that was 1.33 times higher than the level of normal subjects. Also, 18 of the 23 patients with vascular disease who had hyperhomocysteinemia had confirmed cystathionine β-synthase.

Conclusions.—Hyperhomocysteinemia is an independent risk factor for the development of vascular disease, including coronary disease, and in most cases it is probably a result of cystathionine β-synthase deficiency.

▶ From nearly halfway around the world comes corroboration of the University of Orgeon study in which hyperhomocyst(e)inemia was detected in one third of the patients with peripheral arterial occlusive disease and coronary arterial occlusive disease. The relationship with cerebrovascular occlusive disease was even higher, thus establishing hyperhomocyst(e)inemia as a risk factor in peripheral arterial occlusive disease.

Early Signs of Vascular Disease in Homocystinuria: A Noninvasive Study by Ultrasound Methods in Eight Families With Cystathionine-β-Synthase Deficiency
Rubba P, Faccenda F, Pauciullo P, Carbone L, Mancini M, Strisciuglio P, Carrozzo R, Sartorio R, del Giudice E, Andria G (Univ of Naples, Italy)
Metabolism 39:1191–1195, 1990   1–10

Background.—Homocystinuria resulting from cystathionine-β-synthase (CBS) deficiency is inherited as an autosomal recessive trait. Some patients with peripheral or cerebrovascular arterial disease may be heterozygotes for homocystinuria. About half of the patients with homocystinuria respond to high-dose pyroxidine therapy with improved clinical condition and normalization of biochemical signs. Early screening of homozygotes and heterozygotes may detect signs of vascular disease before a crisis.

Methods.—A group of 14 pyroxidine-responsive homozygotes for CBS deficiency (mean age, 20 years) and 14 of their obligate heterozygote first-degree relatives (mean age, 46 years) underwent biochemical tests and vascular examinations using continuous-wave and echo-Doppler techniques. The control groups included 47 normal men and women, and 14 of their young relatives, who were age- and gender-matched to the CBS homozygotes.

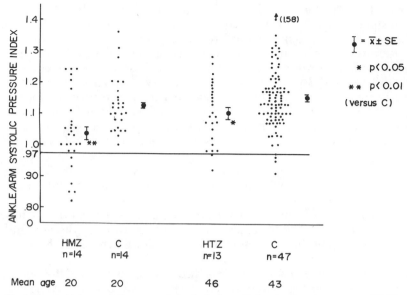

Fig 1–3.—Ankle/arm systolic pressure index in the lower limbs of patients homozygous *(HMZ)* and heterozygous *(HTZ)* for CBS deficiency compared with controls. (Courtesy of Rubba P, Faccenda F, Pauciullo P, et al: *Metabolism* 39:1191–1195, 1990.)

Results.—In both heterozygotes and homozygotes, continuous Doppler scanning showed that ankle/arm systolic pressure was significantly lower than in controls (Fig 1–3). The index was less than .9% but in 21% of the homozygotes compared with no controls, indicating that early, non-flow-reducing arterial lesions iliac arteries were more frequent in homozygotes. In the iliac arteries, echo-Doppler scanning showed non-flow-reducing lesions caused by wall anomalies or mild stenoses in half of both the heterozygotes and the homozygotes, significantly more than in their respective age-matched controls. The early internal carotid lesions were seen in significantly more heterozygotes than controls; for technical reasons, the younger groups could not be accurately assessed. Neither CBS-deficient group had venous anomalies.

Discussion.—These sensitive ultrasonographic screening techniques were successful in showing the early stages of premature vascular disease. Arterial disease appeared with almost the same frequency in young CBS-deficient homozygotes and middle-aged heterozygotes, although they appeared more severely in the younger group. It is possible that the disease occurs later in life in the heterozygote condition; however, only a prospective study can address this question.

▶ Why arterial occlusive disease symptomatology does not appear at a younger age in patients with hyperhomocyst(e)inemia than in those without was investigated. In this study it was shown conclusively that noninvasive techniques can detect more occlusive lesions in younger individuals with hyperhomocyst(e)inemia than in controls. This finding suggests that the end point of symptoms in arterial occlusive disease is too broad to detect differences in the age of onset. Noninvasive testing provides a more precise end point.

Occlusive Vasculopathy in Systemic Lupus Erythematosus: Association With Anticardiolipin Antibody
Greisman SG, Thayaparan R-S, Godwin TA, Lockshin MD (St Luke's-Roosevelt Hosp Ctr; New York Hosp-Cornell Univ Med Ctr; Hosp for Special Surgery, New York)
Arch Intern Med 151:389–392, 1991   1–11

Background.—Sudden vascular occlusion may occur in patients with systemic lupus erythematosus (SLE). Antiphospholipid antibody (aPL) is prevalent in SLE patients and is often associated with thrombosis. Acute, catastrophic, widespread noninflammatory visceral vascular occlusions in SLE patients with high-titer aPL were evaluated.

Case Report.—Woman, 37, was admitted with progressive pain and ischemia of the distal extremities. She had a 20-year history of SLE with Raynaud's phenomenon and other associated disorders. The patient was healthy until several months before admission, when fixed cyanosis of several digits and toes occurred with auto-amputation of a distal finger tuft. Ischemia progressed despite vasodilator treatment. Blood pressure at admission was 190/130 mm Hg. She had livedo reticularis on the upper extremities, acrocyanosis of several fingers, and ischemic ulcers of the toes. The laboratory results included mild anemia, an elevated white cell count, a normal platelet count, and high levels of IgG and IgM cardiolipin antibody. The chest radiograph showed mildly increased bibasilar markings, and the ECG was normal. The patient's condition deteriorated despite treatment with Solu-Medrol, aspirin, dipyridamole, antibiotics, and vasodilators; she was intermittently confused and had oliguria and progressive acrocyanosis. Congestive heart failure responded to furosemide, and the ECG showed a small pericardial effusion and a hyperdynamic ventricle. "Pulse" doses of Solu-Medrol failed to improve her condition, and after several days the patient died of cardiopulmonary arrest. Autopsy revealed an acute and remote myocardial infarct with bland fibrin thrombi in the coronary arteries that were associated with neutrophilic infiltrates in the soft tissue. These thrombi were also found in the brain and liver, and the kidneys had diffuse proliferative glomerulonephritis and fibrin thrombi in the afferent arterioles.

Discussion.—Patients with SLE and high-titer aPL may have acute noninflammatory occlusive vasculopathy with marked tissue injury. The histopathological features are distinct from those of classic SLE vasculitis. The pathogenesis of this disorder may be related to the aPL antibody; this and the noninflammatory nature of the occlusion suggest that steroids and other immunosuppressive drugs are of limited value. The therapeutic options include plasmapheresis and anticoagulant therapy.

▶ When faced with young patients who have severe vasculopathy, the vascular surgeon must accept the challenge of finding the cause of the condition. Among the laboratory tests that must be ordered are assessment of the homo cyst(e)ine levels (as indicated in the previous abstracts) and antiphospholipid antibody testing (as suggested in this abstract). Although the cause of the syndrome is unknown, its prevalence is widespread and will be manifested in obstetric practice as a tendency toward spontaneous abortion. In internal medicine, cardiology, and vascular surgical practices it will be manifested as recurrent venous and arterial thromboses. An excellent review of this syndrome is found in a study by Sammaritano et al. (1).

Reference

1. Sammaritano LR, et al: *Semin Arthritis Rheum* 20:81, 1990.

Prevention of Microvascular Thrombosis With Controlled-Release Transmural Heparin
Jones NS, Glenn MG, Orloff LA, Mayberg MR (Guy's Hosp, London; Univ of Washington)
Arch Otolaryngol Head Neck Surg 116:779–785, 1990   1–12

Objective.—In microvascular surgery local irrigation with heparin is useful in preventing thrombosis. It is possible that a more prolonged effect may be achieved by using local, transmural delivery of controlled-release heparin from a substance placed around the outside of the vessel wall immediately after the anastomosis. The efficacy of the transmural delivery of controlled local-release heparin in preventing thrombosis in microvascular surgery was evaluated using a rat arterial inversion graft model.

Method.—Polyvinyl alcohol (PVA) embedded with heparin was placed around the outside of inversion graft anastomoses in 16 animals. The control group consisted of animals in which PVA alone was placed around the graft or systemic heparin was given.

Results.—The patency rates were significantly higher in the inverted grafts treated with systemic heparin or PVA-heparin (69%), compared with untreated inversion graft controls (6%). Although the patency rates were similar in the systemic heparin and PVA-heparin groups, controlled-release transmural heparin caused no measurable anticoagulation. The incidence of local hematoma formation was similar in the systemic heparin and PVA-heparin groups.

Conclusion.—Controlled-release transmural heparin is as effective as systemic heparin in maintaining microvascular patency in an exceedingly thrombogenic model. Clinical studies of controlled-release heparin are worth undertaking.

▶ Because the cellular proliferative response of the arterial wall to injury currently limits the expansion of endovascular therapy, attention is turning toward the suppression of that response. One approach is the local delivery of antiproliferative agents. Therefore, this study takes on a greater importance than the limited application that was assessed.

Development of Gangrene During Sleep
Jelnes R (Aalborg Sygehus, Aalborg, Denmark)
Scand J Clin Lab Invest 50:351–361, 1990   1–13

Introdction.—Nondiabetic patients with arteriosclerosis of the arteries supplying the lower limbs typically have ischemic foot pain during sleep. The pain is usually severe enough to awaken the patient and is relieved on dependency of the foot. The mechanisms that cause ischemic rest pain are not clearly understood. Continuous measurement was made of the subcutaneous blood flow (SBF) in adipose tissue in the forefoot.

Methods.—The method was based on the radioisotope washout principle. Xenon-133 in isotonic saline was injected as a local depot into the subcutaneous adipose tissue in the forefoot. The measuring equipment consisted of a semiconductor detector placed just above the local isotope depot and a data memory unit carried in a belt around the waist. The dynamic SBF in the forefoot was measured for 24 hours in 24 individuals with normal peripheral circulation, in 55 patients with intermittent claudication but no rest pain, and in 43 patients with nocturnal ischemic rest pain.

Findings.—In normal controls, the SBF doubled during sleep in the supine position. The increase in SBF was attributed to the local venoarteriolar sympathetic axon reflex, that induces vasoconstriction when the transmural pressure of the veins exceeds approximately 25 mm Hg. In patients with nocturnal rest pain, the SBF was reduced by an average of 37% during sleep (Fig 1–4). The reduction in SBF was ascribed to nocturnal hypotension that was reflected proportionally in the foot. In feet

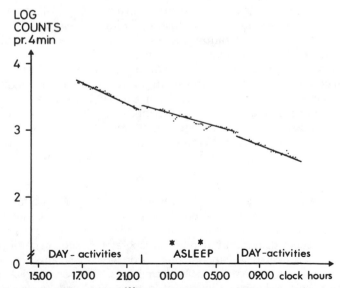

Fig 1–4.—An elimination curve of ^{133}Xe from a patient experiencing ischemic rest pain *(asterisks)* during night hours. (Courtesy of Jelnes R: *Scand J Clin Lab Invest* 50:351–361, 1990.)

with rest pain, the resistance vessels are probably fully dilated. The blood pressure drop during sleep causes the perfusion pressure, and thus the blood flow, to drop below a certain critical limit. A pronounced correlation was found between the reduction in the mean systemic arterial blood pressure and the SBF. In patients with intermittent claudication, the SBF showed a variety of changes from day to night, that were consistent with the continuous spectrum of arteriosclerotic disease.

Conclusion.—The low blood flow in patients with ischemic nocturnal rest pain can be attributed to reduced systemic blood pressure during sleep. This indicates that gangrene occurs during sleep.

▶ The cause of rest pain has been explained in the past by decreased peripheral perfusion resulting fom a combination of decreased cardiac output and lowered systemic pressure during sleep. To this can be added the proof that SBF decreases or 4-extremity sympathetic ablation occurs during sleep. The most ischemic extremity receives the least blood flow. In turn, this causes the ischemic peripheral neuropathy that the patient perceives as aching pain and that causes him to sit up, dangle his extremity, and smoke a cigarette.

Myointimal Hyperplasia: Pathogenesis and Implications. 1. In Vitro Characteristics
Painter TA (Northwestern Univ)
Artif Organs 15:42–55, 1991   1–14

Background.—Myointimal hyperplasia (MIH) constitutes a significant impediment to long-term arterial and graft patency. The pathogenesis of this lesion may be related to the normal arterial responses to an injury. Various pathogenetic factors and histopathological feature of MIH were reviewed, and the proliferation and modulation of smooth muscle and endothelial cell cultures in vitro were analyzed.

Discussion.—The role of MIH in causing the failure of human arterial reconstruction is underscored in the literature. In vitro data suggest intricate biochemical cellular interaction, particularly between smooth muscle cells and endothelial cells. The production, secretion, transportation, and effect of smooth muscle mitogens can be modified by biochemical and mechanical factors in vitro. Although this has not been successful in in vivo experimentation, it may be a fundamental factor in understanding MIH and its effects.

▶ This review of myointimal hyperplasia highlights the importance of the smooth muscle cell in the formation of the intimal lesion and the interaction of endothelial cells with the smooth muscle cells to produce the proliferative response. Recent data from a number of laboratories support the hypothesis that the factors that drive smooth muscle proliferation come not only from platelets, but from the intimal cells themselves. Both endothelial cells and smooth muscle cells are capable of synthesizing and releasing growth factors. The recent data from Reidy's laboratory support the conclusion that basic fibroblast growth factor, derived from smooth muscle cells, stimulates the initial wave of smooth muscle proliferation in the injured artery. The studies of Jawien in Clowes' laboratory, as well as studies in Ross's laboratory, indicate that platelet derived growth factor, released either from the cells or from platelets, stimulates the migration of smooth muscle cells from the media to the intima. In sum, the factors that have been identified in vitro for their growth promoting properties are now being shown to have similiar or sometimes surprisingly different effects in vivo—A.W. Clowes, M.D.

Differential Histopathology of Primary Atherosclerotic and Restenotic Lesions in Coronary Arteries and Saphenous Vein Bypass Grafts: Analysis of Tissue Obtained From 73 Patients by Directional Atherectomy
Garratt KN, Edwards WD, Kaufmann UP, Vlietstra RE, Holmes DR Jr (Mayo Clinic and Found, Rochester, Minn)
J Am Coll Cardiol 17:442–448, 1991   1–15

Objective.—The tissue effects of balloon angioplasty have been described in animal and autopsy studies. By using a directional percutaneous atherectomy device, vascular tissue was obtained from the coronary arteries and saphenous vein grafts of living patients (Fig 1–5).

Study Design.—Microscopic and immunohistochemical studies were performed on tissue specimens from 80 vascular segments, including 31 coronary arteries without prior instrumentation (primary lesions), 8 aortocoronary saphenous vein bypass grafts with primary lesions, 30 coronary arteries with lesions that developed after previous balloon angioplasty or mechanical atherectomy (restenotic lesions), and 4 vein bypass grafts with restenotic lesions.

Findings.—In primary lesions of the coronary artery and saphenous vein graft, dense fibrosis and necrotic tissue accounted for 83% of the intima with associated cholesterol crystals and foam cells. Hyperplasia accounted for 17% of the intima. In contrast, restenotic lesions were characterized not only by these chronic atherosclerotic features (56%) but also by an increased proportion of loose fibroproliferative tissue that accounted for 44% of the intima. Comparison of the resected tissues in-

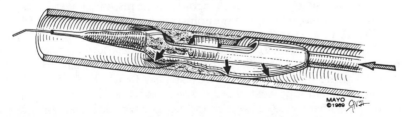

Fig 1–5.—Directional percutaneous coronary atherectomy device. Window on the side of the metallic housing is directed to face an obstructing vascular lesion. A low pressure balloon is inflated (*filled arrows*) to engage the lesion, and the cutter is advanced (*striped arrow*) across the lesion to "shave" tissue that has prolapsed into window. (Courtesy of Garratt KN, Edwards WD, Kaufmann UP, et al: *J Am Coll Cardiol* 17:442–448, 1991.)

dicated that dense fibrosis and necrosis were significantly more common in primary lesions, whereas smooth muscle hyperplasia was significantly more common in restenotic lesions. The immunohistochemical staining of the atheromatous intima and neointima confirmed that the proliferative tissue was primarily smooth muscle. The incidence of partial-thickness resection of medial tissue or full-thickness resection of media with associated adventitial tissue die not differ significantly between the primary and restenotic lesions.

Summary.—The histopathological characteristics of the neointimal layer of restenotic lesions differ from those of the intimal layer of primary atherosclerotic lesions. These findings confirm previous observations made in animals or autopsy studies; early restenosis is associated with acute platelet deposition and thrombosis, whereas late restenosis appears to be related to intimal hyperplasia and fibrosis.

▶ Modern studies sometimes simply uncover the obvious. In this presentation, restenotic lesions were found to be characterized by smooth muscle hyperplasia. The surgical specimens obtained from reoperations on the carotid artery that were performed many years ago revealed the same finding, and they further showed that the older the lesion, the higher its cholesterol content.

Time Course of Smooth Muscle Cell Proliferation in the Intima and Media of Arteries Following Experimental Angioplasty
Hanke H, Strohschneider T, Oberhoff M, Betz E, Karsch KR (Univ of Tübingen, Germany)
Circ Res 67:651–659, 1990   1–16

Introduction.—Smooth muscle cell proliferation (SMC) is an important factor in the development of restenosis after percutaneous transluminal coronary angioplasty. Using an experimental model of angioplasty, the time course of intimal and medial SMC proliferation and morphological changes after angioplasty were assessed.

Study Design.—An intimal atheroma was produced by repeated weak electrical stimulations in the right carotid artery of 45 male New Zealand white rabbits fed with a cholesterol-enriched diet. After 28 days, 35 rabbits underwent angioplasty and the proliferative responses were analyzed with histomorphological and immunohistological criteria at 3, 7, 14, 21, 28, and 42 days after intervention. The incorporation of bromodeoxyuridine (BrdU) 18 hours before excision of the vessels allowed determination of the percentage of cells undergoing DNA synthesis in the intima and media using monoclonal antibody against BrdU. The other 10 rabbits served as sham-operated and control animals.

Findings.—There was a significant progressive increase of intimal thickening in all dilated arteries, from 13 intimal cell layers after electrical stimulation to 33 cell layers at 4 weeks after angioplasty. Thereafter, there was no additional increase in the number of intimal SMC layers. Eight dilated arteries showed hemodynamically relevant stenosis caused by intimal SMC proliferation in 3 and a mural thrombus in 5. Quantification of intimal SMC proliferation by BrdU labeling showed a significant increase in the number of cells undergoing DNA synthesis within the first 7 days after angioplasty, whereas medial SMC proliferation was delayed and showed a small but significant increase 21 days after angioplasty. At 28 days after angioplasty, both intimal and medial SMC proliferation were normalized and were comparable to the control group.

Summary.—A high level of intimal SMCs undergoing proliferation are shown during the first 7 days after transluminal angioplasty and prolonged increase of SMC proliferation in the media. This experimental model of angioplasty may be useful in the further analysis of new interventional and pharmacological treatments to reduce the incidence of restenosis after angioplasty.

▶ The uniform response of the arterial wall to injury appears to be mediated during the first 30 days after injury, thus suggesting that local treatment during this period of time might suppress restenosis and allow minimally invasive therapy to succeed in the future where it has failed in the past.

Effect of Controlled Adventitial Heparin Delivery on Smooth Muscle Cell Proliferation Following Endothelial Injury
Edelman ER, Adams DH, Karnovsky MJ (Harvard Med School; Massachusetts Inst of Technology, Cambridge)
Proc Natl Acad Sci USA 87:3773–3777, 1990   1–17

Background.—High failure rates caused by abrupt vessel closure and arterial restenosis have been associated with angioplasty, intravascular stents, and laser angiosurgery. These events seem to be a result of smooth muscle cell (SMC) proliferation within the intima of the involved vessel. Although heparin and various other agents may inhibit this proliferation, the required dosage usually results in unwanted side effects such as hypotension and thrombocytopenia. In the case of heparin, modifications have reduced its anticoagulant properties, but it can still induce bleeding and other systemic complications. The effects of ethylene-vinyl acetate copolymer matrices containing heparin that were placed adjacent to rat carotid arteries after endothelial denudation by a balloon catheter were evaluated.

Results.—When matrices containing both standard and modified heparin were implanted, the SMC proliferation was significantly reduced compared with blank matrices. Using standard heparin, luminal occlusion was reduced to 9.4% of the matched controls, compared with 16.8% occlusion when heparin was infused intravenously. The modified heparin was not effective when administered intravenously, but it did result in significant reductions (to 17.7% of control values) when released periadventitially at 5 times the dosage used for standard heparin. Only standard heparin administered intravenously resulted in systemic anticoagulation.

Conclusions.—These experiments provide evidence that SMC proliferation after vascular injury might be regulated by local, site-specific therapy. Polymer-based drug delivery systems may permit efficient control of local drug levels and may be useful for the management of accelerated atherosclerotic states.

▶ Very few modes of therapy affect the myointimal proliferative response of arterial injury. However, heparin and its fractions have been promising modes of therapy in the recent past, and they may appear to be useful in the near future. As indicated in Abstract 1–16, such therapy can be delivered for a very short period of time and may have a long duration of effect.

Cyclosporine Inhibits the Development of Medial Thickening After Experimental Arterial Injury
Wengrovitz M, Selassie LG, Gifford RRM, Thiele BL (Pennsylvania State Univ)
J Vasc Surg 12:1–7, 1990   1–18

Background.—Vascular proliferative lesions such as myointimal hyperplasia often follow arterial injury; the lesions consist of inflammatory cells and proliferating smooth muscle cells. The T lymphocytes have also been shown in these lesions, suggesting involvement of immune mechanisms. Whether response to arterial injury might be modulated by inhibiting lymphocyte function with the immunosuppressive agent cyclosporine (CYA) was assessed.

Methods.—Arterial injury was experimentally produced in 90 anesthetized male rats by rotating a 1-mm coronary dilator around inside the right iliac artery. Heparin was never used. Six animals were sacrificed after 6 hours to verify early arterial injury; the remaining animals were given either saline solution or 2 mg/kg/day or 5 mg/kg/day of subcutaneous CYA for 1, 2, 4, or 6 weeks. After sacrifice by perfusion, the right and left iliac arteries were analyzed with standard and muscle-specific histologic stains.

Results.—Both the control and the CYA-treated arteries showed significant edematous thickening of the injured artery at 24 hours. After 14 days, the medial thickening in controls was demonstrably caused by smooth muscle proliferation rather than edema. At 2, 4, and 6 weeks, the rats treated with 5 mg/kg/day of CYA had significantly less medial thickening than the controls, and they also had a quantitative decrease in the infiltration of the arterial wall by monocytes and macrophages compared with controls. Similar effects were seen with the 2 mg/kg/day dose at 2 weeks, but these effects were not maintained at 4 and 6 weeks.

Discussion.—In an experimental setting, CYA may now be added to Verapamil, heparin, and endothelial cell seeding as an in vivo treatment that protects against the occurrence of vascular proliferative lesions. The mechanism by which this particular effect is accomplished is not known, but it may entail quelling the injury-induced inflammatory infiltrates of the arterial wall. Cyclosporine acts by suppressing the production of the lymphokines (that affect monocyte and macrophage activity), including chemotactic factor derived from the lymphocytes. The stimulus for medial thickening may last longer than 2 weeks after injury; this is implied by the finding that the low 2 mg/kg/day dose of CYA was only effective for the first 2 weeks—a higher, prolonged dose may be required for effective inhibition.

▶ The search for effective prevention of myointimal hyperplasia continues and extends from relatively safe agents such as heparin and its fractions to relatively dangerous agents such as immunosuppressive drugs.

Models of Arterial Aneurysm: For the Investigation of Pathogenesis and Pharmacotherapy—A Review
Powell J (Charing Cross and Westminster Med School, London)
Atherosclerosis 87:93–102, 1991   1–19

Background.—Arterial aneurysms are still a clinical challenge. The pathogenesis, growth, rupture, and treatment of these aneurysms were reviewed in many different animal models.

Discussion.—The appropriate choice of animal models is important. Experimental and aortic graft–induced arterial aneurysms have underscored the role of the medial connective tissue in resisting arterial dilation. The viable smooth-muscle cells may be needed to support the integrity of the media. In addition, the disruption of the normal medial architecture in animal models of cerebral, aortic, or femoral aneurysm is common and may be secondary to immunologic rejection, cellular damage, traumatic lesions, or genetic susceptibility. In many of these models, intimal damage, thickening, and other features of atherosclerosis are evident. Vein patch models support the hypothesis that hemodynamic changes lead to the atherosclerotic changes. Ligation of the internal carotid artery in hypertensive animals apparently produces hemodynamical and physiological changes that give rise to saccular aneurysms with histologic features resembling those in humans. Such animal models could be used to study the control and effect of genes, risk factors for atherosclerosis, and pharmacologic reagent. Spontaneously hypertensive rat models and selective medial excision or laser ablation may also be useful in the study of the effects of genetics, drugs, physiological and environmental factors on cerebral aneurysm growth, rupture, and vasospasm. The best animal models of fusiform arterial aneurysms in the middle aged and elderly appear to be the periarterial application of calcium chloride, laser damage of femoral arteries, and the blotchy mouse.

Conclusions.—The management of aneurysms may be improved through further research using the best experimental models and the development of new transgenic models.

▶ This abstract may be of little interest to the community-practicing vascular surgeon, but it was included for the academic vascular surgeon beginning his investigative career. The article itself describes the various experimental aneurysms, correctly starting with the work of John Hunter and including the author's updated presentations in 1991.

2 New Developments

A Clinical Trial of Laser Thermal Angioplasty in Patients With Advanced Peripheral Vascular Disease
White RA, White GH, Mehringer MC, Chaing FL, Wilson SE (Harbor-Univ of California, Los Angeles Med Ctr, Torrance, Calif)
Ann Surg 212:257–264, 1990   2–1

Background and Methods.—Few applications have been identified for laser angioplasty that go beyond those of conventional surgical procedures or transluminal balloon angioplasty. Of 28 patients who were enrolled in a 3-year prospective trial of laser thermal-assisted balloon angioplasty, 27 had advanced peripheral vascular disease, with severe tissue loss, gangrene, infection, and rest pain; 7 had failed either surgery of thrombolysis; and 4 were at high risk for surgery because of myocardial infarction within 6 weeks and/or ejection fractions of 20% or less. Of the 27 patients with advanced peripheral vascular disease, 17 were diabetic. A surgeon-radiologist team performed laser angioplasty through a groin incision.

Results.—Recanalization of the native vessel was successful in 16 patients with advanced peripheral vascular disease. Also, patency was restored in 2 chronically occluded polytetrafluorethylene (PTFE) grafts. However, 5 amputations were required within 1 month in these 18 successfully recanalized patients. Another 6 amputations were performed 8–12 months after recanalization. Failure of wound healing made early amputation necessary, even though the angioplasty sites remained patent. In 5 of the 6 patients requiring late amputations, the treated site reoccluded. Limbs had healed at 6–24 months in 5 of the remaining patients in whom laser angioplasty alone was successful. The other 2 patients were incompletely healed but functional. Patency for successful recanalization ranged from 48 hours to 25 months. According to life-table analysis, cumulative patency was 55.5% at 3 months, 38.8% at 6 months, and 11.1% at 1 year. None of the patients died of procedure-related complications, but there were 7 arterial-wall perforations caused by the laser probe.

Conclusions.—The role of laser angioplasty is limited in patients with advanced peripheral vascular disease. However, the procedure may provide an interval of patency that permits the postponement of surgery in high-risk patients until their medical condition improves. Laser angioplasty may also be used to correct local tissue necrosis or infection in the operative field before reconstruction and to restore patency in occluded PTFE grafts.

▶ Annual meetings of the American Surgical Association are characterized by presentations that are, in effect, status reports for surgical procedures. This report is such a presentation. Its authors stress the potential of laser-assisted transluminal angioplasty and further emphasize the limited potential of the procedure as it is performed today. Of particular value is the fact that this author, with his enormous experience, is stressing improvements in technology such as guidance systems and increased precision in tissue ablation. Other investigations not referred to in this study will allow suppression of the myointimal proliferative response and open this entire field once again.

Angiographic Follow-Up and Clinical Outcome of 126 Patients After Percutaneous Directional Atherectomy (Simpson AtheroCath™) for Occlusive Peripheral Vascular Disease
Dorros G, Iyer S, Lewin R, Zaitoun R, Mathiak L, Olson K (St Luke's Med Ctr; William Dorros-Isadore Feuer Found for Cardiovascular Disease, Milwaukee)
Cathet Cardiovasc Diagn 22:79–84, 1991   2–2

Introduction.—The preliminary experience with percutaneous directional atherectomy for occlusive peripheral vascular disease has been promising.

Patients.—Follow-up data were obtained in 115 of the 126 patients with symptomatic occlusive peripheral arterial disease who underwent percutaneous directional atherectomy with the Simpson AtheroCath™. These initially successful atherectomy patients had follow-up involving 182 lesions (Fig 2–1). Of these patients, 74 were followed with angiography at a mean 5.4 months and 41 had clinical data.

Findings.—Of the 128 lesions with angiographic follow-up, 52% of the stenoses and 65% of the occlusions recurred, for an overall recurrence rate of 55%. Of the lesions that recurred, approximately two thirds occurred as stenoses and one third occurred as occlusions. The lesion distribution did not differ between angiography and clinical follow-up groups, with nearly 85% of the lesions involving the superficial femoral

Patient Follow-up

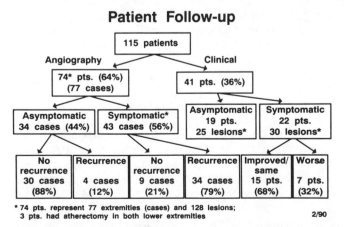

Fig 2–1.—Follow-up of 115 successful atherectomy patients. (Courtesy of Dorros G, Iyer S, Lewin R, et al: *Cathet Cardiovasc Diagn* 22:79–84, 1991.)

or popliteal arteries. There was a trend toward a higher recurrence rate in tibioperoneal vessels (80%) compared with superficial femoral lesions (54%). Among the latter lesions, the recurrence rate was significantly higher in lesions 10 cm or more in length compared with shorter lesions.

Conclusion.—Although directional atherectomy has excellent primary success and few complications, follow-up angiography shows a higher lesion recurrence rate than is seen with conventional balloon angioplasty.

▶ Even an enthusiastic interventional group such as this one is now reporting an unacceptable rate of restenosis and occlusion after present applications of minimally invasive devices in the treatment of atherosclerotic occlusive disease.

Laser Angioplasty: Results of a Prospective, Multicenter Study at 3-Year Follow-Up

Lammer J, Pilger E, Karnel F, Schurawitzki H, Horvath W, Riedl M, Umek H, Klein GE, Schreyer H, Kretschmer G, Haidinger D, Partsch H (Karl Franzens Univ, Graz, Austria; Univ of Vienna; Krankenhaus der Barmherzigen Brüder, Linz, Austria; Wilhelminenspital, Vienna)
Radiology 178:335–337, 1991   2–3

Introduction.—The development of contact probes has markedly improved the intravascular applicability of lasers. The efficacy and safety of laser angioplasty were evaluated in a large prospective, multicenter clinical trial.

Patients-Method.—A group of 338 patients with arteriosclerotic femoropopliteal artery occlusions underwent laser recanalization. A neodymium-yttrium-aluminum garnet laser with a sapphire contact probe was used. The average length of the occlusions was 8.5 cm (range, 2 cm to 26 cm). During the 3-year follow-up period, all of the patients underwent both Doppler ultrasound for calculation of the ankle-arm systolic pressure index and an intravenous digital subtraction angiography.

Results.—Laser recanalization was initially successful in 85% of the patients. Complications occurred in 14% of patients, the most common being a painful heat sensation. Vascular spasm occurred in only .6% of the patients and only 1.5% required emergency surgery. Life-table analysis showed that the cumulative patency rate of successfully recanalyzed arteries was 80% at 6 months, 70% at 1 year, 62% at 2 years, and 57% at 3 years. The 3-year patency rate was significantly better in patients with a normal runoff than in those with a reduced runoff (63% versus 52%). The length of the occlusion and treatment with long-term platelet inhibition or anticoagulation did not influence patency rates.

Conclusion.—Laser angioplasty is safe and at least as effective as conventional angioplasty in the treatment of arteriosclerotic femoropopliteal occlusions.

▶ Current methods of platelet inhibition and anticoagulation do not have an effect on the myoproliferative restenotic response of the arterial wall to injury.

Intravascular Sonography in the Detection of Arteriosclerosis and Evaluation of Vascular Interventional Procedures

Engeler CE, Yedlicka JW, Letourneau JG, Castañeda-Zúñiga WR, Hunter DW, Amplatz K (Univ of Minnesota)
AJR 156:1087–1090, 1991   2–4

Background.—Miniaturized sonographic transducers with crystal thicknesses less than .1 mm have been produced. This technology was evaluated in the detection of arteriosclerosis by intravascular sonography (Fig 2–2). The effects of vascular interventional procedures on the arterial wall were also assessed.

Methods.—The 40 subjects included 13 renal donors (mean age, 38 years), 12 patients with peripheral vascular symptoms, and 15 patients who had undergone 23 interventional vascular procedures. All of the patients underwent intravascular sonography of the aorta and ipsilateral iliac artery in real time under fluoroscopic guidance. A catheter-based miniature sonographic device with a 20-MHz transducer was used. The results of this study were compared with those of angiography.

Results.—Several arterial wall abnormalities in 8 of the 13 renal donors were shown by sonography but not by arteriography, including fatty streaks, diffuse or asymmetric intimal thickening, and focal calcified lesions. In the patients with peripheral vascular disease, more extensive arteriosclerotic changes were evident on sonography than on angiography, especially in the analysis of the composition of the arteriosclerotic abnor-

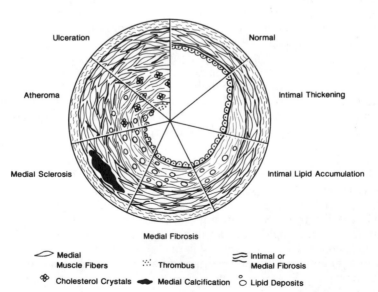

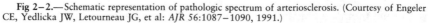

Fig 2–2.—Schematic representation of pathologic spectrum of arteriosclerosis. (Courtesy of Engeler CE, Yedlicka JW, Letourneau JG, et al: *AJR* 56:1087–1090, 1991.)

mality and the determination of the degree of underlying diffuse arteriosclerotic disease. In the patients who had undergone angioplasty or atherectomy, sonography demonstrated plaque fractures, intramural dissections, or atherectomy grooves.

Conclusions.—Intravascular sonography appears to have value in reducing the need for angiography and in monitoring progress or complications of vascular interventions. Intravascular sonography can differentiate the layers of the arterial wall, show vascular calcification, and characterize the diseased vessel and confirm the effect of angioplasty.

▶ As indicated in Abstract 2–1, improved guidance systems and improved monitoring of therapy are directions that must be pursued in developing new methods of successful, minimally invasive intervention.

A Flexible Sutureless Intraluminal Graft That Becomes Rigid After Placement in the Aorta

Matsumae M, Oz MC, Lemole GM (Med Ctr of Delaware, Wilmington; Columbia Univ)
J Thorac Cardiovasc Surg 100:787–792, 1990   2–5

Introduction.—A new sutureless intraluminal graft with a compressible ring made of coiled and overlapping stainless steel spring with ratchets in 1 overlapping end was developed for aortic reconstruction. Although this graft is flexible during insertion, it becomes rigid after placement in the aorta, allowing easier implantation of larger-size grafts and prevents spool dislodgement.

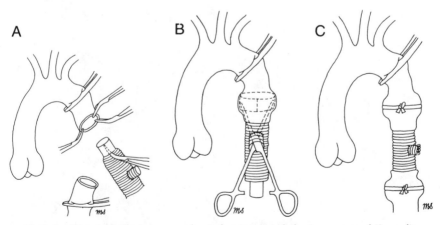

Fig 2–3.—Proposed implantation procedure in humans. **A,** with the ring compressed (8-mm diameter) by pinching overlapping sections with a clamp, the graft is introduced into the aorta until the proximal spool is covered entirely with aortic tissue. **B,** after insertion to the appropriate level, a clamp is passed through the sidearm of the Dacron graft and is used to expand the spool until the ratchets lock. The spool is then secured with a circular tie. **C,** the same maneuver is performed distally, and the sidearm is oversewn. (Courtesy of Matsumae M, Oz MC, Lemole GM: *J Thorac Cardiovasc Surg* 100:787–792, 1990.)

Technique.—The new graft was implanted in the descending aorta of 10 dogs (Fig 2–3). The rings were compressed to 8 mm in diameter by pinching the overlapping ends with a clamp. The prosthesis was then introduced into the aorta until the proximal spool was covered entirely with aortic tissue. The clamp was released and the ring was expanded with a dilating clamp, which was introduced through the short sidearm of the graft, until the ratchets engaged. A circular tie was placed around the ring. The distal spool was inserted similarly, and the sidearm was oversewn.

Findings.—Aortograms at various intervals showed no stenosis nor dilatation at the anastomoses. Autopsies were performed at intervals 8–121 days after placement, and they showed no spool dislodgement, pseudoaneurysm formation, or aortic rupture. In 1 dog, the distal aortic wall was lacerated during expansion of the spool with a dilating clamp. Histologically, the anastomotic lines were smooth, with minimal flow surface irregularities. However, the silk ties caused necrosis of the aortic wall in some dogs and also eroded into the aortic wall.

Conclusion.—This prototype sutureless device is suitable for aortic and peripheral arterial reconstruction, including branches of the transverse aortic arch or thoracoabdominal aorta. This graft requires further improvements to allow for variable spool diameters and to facilitate intraoperative ring expansion.

▶ Various techniques of sutureless repair of aortic problems are being reported. Whether or not this one will survive is conjectural.

3 Nonsurgical Treatments

Percutaneous Intraarterial Thrombolysis in the Treatment of Thrombosis of Lower Extremity Arterial Reconstruction
Seabrook GR, Mewissen MW, Schmitt DD, Reifsnyder T, Bandyk DF, Lipchik EO, Towne JB (Med College of Wisconsin; Clement J Zablocki VA Med Ctr, Milwaukee)
J Vasc Surg 13:646–651, 1991   3–1

Background.—Acute thrombosis of lower extremity vascular bypass grafts can lead to loss of the limb. One alternative to balloon catheter thrombectomy salvage is intra-arterial thrombolytic therapy under angiographic guidance. This study assesses fifteen patients with 30 acute occlusions of an autologous or prosthetic vascular graft were treated with intra-arterial urokinase.

Results.—The origins of the graft occlusions were morphological defects, pseudoaneurysm, disease progression distal to the graft, or coagulation disorders. In 13 cases a cause could not be determined. Patency was restored initially in all cases. However, in 6 cases adjunctive surgical thrombectomy was required to remove persistent thrombus. One graft could not be salvaged and amputation was performed. Five significant hemorrhagic complications occurred, and 1 patient died.

Conclusion.—Percutaneous intraarterial thrombolysis allows the salvage of some grafts that would not remain patent after balloon catheter thrombectomy. Thrombolytic therapy is associated with serious complications and should only be utilized if the benefits of graft salvage outweigh the risk of hemorrhage.

▶ This study is one of many that has described the treatment of acute arterial occlusion by thrombolytic agents. Other studies were rejected for inclusion in this YEAR BOOK in favor of this one simply because of the quality of work performed by this vascular group from Milwaukee and the objective methods of presentation that they have exhibited in previous reports. After reviewing this report presented to the Midwestern Vascular Surgical Society meeting, one cannot help but believe that local lytic therapy is useful for uncovering the cause of the acute arterial occlusion, and that coagulopathies may be uncovered by appropriate investigation of the patients.

The Role of Duplex Scanning in the Selection of Patients for Transluminal Angioplasty

Edwards JM, Coldwell DM, Goldman ML, Strandness DE Jr (Univ of Washington)
J Vasc Surg 13:69–74, 1991   3–2

Introduction.—The current gold standard for the selection of patients for transluminal angioplasty (TLA) is arteriography. A noninvasive test that can predict with high accuracy the lesions that may be treatable with TLA is highly desirable. Between July 1987 and March 1990, arterial duplex examinations were performed as part of the initial evaluation of patients with lower extremity ischemia who were considered candidates for some intervention.

Patients.—Of the 134 arteriograms performed for the evaluation of lower extremity ischemia in 122 patients, 110 (82%) were preceded by a lower extremity arterial duplex examination. Fifty patients were considered candidates for TLA based on the findings of duplex examination showing isolated, short lesions that were, for the most part, not occlusions.

Results.—Transluminal angioplasty was performed in 47 (94%) of the 50 patients in whom arterial duplex examination predicted a lesion that would be amenable to TLA. Age, sex, and frequency of diabetes did not differ significantly between the patients who were referred for TLA and those who were not. The need for operative intervention was markedly reduced in patients who underwent TLA (15%) compared with those who did not undergo TLA (75%).

Summary.—Duplex scanning of the lower extremities allows the detection of lesions that are treatable with TLA. Duplex scanning should be the standard screening tool for detection of treatable lower extremity lesions.

▶ Because TLA is useful in the treatment of certain lesions, it is important to know that the pathway of the patient with early symptoms of arterial occlusive disease can be from the clinic or office to the noninvasive laboratory; it can then progress to invasive corroboration of diagnosis and therapy. All of this can be accomplished on an outpatient basis.

How Does Lower Limb Balloon Angioplasty Affect Vascular Surgical Practice?

Vallance R (Gartnavel Gen Hosp, Glasgow)
J Intervent Radiol 6:5–9, 1991   3–3

Objective.—The impact of the introduction of lower limb percutaneous balloon angioplasty (PTA) was assessed retrospectively on a well-established vascular surgical service. Whether PTA provided a significant alternative to surgery, was used only for patients with inoperable vascular disease, or added a new group of mildly or moderately affected patients for whom surgery would entail unjustifiable risk and expense was determined.

GARTNAVEL GENERAL HOSPITAL

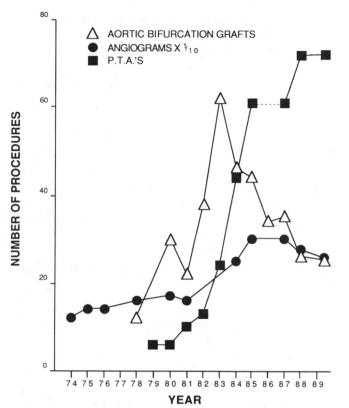

Fig 3–1.—Between 1978 and 1983 the number of aortic bifurcation grafts rose rapidly to a maximum of 62 operations. However, it has fallen almost every year since then (with the exception of 1987, in which there were 35 operations performed—1 more than in 1986). In 1988, 1 aortic bifurcation graft was performed per fortnight, compared with 62 in 1983. This occurred despite an overall increased prevalence of peripheral vascular disease according to the number of angiograms and vascular clinic new patients. (Courtesy of Vallance R: *J Intervent Radiol* 6:5–9, 1991.)

Study Design.—For the years 1981, 1985, 1986, 1987, 1988, and 1989, the number of new patients who registered at the vascular clinics was extracted from hospital records; these cases were predominantly, although not exclusively, patients with lower limb peripheral vascular disease. The number of PTAs performed each year, as well as the number and type of vascular reconstructive surgeries and amputations, were also analyzed.

Results.—Beginning in 1983, increasing numbers of PTAs were associated with a marked decrease in the numbers of aortic bifurcation grafts (Fig 3–1) and a moderate decrease in the number of femoro-popliteal bypass grafts beginning in 1985 (Fig 3–2). Although the number of surgical procedures declined, there was a dramatic increase in the prevalence of peripheral vascular disease, and a sixfold increase in the total number of

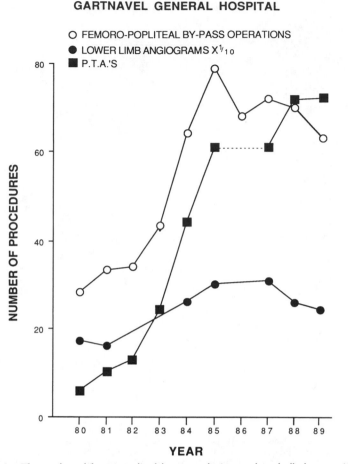

GARTNAVEL GENERAL HOSPITAL

○ FEMORO-POPLITEAL BY-PASS OPERATIONS
● LOWER LIMB ANGIOGRAMS $X^{1/10}$
■ P.T.A.'S

Fig 3−2.—The number of femoro-popliteal bypass grafts increased markedly between 1978 and 1985, thereafter falling slightly. Almost identical numbers of operations were performed in 1986 (68), in 1987 (72), and in 1988 (70). This occurred despite an increase in the prevalence of peripheral vascular disease. A further reduction to 62 operations was observed in 1989; however, compared with the falling numbers of aortic bifurcation grafts, the reductions in numbers of femoro-popliteal grafts have been much less dramatic. (Courtesy of Vallance R: *J Intervent Radiol* 6:5−9, 1991.)

patients receiving PTAs or surgical procedures or both during the period from 1978 to 1989. The number of amputations decreased slightly.

Conclusions.—Percutaneous balloon angioplasty is an important alternate treatment option for patients with peripheral vascular disease of the lower limbs, particularly those who would have had vascular reconstructive procedures of the aorto-iliac segments. It can be followed by surgery if necessary. Although the numbers of patients increased dramatically during the study decade, the increase was not attributable to the introduction of a new population of mildly diseased patients to PTA.

▶ Unfortunately, new interventional techniques increase the cost of medical care. However, these techniques allow more patients to be treated and offer relief to a greater number of patients with severe symptomatology. This is the objective of medical care. Vascular surgeons should recall that effective interventions, whether performed in the radiology suite or in the operating room, merely increase the number of patients who come under care. They do not decrease surgical practice.

Fate of Patients Undergoing Transluminal Angioplasty for Lower-Limb Ischemia

Jeans WD, Armstrong S, Cole SEA, Horrocks M, Baird RN (Bristol Royal Infirmary, Bristol, England)
Radiology 177:559–564, 1990   3–4

Background.—The indications for percutaneous transluminal angioplasty (PTA) of lower limb ischemia have included the extremes of the clinical spectrum.

Study Design.—In a 7-year prospective study, 500 PTAs for lower limb ischemia were performed in 370 patients. Of these patients, 97% were evaluable during a follow-up period of 2–9 years.

Outcome.—There were 51% successful PTAs and 49% failures, for a 5-year cumulative patency rate of 49%. The 30-day mortality rate was 3%, with 1% of the deaths attributable to PTA. Of the PTA failures, 31% were failed attempts at dilation and 73% occurred within 1 month of intervention. Bypass surgery was performed in 39% of the failed PTAs and amputation was performed in 24%. Log rank tests on the life-table data showed that outcome was significantly better in patients with claudication compared with patients with critical ischemia (5-year cumulative patency rates, 54% vs. 43%) and in those with iliac lesions compared with those with femoropopliteal lesions (5-year cumulative patency rates, 57% vs. 41%). Furthermore, in a subgroup of patients with femoropopliteal stenoses, the outcome was significantly better in patients with 2 or 3 patent vessels compared with those with no or 1 patent vessel (3-year cumulative patency rates, 78% vs. 25%). Deaths at 5 years were twice as frequent in patients with failed PTAs.

Conclusion.—These data show that PTA is safe and should be the first treatment of choice in suitable patients. The outcome of PTA is better in patients with iliac stenoses, those with claudication, and those with 2 or more patent calf vessels. Furthermore, in patients with little chance of surgical treatment (those with occlusions and 1 or more patent vessels), PTA is a valuable addition to the therapeutic options, that results in a 3-year cumulative patency rate of 25%.

▶ Although this study does not provide particularly new or startling information regarding the fate of transluminal angioplasty, it does uncover the interesting finding that the 5-year mortality rate was twice as great in patients with failed PTAs as it was in patients with successful treatment. There is a truth in this finding that is waiting to be revealed.

4 Nonatherosclerotic Conditions

Acrocyanosis in Anorexia Nervosa
Bhanji S, Mattingly D (Univ of Exeter Postgraduate Med School; Royal Devon and Exeter Hosp, Exeter, England)
Postgrad Med J 67:33–35, 1991   4–1

Background.—Acrocyanosis, a rare disorder of the peripheral circulation characterized by cyanosis and coldness of the hands and feet, is prevalent in patients with anorexia nervosa. The reason for this association is unknown. A series of patients with anorexia, many of whom had acrocyanosis, was studied.

Methods.—A group of 155 patients with anorexia nervosa, all but 4 of whom were female, were referred during a 20-year period. The age range was 13–67 years; most patients were younger than 25 years and had been losing weight for less than 2 years. A total of 32 patients (21%) had acrocyanosis. The correlations between this disorder and other clinical findings were assessed retrospectively.

Results.—The mean weight of the acrocyanosis group, expressed as a percentage of the calculated optimum, was 66.7% compared with 74.5% in the other patients with anorexia. The acrocyanosis patients were more likely to be emaciated, to have pallor of the face and trunk, and to have a lower pulse rate. There were no significant differences in eating or exercise behavior. The only significant difference in laboratory tests was a significantly higher fasting serum glucose level in the acrocyanosis patients. Comparison of chest radiographs and brain CT scans showed no significant differences.

Conclusions.—Acrocyanosis is not uncommon in anorexia nervosa patients and may be more prevalent in more severely affected patients. This condition may be a more extreme type of the heat conserving mechanism sometimes observed in anorexic patients. The association between acrocyanosis and plasma glucose levels warrants further study.

▶ The entire subject of acrocyanosis is fascinatingly obscure; however, vascular surgeons acting as vascular authorities must be aware of it as a condition, at least for diagnosis if not for effective treatment. Older textbooks on vascular surgery recognized the hypometabolic state, menstrual disturbances, and a flat glucose tolerance curve, but they failed to draw the association with anorexia even though virtually all of the patients with acrocyanosis were young women.

Anticardiolipin Antibodies in Polymyalgia Rheumatica-Giant Cell Arteritis: Association With Severe Vascular Complications

Espinoza LR, Jara LJ, Silveira LH, Martínez-Osuna P, Zwolinska JB, Kneer C, Aguilar JL (Univ of South Florida, Tampa)
Am J Med 90:474–478, 1991   4–2

Background.—Antiphospholipid antibodies (APA) induce vasculopathy and thrombosis in a variety of connective tissue diseases, autoimmune disorders, and infections. In addition, APA may have a role in the pathogenesis of giant cell arteritis (GCA) in patients with polymyalgia rheumatica (PMR). A group of PMR patients with and without GCA were studied to determine the prevalence of anticardiolipin antibodies (aCL) and their association with vascular complications.

Methods.—Fifty patients, 34 women and 16 men, were studied. Of these patients, 30 (mean age, 71.2 years) had PMR alone, and 20 patients (mean age, 72.4 years) had associated GCA. An enzyme-linked immunosorbent assay was done to detect IgG and IgM aCL in stored sera in all of the patients. The sera from 50 age- and sex-matched healthy control subjects were also investigated. The von Willebrand factor (vWF) antigen, C-reactive protein, and erythrocyte sedimentation rate were also measured.

Results.—The presence of aCL was noted in 24 of the 50 patients, 11 of whom were positive for IgG, 5 for IgM, and 8 for both. In the PMR-only group, 26.6% had aCL, compared with 80% of patients in the PMR/GCA group. Ten of 50 controls had aCL. This was significant only in comparison with the GCA group. Both aCL isotypes were found mostly in GCA patients; severe vascular complications were present in 6 of these patients. Patients in the PMR/GCA group had a mean vWF antigen level of 384 U/dL, compared with 166.9 U/dL in the PMR-only group. However, the highest titers did not correlate with vascular complications. Both groups of PMR patients had comparably high erythrocyte sedimentation rate and C-reactive protein.

Conclusions.—The presence of aCL is common in PMR patients with GCA. Their presence may imply severe vascular damage and may be partly responsible for the vasculopathy seen in GCA. Anticardiolipin antibodies found in association with elevated vWF antigen may suggest the presence of arteritis, even if it is not clinically evident.

▶ The aCLs are terribly important to vascular surgeons. Although this study focuses on the polymyalgia/giant-cell arteritis syndromes, other forms of collagen vascular diseases that may be associated with vascular thromboses often are seen by vascular surgeons. Further comments on this subject may be found in Chapter 1 of this volume.

Vasculo-Behçet's Disease: A Pathologic Study of Eight Cases

Matsumoto T, Uekusa T, Fukuda Y (Juntendo Univ School of Medicine, Tokyo)
Hum Pathol 22:45–51, 1991   4–3

Background.—Behçet's syndrome, prevalent in the Mediterranean, Middle East, and Japan, is a multisystemic disorder signaled by aphthous stomatitis, genital ulcerations, and skin and eye lesions, and is divided into neuro-, entero-, and vasculo-Behçet's subtypes. The latter may be manifested as various large vascular lesions, principally aneurysms, and occlusions of arteries or veins. Large arteries are rarely involved in this disorder. Eight autopsy cases of vasculo-Behçet's disease identified from the Japanese national autopsy registry.

Methods.—Clinical histories were reviewed and standard histological samples analyzed. The interval between diagnosis of the disease and death ranged from 5 to 25 years; the 5 men and 3 women ranged image from 31 to 56 years at the time of death.

Results.—Saccular (n = 0.4) or dissecting aneurysms (n = 0.1) were the most common manifestation; they were accompanied by arterial and/or venous blockage in 2 cases, and venous occlusion without aneurysm in 2 cases. Active aortitis, evidenced by focused infiltration of inflammatory cells around the vasa vasorum and into the media was observed in the aortic arch of 2 patients. The entire aorta showed scarred aortitis in 4 cases, the aortic arch in 1, and the abdominal and descending thoracic aorta in 1; 2 patients had both scar and active aortitis. There was evidence of loss of elastic and muscle fibers, fibroblast propagation, and an infiltrate comprising eosinophils, histiocytes, lymphocytes, plasma cells, and neutrophils. Five patients also had scarred arteritis of major aortic branches.

Discussion.—The observation of inflammatory activity centered on the proliferating vasa vasorum in 2 cases of active aortitis implies that that is the site of active inflammation. Severe medial destruction is probably the cause of the saccular aneurysms, whereas the venous lesions are thrombophlebitis. Although a granulomatous lesion typical of the active phase of Takayasu's arteritis was seen in 1 patient with active aortitis, the clinical manifestations of the 2 syndromes are quite distinct.

▶ The manifestations of Behçet's disease are being seen in increasing numbers in this country, and vascular surgeons must be aware of the difficulties in managing these patients. Repeated total body surveillance by imaging must be carried out in each patient with this diagnosis.

Recognition and Embolic Potential of Intraaortic Atherosclerotic Debris
Karalis DG, Chandrasekaran K, Victor MF, Ross JJ Jr, Mintz GS (Hahnemann Univ Hosp, Philadelphia)
J Am Coll Cardiol 17:73–78, 1991   4–4

Objective.—Atherosclerotic debris within the thoracic aorta can cause cerebral and peripheral embolism, but it is not frequently considered a source of systemic embolism. The prevalence, clinical significance, and embolic potential of intraaortic atherosclerotic debris as detected by transesophageal echocardiography were evaluated in 556 patients.

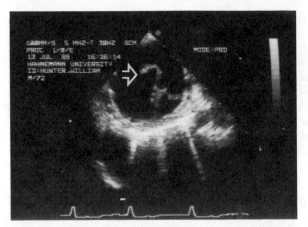

Fig 4–1.—Transesophageal echocardiographic short-axis view at the level of the descending thoracic aorta in a patient with intraaortic atherosclerotic debris. There is a narrow base of attachment to the intima. Debris *(arrow)* is pedunculated and protruding into lumen. Although not demonstrable on still image, the debris was highly mobile. (Courtesy of Karalis DG, Chandrasekaran K, Victor MF, et al: *J Am Coll Cardiol* 17:73–78, 1991.)

Findings.—Intra-aortic atherosclerotic debris was identified in 38 patients (7%), particularly in the arch and descending thoracic aorta. An embolic event occurred in 11 of 36 patients (31%), all within 1 month of recognition of the debris. In all but 2 patients, intraaortic atherosclerotic debris was the only potential cardiac source of systemic emboli. The incidence of an embolic event was significantly higher when the debris was pedunculated and highly mobile (73%) (Fig 4–1), than when it was layered and immobile (12%) (Fig 4–2). Among the 15 patients who underwent an invasive procedure after recognition of the intra-aortic atherosclerotic debris, the incidence of embolic events was 27% and occurred in

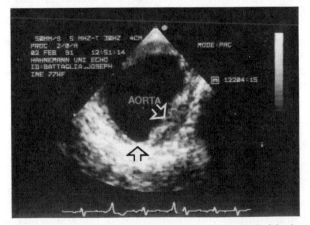

Fig 4–2.—Transesophageal echocardiographic short-axis view at the level of the descending thoracic aorta in patient with intraaortic atherosclerotic debris. Debris *(open arrow)* is layered. There is broad base of attachment to the intima *(filled arrow)* and the debris is immobile. (Courtesy of Karalis DG, Chandrasekaran K, Victor MF, et al: *J Am Coll Cardiol* 17:73–78, 1991.)

patients with pedunculated and highly mobile intra-aortic atherosclerotic debris.

Conclusion.—The thoracic aorta should be considered a potential source of systemic embolism. Intraaortic atherosclerotic debris can be identified reliably by transesophageal echocardiography. When debris is detected, particularly if it is pedunculated and highly mobile, an invasive aortic procedure should be avoided if possible.

▶ In the search for a source of atheroembolization, the thoracic aorta must not be forgotten.

Protruding Atherosclerotic Plaque in the Aortic Arch of Patients With Systemic Embolization: A New Finding Seen by Transesophageal Echocardiography
Tunick PA, Kronzon I (New York Univ Med Ctr)
Am Heart J 120:658–660, 1990   4–5

Introduction.—Patients with unexplained stroke or other neurological events who undergo echocardiography to search for a possible cardiac embolization source have often negative findings on routine transthoracic investigation. Three patients with embolic events who had unusual findings on transesophageal echocardiography are studied.

Case 1.—Woman, 68, with atrial fibrillation, bilateral carotid bruits, an episode of transient dysarthria, and an embolus to 1 toe had negative findings on transthoracic echocardiography. Transesophageal echocardiography showed a normal heart except for mild-to-moderate mitral regurgitation. However, the descending thoracic aorta and aortic arch had protruding, large atherosclerotic plaques with flail projections that were moving freely in the lumen with the blood flow (Fig 4–3).

Case 2.—Woman, 77, with increasing angina pectoris, had severe circumflex coronary obstruction, moderate right coronary obstruction, and mild disease in the left anterior descending coronary artery on cardiac catheterization. At the end of the procedure, she had a cerebellar infarction. Transthoracic echocardiography was unremarkable. However, transesophageal echocardiography showed large, protruding atherosclerotic plaques in the aortic arch, with 1 plaque showing a small, mobile projection.

Case 3.—Man, 70, who had experienced a transient neurological event had normal transthoracic echocardiographic findings except for mild mitral regurgitation. Transesophageal echocardiography also showed a normal heart, but the aortic arch and descending aorta revealed large atherosclerotic plaques with freely mobile projections.

Summary.—Routine transthoracic echocardiography for the investigation of a possible cardiac embolization source in 3 patients with unexplained neurologic events was essentially negative. However, transesophageal echocardiography revealed striking, large protruding atheroscle-

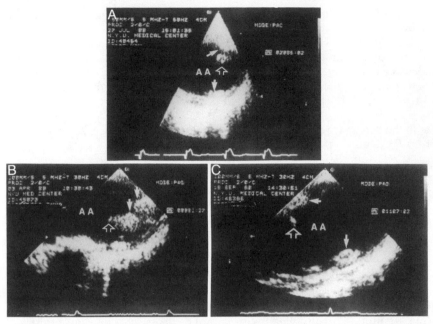

Fig 4–3.—Transesophageal echocardiogram that shows the aortic arch. **A,** patient 1; **B,** patient 2; **C,** patient 3. *AA,* aortic arch; *solid arrows,* projecting atherosclerotic plaque; *open arrows,* mobile projections from plaques. (Courtesy of Tunick PA, Kronzon I: *Am Heart J* 120:658–660, 1990.)

rotic plaques in the aortic arch and the descending thoracic aorta with mobile components that could have caused the clinical syndromes in these 3 patients.

▶ Fortunately, this simple technique of evaluation of the thoracic aorta is available in most hospitals; it may reveal an occult source of peripheral atheroembolic disease.

Medical Treatment of Cholesterol Crystal Embolization
Hachulla E, Devulder B (CHU-Hôpital Claude Huriez, Lille, France)
Presse Med 20:215–219, 1991   4–6

Background.—The mortality associated with cholesterol crystal embolism (CCE) syndrome is very high, particularly in the elderly. Because only a small proportion of patients with CCE become symptomatic, the frequency of CCE is underestimated. In a recent autopsy study, cholesterol crystals were found in the kidneys of 77% of the patients who had been operated on for severe aortic atherosclerosis.

Diagnosis.—The diagnosis of CCE is difficult to establish because the clinical picture is polymorphic. The syndrome is often first diagnosed at autopsy. In some patients, the clinical picture resembles that of vasculitis. The most common clinical findings are the triad of skin involvement, including livedo reticularis, purple toes syndrome and gangrene, malignant arterial hypertension, and acute renal insufficiency. The most common predisposing factors are surgical intervention, interventional vascular procedures, and the use of anticoagulants. Several authors have implicated streptokinase therapy as a cause of CCE, but it is difficult to separate the causative role of streptokinase from that of the aortic manipulation itself. Similarly, CCE after treatment with tissue plasminogen activator has been reported. The diagnosis of CCE may be confirmed by skin, muscle, or renal biopsy.

Treatment.—There is controversy over the optimal treatment of CCE, and controlled clinical studies are not available. The use of anticoagulant therapy in the treatment of cutaneous ischemic symptoms should be avoided. The use of heparin or antiplatelet drugs seems to precipitate acute renal failure. The use of vasodilators, low molecular weight dextran, or sympathectomy occasionally results in the transient improvement of certain symptoms, but none of these therapies alter the prognosis. Beta-blockers and enzyme conversion inhibitors are recommended as the drugs of choice in the treatment of arterial hypertension. In a recent study, 2 of 3 patients had improved renal function after treatment with minoxidil. Hemodialysis is usually the only available option for patients with acute renal failure. The efficacy of corticosteroids has not been conclusively demonstrated. Whereas some patients treated with prednisone had dramatic clinical improvement, others had no improvement after prednisone therapy. Although surgical eradication of the CCE source with vascular repair would be the only effective treatment, most patients with CCE are too ill to tolerate either the operation or the required preoperative aortography.

Conclusion.—The treatment of CCE remains symptomatic at best, and prevention remains the only effective option.

▶ Although this study recommends diagnosis of atheroembolic disease by skin or muscle biopsy, the clinical syndrome creates its own diagnosis and biopsies are to be avoided. The source of this confusion comes from the literature of pathology in which cholesterol crystals have been seen in muscle biopsy specimens or in muscle sections taken from autopsy.

Medical treatments advocated in this study may prove to be useful, but surgeons must concern themselves with finding the source of the problem and eliminating that source from the circulation.

The Role of Extraanatomic Exclusion Bypass in the Treatment of Disseminated Atheroembolism Syndrome

Kaufman JL, Saifi J, Chang BB, Shah DM, Leather RP (Albany Med College; Albany VA Med Ctr, Albany, NY)
Ann Vasc Surg 4:260–263, 1990   4–7

Background.—The treatment of patients with extensive degenerative aortic atherosclerosis is difficult when disseminated atheroembolism occurs. The majority of these patients have severe cardiopulmonary dysfunction that makes total replacement of the offending thoracoabdominal arterial segment impossible.

Patients and Management.—Six patients with ongoing disseminated atheroembolism complicated by severe and unremitting pain from bilateral foot lesions assessed. They were treated with axillobifemoral bypass with exclusion-ligation of the external iliac arteries. One patient had a recent myocardial infarction, 6 had renal failure, and 3 were undergoing hemodialysis, thus precluding definitive aortic reconstruction. All patients had failed to achieve relief with antiplatelet drugs and all required significant doses of narcotic analgesics for pain.

Results.—There were no operative complications. Healing of the wounds was achieved in 11 of the 12 limbs at risk. One patient with progressive necrosis in 1 foot had below-knee amputation; lesions of the other foot healed spontaneously. Pain was reduced in all patients within a few days after surgery.

Conclusions.—Exclusion-ligation bypass is an effective and safe alternative for the management of severe disseminated atheroembolism in patients with severe cardiopulmonary disease and short life expectancy.

▶ The principle of excluding the embolizing source from the circulation is a good one, but new problems are introduced by the construction of complex extra-anatomical reconstructions.

Infected Aortitis Masquerading as Bronchogenic Carcinoma
Paradowski LJ, Hajdu I, Coli L, Loewen G (State Univ of New York, Buffalo)
NY State J Med 90:415–416, 1990   4–8

Introduction.—Aortobronchial fistula is an uncommon, usually fatal complication of thoracic aortic aneurysm. It is often diagnosed on postmortem examination. Infected aortitis complicated by aortobronchial fistula was diagnosed and assessed in a patient.

Case Report.—Man, 72, had generalized malaise, night sweats, and bloodstreaked sputum. He was a smoker. A chest radiograph showed a left hilar mass and volume loss. Bronchoscopy showed a patent left upper lobe and a left lower lobe obscured by blood. A CT scan showed a posterior mediastinal soft tissue mass that was contiguous with the descending thoracic aorta. This was confirmed on aortography as a large saccular aneurysm of the descending thoracic aorta. Surgery revealed erosion of the aneurysm into the left lower lobe of the lung. Pathological examination showed focal acute aortitis with atherosclerotic plaques. Small aggregates of gram-positive cocci were found in the aortic media. A left lower lobectomy with interposition of a dacron graft was performed, and antibiotic therapy was given. The patient improved but died 4 months later of massive hemoptysis.

Summary.—Involvement of the lung in infected aneurysm is not common. The aortobronchial communication almost always occurs with the left lung, particularly with the left lower lobe. Diagnosis requires a high index of suspicion because the presentation is usually insiduous. Treatment consists of surgical resection of all aneurysmal inflammatory tissue followed by prolonged antibiotic therapy.

▶ Aortobronchial fistulas are an accompaniment of dissecting aneurysms; however, even in that condition, they are found in less than 10% of patients.

An Easy Method for Diagnosis of Lymphedema
Richards TB, McBiles M, Collins PS (Letterman Army Med Ctr, Presidio of San Francisco)
Ann Vasc Surg 4:255–259, 1990   4–9

Purpose.—Lymphoscintigraphy has proven useful for studying the lymphatic component of a swollen limb. However, the radioactive isotopes used in lymphoscintigraphy have been investigational and are difficult to obtain. The use of technetium-99m sulfur minicolloid (99mTc) in patients undergoing lymphoscintigraphy for edema of the extremities was evaluated.

Patients.—During a 1-year period, 20 patients aged 22–81 years with edema of 1 or both lower extremities underwent 99m-Tc lymphoscintig-

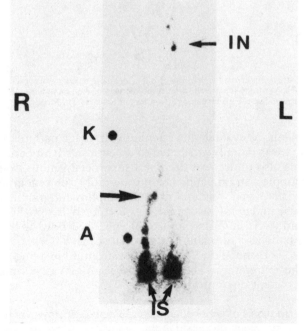

Fig 4–4.—Obstructed pattern. *Large arrow* identifies point of lymphatic obstruction secondary to trauma. *K* indicates knees; *A*, ankle; *IS*, injection site; *IN*, inguinal nodes. (Courtesy of Richards TB, McBiles M, Collins PS: *Ann Vasc Surg* 4:255–259, 1990.)

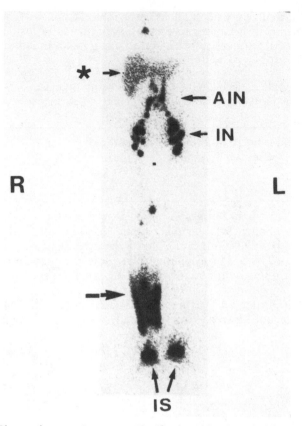

Fig 4–5.—Obstructed pattern. *Large arrow* identifies dermal lymphatic backflow pattern after saphenous vein harvesting for lower extremity arterial reconstruction. *Asterisk* indicates liver; *IS*, injection site; *AIN*, aortoilliac nodes; *IN*, inguinal nodes. (Courtesy of Richards TB, McBiles M, Collins PS: *Ann Vasc Surg* 4:255–259, 1990.)

raphy of 40 limbs to evaluate the lymphatic drainage patterns. Lower extremity edema was initially attributed to a venous or lymphatic cause. All of the patients also underwent deep and superficial venous examinations by venous Doppler, strain gauge plethysmography, or venography.

Results.—There were bilateral normal lymphoscintigraphical patterns in 12 patients, unilateral decreased or obstructed lymph flow patterns (Figs 4–4 and 4–5) in 7, and unilateral enhanced flow of lymphs in 1. None of the patients had bilateral abnormal scans.

Conclusion.—Technetium 99m provides accurate imaging of the lymphatics in the extremities. The procedure is noninvasive and causes a minimum of patient discomfort.

▶ The clinical diagnosis of lymphedema usually suffices. However, in questionable cases, the technique described in this study may prove to be useful.

5 Claudication

The Fate of the Claudicant—A Prospective Study of 1969 Claudicants
Dormandy JA, Murray GD (St George's Hosp, London; Western Infirmary, Glasgow)
Eur J Vasc Surg 5:131–133, 1991   5–1

Background.—Short-term morta′lity and cardiovascular disease were assessed in a randomly selected group of patients with intermittent claudication who were not treated for the condition. The complications that occurred were documented, and the risk factors that best predicted the various complications were identified.

Methods.—A group of 1,969 patients from 147 hospitals in 14 countries were studied; these patients were the placebo-control subjects in the double-blind Prevention of Atherosclerotic Complications with Ketanserin (PACK) trial. All evaluated patients had an ankle-arm pressure ratio of less than .85 in the ankle arteries of 1 or both legs and a history of intermittent claudication resulting from atherosclerosis. Those patients who received β-blockers or platelet-active drugs and those with gangrene or rest pain were excluded. However, those who no longer fulfilled the criteria because of a successful arterial reconstruction were included. The follow-up for myocardial infarct, major stroke, amputation, and definite vascular or nonvascular death continued for at least a year.

Results.—The annual mortality was 4.3%. There were 36 myocardial infarcts (12 fatal), 27 major strokes (8 fatal), 32 above-ankle amputations (1 fatal), 28 nonvascular deaths, and 43 other vascular deaths. A total of 111 patients required intervention for worsening ischemia of the leg. An ankle-arm ratio of less than .5, age, and a history of coronary morbidity were significant predictors of overall mortality. These factors plus diabetes, hypertension, and white cell count were significant hazards in a multivariate analysis of the predictors of vascular deaths, nonfatal stroke, and myocardial infarction. Both ankle-arm ratio and previous vascular surgery predicted the likelihood of worsening leg ischemia.

Discussion.—The study produced some surprising results. Mortality was not higher among smokers or patients who had undergone previous arterial surgery. Expected classic risk factors such as diabetes, smoking, hypertension, and plasma cholesterol did not predict total mortality or cardiovascular events as well as an ankle-arm pressure ratio less than .5; the latter measure portended mortality and morbidity as reliably as a history of previous coronary artery disease. It is possible that the classic risk factors that foreshadow the progression and early stages of atherosclerosis have less value in predicting the end result of the disease.

▶ Claudication is acknowledged as an important symptom in peripheral arterial occlusive disease. Although claudication is not treated regularly by surgical intervention when the occlusion is distal to the femoral artery, the lesion is treated regularly by intervention when the occlusive lesion is in the aortoiliac segment. Furthermore, when the lesion is stenotic, it should be treated by percutaneous techniques to prevent the occlusion that would demand surgical care. The natural history of claudication and its treatment by modification described in this chapter are important. This study uncovers the amazing fact that acknowledged risk factors that are commonly treated by our medical colleagues have little value in predicting the end results of occlusive arterial disease. The abstracts in Chapter 1 that dealt with basic considerations in arterial disease may prove to be more informative concerning the prediction of outcome than our current concepts have been.

Important Predictors of the Outcome of Physical Training in Patients With Intermittent Claudication
Rosfors S, Arnetz BB, Bygdeman S, Sköldö L, Lahnborg G, Eneroth P (St Göran's Hosp, Stockholm; Natl Inst for Psychosocial Factors and Health, Stockholm; Huddinge Hosp, Huddinge, Sweden)
Scand J Rehabil Med 22:135–137, 1990   5–2

Purpose.—The overall benefits of structured physical training in improving the walking distance in patients with intermittent claudication have been well documented. However, specific physiological factors or mental factors that could predict the extent of improvement after training have not been identified. A study was designed to find the variables of relative improvement in walking distance in patients with intermittent claudication who were undergoing structured training.

Patients.—A group of 15 men and 10 women (age, 55–76 years) with confirmed peripheral occlusive disease were evaluated. All of the patients participated in a 6-month training program that consisted of 2 training sessions of 30 minutes each twice a week at the hospital, combined with daily training at home. Each patient completed a standardized questionnaire at the start of the study to assess their level of worry concerning the disease, emotional stress, motivation, and personal belief that training is beneficial to the condition. Treadmill testing was performed at baseline and at the completion of the training program.

Results.—After 6 months of training the mean walking distance improved from 575 m to 924 m. There was no relationship between walking improvement and hemodynamic parameters, including ankle pressures, as recorded before and after training. The basal levels of hormonal and metabolic factors did not predict the outcome of the training program. However, short initial walking distance, the belief that training would have a beneficial effect, and the number of years the patient smoked were predictive of the percentage increase in walking distance. Patient age and gender were not significantly predictive of outcome.

Conclusion.—A patient with a short initial walking distance, extensive smoking habits, and a belief that training has a positive effect will most likely benefit from training—if he stops smoking.

▶ In North America exercise is commonly advised in the management of claudication; however, few vascular surgeons avail themselves of supervised exercise programs. There is vast literature on this subject, much of which has been abstracted in previous YEAR BOOKS. The best of these studies has shown a marked improvement in the overall walking distance in patients with supervised physical training. This study stresses the cognitive aspects of predicting improvement and also serves to remind us that structured programs are better than simple advice given in the clinic or office.

Evaluation of Non-Invasive Haemodynamic Parameters in Patients With Intermittent Claudication Subjected to Physical Training
Binaghi F, Fronteddu PF, Carboni MR, Onnis A, Astara C, Pitzus F (Univ of Cagliari, Italy)
Int Angiol 9:251–255, 1990   5–3

Background.—Although physical training is beneficial for patients with intermittent claudication, the mechanism of this effect is unclear. Hemodynamic parameters were evaluated in a group of patients before and after physical training, and modification of walking ability and hematological parameters were studied to assess the correlation between these findings and the hemodynamic parameters.

Methods.—Twenty-six patients with intermittent claudication caused by arterial obliterative disease were studied. Their mean age was 56.9 years; all were smokers. The hemodynamic, hematological, and clinical parameters were investigated before and 3 months after a program of physical training. The patients were instructed to walk at least 1 hour every day for 3 months, in addition to their normal activities. They were instructed to walk until pain began to occur and to resume walking after the pain disappeared. The patients received no vasoactive, anticoagulant, anti-aggregant or other drugs that might have affected blood lipids during the study period.

Results.—Physical training improved claudication pain distance by 65%. It also improved maximal walking distance (determined during a treadmill test at 2 mph up 12%) by 82%. The t/2 peak flow improved from 30 seconds to 46.3 seconds, as determined by plethysmographic venous occlusion strain-gauge studies. Fibrinogen decreased from 328 mg% to 302 mg%; this difference was important but not significant. No significant differences were found for the more important hemodynamic parameters, including Widsor index, peak flow, and time to peak flow. Neither were there any significant differences in total cholesterol and hematocrit.

Conclusions.—In patients with intermittent claudication, physical training significantly increases walking tolerance, but it does not increase peripheral blood flow measured by plethysmographic and Doppler techniques. Training may result in better muscle perfusion because of increased aerobic capacity and decreased production of vasodilator catabolites.

▶ Contrary to the opinion expressed in this abstract, the mechanism for improvement of walking distance in patients with claudication is known to be more efficient anaerobic muscle metabolism. Hemodynamic parameters change very little as patients' walking distance is improved. Previous studies have proven this fact. From a practical point of view, the patient is not interested in an explanation of mechanisms, but is only hopeful of an improvement in walking distance. This can be achieved through a structured, supervised exercise program.

6 Preoperative Considerations

Progression of Peripheral Occlusive Arterial Disease in Diabetes Mellitus: What Factors Are Predictive?
Palumbo PJ, O'Fallon M, Osmundson PJ, Zimmerman BR, Langworthy AL, Kazmier FJ (Mayo Clin and Mayo Found, Rochester, Minn)
Arch Intern Med 151:717–721, 1991   6–1

Background.—Four years ago, 700 patients were evaluated in a follow-up study of peripheral occlusive arterial disease (POAD). Previous reports described the baseline characteristics of these patients. The clinical and laboratory variables measured at baseline that might be considered risk factors for the occurrence or progression of POAD were investigated.

Methods.—During the 4-year period, 110 normal controls, 112 patients with POAD without diabetes mellitus, 240 patients with diabetes mellitus without POAD, and 100 patients with diabetes mellitus and POAD were evaluated. In addition, the clinical, biochemical, and vascular laboratory measurements were recorded.

Results.—The progression of POAD was associated with age, a history of hypertension or coronary heart disease, a history of cigarette smoking, the presence of POAD, systolic blood pressure, and β-thromboglobulin levels. According to a multivariate logistic regression model, the presence of diabetes mellitus and/or POAD at baseline, a reduction in the post-exercise ankle-brachial index, an elevated arm systolic blood pressure, and current smoking were associated independently with POAD progression.

Conclusions.—This study confirms the clinical impression that smoking, hypertension, and evidence of POAD are related to the progression of POAD. Quitting smoking and controlling hypertension are therefore essential to reduce the risk of the progression of this disease in diabetic patients.

▶ It must be disappointing to some individuals that there is a lack of association between the occurrence and progression of POAD and serum lipid levels, platelet function measurements, elevated levels of platelet-derived factors, von Willebrand antigen, and glycosylated hemoglobin. Instead, the more obvious risk factors of smoking, hypertension, and peripheral arterial occlusive disease are markers of severity progression.

Transcutaneous Oxygen Tension in Normal Subjects and in Patients With Critical Ischemia During Orthostatic Blood Pressure Changes
Jensen FB, Utzon NP, Aabech J, Paaske WP (Rigshospitalet, Univ of Copenhagen)
Surg Res Comm 9:243–247, 1990   6–2

Introduction.—In normal individuals, 2 discrete microcirculatory phenomena exist when the arterial and venous pressures are changed by the passive elevation or lowering of an extremity in relation to the reference heart level. These phenomena include the autoregulation of cutaneous blood flow and a local vasoconstrictor response. In patients with severe ischemia of the peripheral vascular bed, these responses are abolished. Experimental studies suggest a correlation between transcutaneous oxygen tension (tc-PO_2) and cutaneous blood flow.

Methods.—The effect of passive orthostatic blood pressure changes on tc-PO_2 of the feet was studied in 8 normal individuals and 6 patients with critical ischemia of the foot. During orthostatic blood pressure changes, the tc-PO_2 was measured at 41° C on the back of the forefoot between the extensor tendons of first and second toe.

Findings.—In normal individuals, the tc-PO_2 remained relatively constant from about 20 cm above to about 25 cm below the heart level. Beyond this interval, the tc-Po_2 decreased in parallel with the decrease in arterial pressure. However, in patients with critical ischemia, the relative tc-PO_2 was 0 from 60 cm above the heart level. When the ischemic foot was lowered, there was a dramatic increase in the tc-Po_2 by a factor of 1.5–8 times the heart level values, suggesting that neither autoregulation nor vasoconstrictor response was operating in critically ischemic areas.

Conclusion.—It is possible to identify patients with critical ischemia on the basis of characteristic tc-PO_2 responses to orthostatic blood pressure changes.

▶ Although the measurement of tc-Po_2 has been possible for many years, it seems to be a technique looking for an application. This study is important because it explains the mechanism of relief of rest pain in patients with critical ischemia.

The Effect of Femoral Arteriography on the Incidence of Groin Contamination and Postoperative Infections
Ameli FM, Knackstedt J, Provan JL, St Louis EL (Univ of Toronto)
Ann Vasc Surg 4:328–333, 1990   6–3

Background.—Previous studies have suggested that bacterial contamination of the punctured groin after preoperative transcutaneous arteriography may be 1 cause of the high rate of infections involving synthetic grafts with a femoral anastomosis. In this prospective study, the relationship of the side of arteriography to the site and incidence of bacterial infections and the relationship of the postoperative wound complications to preceding positive bacterial cultures were assessed.

Patients.—Aortobifemoral bypasses were done on 44 patients, all of whom had preoperative femoral arteriography; 77% had the test within 48 hours of surgery. The average age of the 26 men and 18 women was 63 years; postoperatively, they were seen annually for an average follow-up period of 28.4 months. The patients were prepared by standard

Summary of Postoperative Groin Wound Complications

Complication	Side	Bacteriological data	Arteriography
Lymph leak	Control	Positive arteriography: Streptococcus Negative control	Routine
Gaping, drainage groin incisions	Bilateral	Positive arteriography: Staphylococcus epidermidis negative control	Routine
Lymph leak	Control	Bilateral positive: Staphylococcus aureus	Routine
Lymph leak	Arteriography	Bilateral positive: Streptococcus Staphylococcus epidermidis	Difficult
Wound infection	Arteriography	Positive arteriography: streptococcus	Difficult
Draining groin incision	Control	Bilateral negative	Routine
Wound infection	Arteriography	Bilateral negative	Routine

(Courtesy of Ameli FM, Knackstedt J, Provan JL, et al: *Ann Vasc Surg* 4:328–333, 1990.)

aseptic procedures. The intraoperative aerobic and nonaerobic cultures were made with tissue samples taken from the needle tract on the arteriographic side, and from a comparable site along the femoral artery on the opposite side. The difficulty of arteriography, length of surgery, presence of hematoma caused by arteriography, and postoperative infections of the incisions were evaluated.

Results.—Cultures, predominantly of *Staphylococcus epidermidis,* were positive in 30.7% of the 88 operative incisions (43.2% of the patients). Whereas 18.2% of the patients had bilateral positive cultures, the additional 25% were almost equally divided between the control and arteriographic sides. There was no significant relationship between the puncture side and subsequent infection. In the 11.4% of "difficult" arteriographies that involved multiple punctures, cannula manipulation, or persistent bleeding, there were positive culture results in 80% and hematomas in 80%, but no correlation between hematomas and positive cultures. Hematomas evidently did not act as a bed for bacterial colonization. There were significantly more positive cultures in 83.2% of the operations that lasted longer than 4 hours, in contrast to 36.8% of the procedures that lasted for an average of 3 hours. The postoperative problems with groin wound healing in 7 patients are summarized in the table. There is no apparent relationship to the side of arteriography and no significant correlation with positive culture results.

Discussion.—The arteriographic risks of hematoma and bacterial contamination after skin puncture do not affect the incidence of femoral graft infections. Because the incidence of positive cultures increased dramatically as the duration of surgery increased, the high overall incidence is more likely a result of the contamination that occurs during the aortobifemoral bypass surgery itself.

▶ It is important for vascular surgeons to understand that the complications of surgery are in the hands of the surgeon. Wound infection and graft infection that occur during arterial reconstruction do not seem to be functions of the previous arteriographic manipulations.

Renal Dysfunction After Angiography; A Risk Factor Analysis in Patients With Peripheral Vascular Disease

Gussenhoven MJE, Ravensbergen J, van Bockel JH, Feuth JDM, Aarts JCNM
(Univ Hosp Leiden, The Netherlands)
J Cardiovasc Surg 32:81–86, 1991

6–4

Incidence of Induced Renal Dysfunction With Respect to Clinical and Radiological Variables

	Patients with Induced Renal Dysfunction		
	Number of patients	Percent of patients	p value
1. Age:			
— less than 70	7	2.9%	
— more than 70	14	11.0%	<0.005
2. Hypertension:			
— absent	3	1.6%	
— present	18	9.7%	<0.005
3. Antihypertensive medication:			
— not used	3	1.4%	
— used	18	11.5%	<0.0005
4. Renal disease:			
— absent	15	4.4%	
— present	6	20.0%	<0.005
5. Diabetes mellitus:			
— absent	16	5.0%	
— present	5	9.6%	>0.1
6. Diabetes:			
— insulin independent	1	2.6%	
— insulin dependent	4	28.6%	<0.05
7. Serum creatinine level:			
— less than 133 micromol/l	10	3.0%	
— more than 133 micromol/l	11	27.5%	<0.001
8. Site of contrast injection:			
— abdominal angiography	17	5.2%	
— aortic arch angiography	3	7.9%	>0.01
9. Type of contrast medium:			
— Hexabrix 320®	17	5.5%	
— Isopaque 370®	2	8.0%	>0.5
10. Quantity of contrast medium:			
— less than 150 ml	4	1.9%	
— more than 150 ml	15	11.7%	<0.0005

(Courtesy of Gussenhoven MJE, Ravensbergen J, van Bockel JH, et al: *J Cardiovasc Surg* 32:81–86, 1991.)

Background.—Before reconstructive surgery or percutaneous translu-minal angioplasty can be performed, angiography must be done. Al-though the procedure is safe, about 10% of patients have renal dysfunc-tion that is usually transient. The incidence of induced renal dysfunction was determined in a series of 369, Seldinger angiographic procedures, and the risk factors for this complication were identified.

Methods.—An increase in the serum creatinine level of at least 10% within 48 hours after angiography was used as the definition of induced renal dysfunction. The clinical and angiographic variables that were eval-uated as potential risk factors included age, hypertension, use of antihy-pertensive drugs. diabetes mellitus, angiographic technique, and injection site, type, and amount of contrast medium.

Results.—There were 21 cases of induced renal dysfunction, for an in-cidence of 5.7% (table). No patient died or required dialysis. According to univariate analysis, the variables associated with this complication were age 70 years or older, hypertension, use of antihypertensive drugs, renal disease, diabetes mellitus, a serum creatinine level of more than 133 μmol/L, and injection of more than 150 mL of contrast medium. The in-dependent risk factors included renal disease, use of antihypertensive drugs, more than 150 mL of contrast medium, and age over 70 years, but not diabetes mellitus. Two or more risk factors were present in 95% of the patients who had renal dysfunction.

Conclusions.—Induced renal dysfunction occurs at a low, but not neg-ligible, rate after angiography. The identified risk factors can easily deter-mine a patient's risk of renal dysfunction. Appropriate preventive mea-sures, such as creatinine monitoring, intravenous fluid administration, and the use of less than 100 mL of contrast medium, should be taken in patients with 2 or more risk factors.

▶ As imaging techniques move more and more toward minimal invasion and application of techniques without side effects, the role of angiography is pre-dictably going to diminish. At present, it is essential in restricted circum-stances. The future holds for noncontrast imaging without body penetration.

Can Duplex Scanning Replace Arteriography for Lower Extremity Arterial Disease?
Kohler TR, Andros G, Porter JM, Clowes A, Goldstone J, Johansen K, Raker E, Nance DR, Strandness DE Jr (VA Med Ctr, Seattle; Univ of Washington; Ma-son Clinic, Seattle; St Joseph Med Ctr, Burbank, Calif; Oregon Health Sciences Univ, Portland; et al)
Ann Vasc Surg 4:280–287, 1990   6–5

Study Design.—A preliminary study compared the differences in sur-geons' choice of an intervention for the treatment of lower extremity oc-clusive disease when data from either a duplex scan or an arteriogram were provided along with basic clinical information.

Method.—Six vascular surgeons chose a clinical plan for each of 29 patients in a blinded fashion. Information on the degree of stenosis from duplex scans and arteriograms was indicated on an anatomical line drawing along with the ankle blood pressures and a brief clinical description.

Findings.—Each plan was placed into 1 of 8 possible categories for comparison using the kappa statistic. Intraobserver agreement between surgeons' decisions based on duplex scanning versus those based on arteriography was very good, with exact agreement in 76%. The interobserver agreement between different surgeons' decisions based on the same studies was significantly less. Significant disparity among different surgeons' clinical decisions occurred in 43% of patients when there were no significant differences between the duplex scan and arteriogram reports.

Conclusion.—Clinical decisions based on duplex scans are very similar to those made by using arteriograms. As reported in earlier studies, a combination of clinical history and bedside Doppler examination can limit the need for arteriography in assessing patients with lower extremity arterial occlusive disease.

▶ The Washington group investigated the possibility of using ultrasound as the imaging modality that can produce physiological and anatomical information. Their current research efforts will throw further light on this subject. Many forms of arterial reconstruction will most likely be applied without angiography in the future.

Colour-Coded Doppler Sonography for the Investigation of the Morphology and Haemodynamics of the Pelvic and Lower Limb Arteries in Normal Individuals

Luska VG, Risch U, Pellengahr M, von Boetticher H (Zentralkrankenhaus "Links der Weser", Bremen, Germany)
Fortschr Röntgenstr 153:246–251, 1990   6–6

Introduction.—Color-coded Doppler sonography (CCDS) is a new noninvasive diagnostic technique for investigating vascular disorders. However, the diagnostic accuracy of a new technique can be evaluated only when sufficient normal data from healthy individuals are available for comparison. Color-coded Doppler sonography was used with quantitative angiodynography to define the morphology and hemodynamics in the arteries of the pelvis and in the lower extremities of healthy individuals.

Methods.—Twelve women and 8 men, (age range, 18–50 years) with no evidence of arterial vascular disorders were scanned. All measurements were obtained after a 15-minute rest period in a room at constant temperature. A total of 360 morphological measurements and 6,480 hemodynamic measurements were obtained.

Results.—Morphological assessment of the vasculature with CCDS revealed that the common iliac artery, the external iliac artery, the superficial femoral artery in the distal adductor canal, and the fibular artery were visualized poorly. Hemodynamic assessment in the spectral mode was only possible when vascular morphology was adequately visualized. Because of technical limitations, flow velocity measurements were limited in the pelvic area, the thigh, and the knee. Flow velocity measurements in the thigh were obtainable only in superifical vessels. All other measurements gave falsely low readings.

Conclusion.—The quantitative hemodynamic parameters for the pelvic and lower limb arteries obtained with CCDS in normal individuals may serve as a reference for future studies.

▶ This study points out the limitations of duplex scanning and heralds wider application as these limitations are overcome.

Determination of the Extent of Lower-Extremity Peripheral Arterial Disease With Color-Assisted Duplex Sonography: Comparison With Angiography
Polak JF, Karmel MI, Mannick JA, O'Leary DH, Donaldson MC, Whittemore AD
(Harvard Med School; Brigham and Women's Hosp, Boston)
AJR 155:1085–1089, 1990   6–7

Introduction.—Color Doppler flow sonography may be able to facilitate the preangiographic determination of the nature and the extent of segmental arterial disease in the legs. The subjective grading of the narrowing of the arterial lumen by color flow imaging could be combined with Doppler spectral analysis, a method that by itself is accurate but time consuming.

Study Design.—The determination of the extent of lower extremity peripheral arterial disease with color-assisted Duplex sonography was compared with that of angiography (table). A group of 17 consecutive symp-

---

Summary of the Results of Color-Assisted Duplex Sonography Compared With Arteriography for the Detection of Arterial Segment Stenosis and Occlusions

Artery	True Positive		False Positive		True Negative
	Stenosis	Occlusion	Stenosis	Occlusion	
Common femoral	1	0	0	0	32
Profunda femoris	1	0	0	0	30
Superficial femoral					
Proximal	4	5	1	0	24
Mid	7	5	1	0	20
Distal	4	7	0	4	17
Popliteal					
Proximal	3	4	2	0	25
Distal	2	6	1	0	25
Total	22	27	5	4	173

Results of 7 examinations were false negative for stenosis. Of these, 3 resulted from dense calcifications, 1 each in the common femoral and mid and distal superficial femoral arteries. Four lesions were distal to a more proximal high-grade stenosis or occlusion, with 3 in the profunda femoris artery and 1 in the distal superficial femoral artery. No examination results were false negative for occlusion.
(Courtesy of Polak JF, Karmel MI, Mannick JA, et al: AJR 155:1085–1089, 1990.)

tomatic patients who had never had arteriography or surgical revascularization of the lower extremities were assessed sonographically before undergoing arteriography. The mean patient age was 62 years. The results of angiography of the femoropopliteal arteries were graded and localized in 1 of 7 arterial segments that were approximately equal. These were then compared with similar segmental maps done with sonography.

Findings.—For detecting stenosis or occlusion in any of the 238 segments, the sensitivity of the technique was 88%; the specificity was 95%; and the accuracy was 93%. The time needed to survey both limbs was an average of 29 minutes.

Discussion.—Duplex sonography coupled with color flow sonography has a sensitivity for detecting significant stenoses or occluded segments that is at least equivalent to the reported rates for duplex sonography. The major advantage of color-assisted duplex imaging is the time it takes to survey the femoropopliteal arterial system of the lower extremities: the average examination time of 29 minutes compares quite favorably with the 1−2 hours needed for duplex sonography alone. This technique is an improvement over the noninvasive use of segmental Doppler pressure measurements.

▶ At present, duplex evaluation of the peripheral circulation can select patients for transluminal angioplasty. It can then accompany the arteriographic event. In the future, bypass reconstructions may also be based on such techniques.

Peripheral Arterial Occlusive Disease: Prospective Comparison of MR Angiography and Color Duplex US With Conventional Angiography
Mulligan SA, Matsuda T, Lanzer P, Gross GM, Routh WD, Keller FS, Koslin DB, Berland LL, Fields MD, Doyle M, Cranney GB, Lee JY, Pohost GM (Univ of Alabama, Birmingham)
Radiology 178:695–700, 1991   6–8

Objective.—To ascertain how noninvasive methods of assessment of peripheral arterial occlusive disease of the lower extremities compared with conventional angiography, 12 patients with symptomatic peripheral vascular disease were evaluated in a prospective, blinded study.

Data Analysis.—The ability to grade arterial lesions and plan revascularization interventions using 2-dimensional inflow MR angiography, color duplex ultrasound, and conventional angiography were compared. Arterial lesions were defined as nonsignificant in the presence of 0 to 49% diameter reduction or significant with 50% to 99% stenosis or occlusion.

Results.—In the determination of nonsignificant and significant arterial lesions, there was agreement between MR angiography and conventional angiography in 100 (71%) of 140 lesions and between color duplex ultrasound and conventional angiography in 114 (93%) of 123 lesions. The color duplex ultrasound was limited in its evaluation of the iliac segment because of nonvisualization, but it performed well in the evaluation of infrainguinal disease. Although the iliac region was visualized in more patients with MR angiography, the image quality with MR angiography was inconsistent. Ten lesions were underestimated on MR angiography compared with conventional angiography. Of the 21 vascular interventions planned by using conventional angiography, 11 were suggested by color duplex ultrasound and 5 were suggested by MR angiography. These disagreements resulted from differences in the grading and location of stenosis, and from nonvisualization of arterial segments.

Conclusion.—Better and more consistent images with MR angiography and increased experience with color duplex scanning are needed in the evaluation of peripheral arterial occlusive disease.

▶ At present, color duplex ultrasound and MR angiography are complementary rather than competitive. The application of both techniques is advantageous in decreasing the side effects of invasive arteriography.

Penetrating Aortic Ulcers: Diagnosis With MR Imaging
Yucel EK, Steinberg FL, Egglin TK, Geller SC, Waltman AC, Athanasoulis CA
(Massachusetts Gen Hosp, Boston)
Radiology 177:779–781, 1990   6–9

Background.—Magnetic resonance imaging (MRI) has proved its value in the diagnosis of aortic dissection and in the detection of acute and subacute hematoma. Whether MRI can discriminate between an intraluminal clot and a hematoma within the wall of the aorta, and whether it can be used to diagnose a deep aortic ulcer were investigated. Images derived from MRI, CT, and aortography were compared.

Methods.—Seven patients, between the ages of 62 and 81 years, were admitted with acute chest and/or back pain and underwent multiple-plane MRI within 10 days. Six patients had CT studies. Four of these

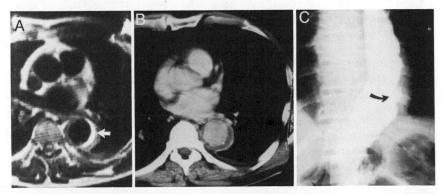

Fig 6–1.—A, T1-weighted (gated first-echo) axial image shows high signal intensity in the aortic wall *(arrow)*; B, contrast material-enhanced CT scan at the same level shows a rim of nonspecific low-attenuation material (note the displaced intimal calcium not seen on the MR image); C, aortogram shows the thickened aortic wall with an ulcer *(arrow)*. (Courtesy of Yucel EK, Steinberg FL, Egglin TK, et al: *Radiology* 177:779–781, 1990.)

studies were done with contrast-enhancement. All 7 patients had biplane aortography, and the results were correlated with surgical observations in 3 patients who underwent thoracic aortic repair.

Results.—In the MRI series, the aortic wall showed localized regions of high signal intensity in T1- and T2-weighted images indicating focal intramural hemorrhage in 4 patients (Fig 6–1); whereas 5 patients had profoundly ulcerated atherosclerotic plaque, and 2 patients had considerably dissected hematoma in the aortic wall. Two patients had localized intramural hematoma 1 of which ruptured. Four patients had both ulceration and increased T1 and T2 signals. One ulcer revealed by angiography was not seen with MRI. In the CT studies, intraluminal clot, atherosclerotic plaque, and intramural hematoma could not be distinguished, and ulcers were identified in only 2 patients. By angiography, penetrating aortic ulcer was verified in all of the patients.

Discussion.—The results indicate that MRI can be an accurate means of diagnosing penetrating aortic ulcer. Although 1 ulcer was missed in the MRI studies, determination of the extent of clotting within the aortic wall was better than that achieved by angiography. In comparison with CT scanning, MRI missed an intimal calcification in 1 case, but was better for distinguishing different types of lesions. Because the risk of iodinated contrast-enhancement need not be taken with MRI, and because it appears to be accurate in this setting, it is recommended as the best noninvasive diagnostic test when penetrating aortic ulcer is suspected.

▶ Penetrating ulcers of the thoracic aortic wall are a source of shredding atheromatous embolization to peripheral circulation. It appears that the syndrome of peripheral small vessel occlusive disease can be investigated well with MR in addition to conventional methods.

Combined Epidural and General Anesthesia in Aortic Surgery

Mason RA, Newton GB, Cassel W, Maneksha F, Giron F (State Univ of New York, Stony Brook)
J Cardiovasc Surg 31:442–447, 1990   6–10

Introduction.—There has been increasing focus on the use of combined epidural and general anesthesia in reducing the cardiac and pulmonary morbidity associated with aortic surgery. The perioperative courses of 144 consecutive patients who underwent elective transperitoneal aortic reconstructive surgery were studied.

Intervention.—Epidural and light general anesthesia (Epi-GA) was employed in 77 patients, and conventional general anesthesia (GA) was used in 67. Age, medical risk factors, preoperative cardiac and pulmonary function, and type of surgical reconstruction did not differ between the groups.

Results.—The groups had similar anesthetic, operative, and clamp times. The rate pressure product, an indicator of myocardial stress, was significantly lower in the Epi-GA group during aortic cross-clamping.

Postoperatively, significantly more patients in the GA group required prolonged ventilatory support and more parenteral narcotics during the first 48 hours. Mortality did not differ significantly between groups; the rate was 3% in the GA group and 5.2% in the Epi-GA group. Pulmonary complications were more common in the GA group (7.5%) than in the Epi-GA group (2.6%), although the difference was not significant.

Implications.—In aortic surgery, Epi-GA provides a stable intraoperative hemodynamic course, allows early weaning from ventilator support, and provides excellent postoperative analgesia. Hence, Epi-GA may be the preferred form of anesthesia for the high-risk pulmonary patient undergoing transperitoneal aortic reconstruction.

▶ Among the important preoperative considerations in patients who are scheduled to undergo aortic surgery is the choice of anesthesia. This choice is linked inextricably to the choice of operative approach. Retroperitoneal aortic exposure is an aid in decreasing ileus in patients undergoing conventional general anesthesia. Epidural anesthesia appears to aid the convalescence of patients with a transperitoneal approach. This report on the combination of the 2 modalities of anesthesia suggests a happy combination.

Prophylactic Antibiotics in Vascular Surgery
Bunt TJ (Maricopa Med Ctr, Phoenix)
Compl Surg 46–52, 1991   6–11

Background.—In vascular surgery, prophylactic antibiotics are used to prevent serious complications of synthetic vascular graft infections such as wound infections, local skin or tissue secondary contamination, or seeding of the graft. Methods of prophylaxis include intravenous perioperative prophylactic or therapeutic regimens, topical or local wound irrigations, or impregnation of the graft matrix with antibiotics.

Findings.—Polytetrafluorethylene grafts were associated with a lower rate of infection for 4 organisms compared with the Dacron velour or woven graft. Antibiotic-impregnated grafts are not yet available commercially, but laboratory models have shown an improved resistance to graft matrix infection. The slow release of antibiotics may confer prolonged bacterial resistance. In cultures of arteriotomy sites, aortic aneurysm clot cultures, and inguinal incisions, *Staphylococcus epidermidis* was the primary bacterium. Typically *S. epidermidis* does not present early in the postoperative period.

Conclusions.—Antibiotic prophylaxis should be determined by the potential sources of graft infection, the expected pathogens, the presence of risk factors such as distal pedal infections, and the theoretical problems of postoperative wound complications. The regimen must provide the appropriate therapeutic ratio and the adequate dose-response curve for the relatively high minimum inhibitory concentration of *S. epidermidis* (table).

Recommendations for Utilization of Antibiotics for Peripheral Vascular Surgery

Type of Case	Recommendations
Clean elective abdominal (Aortorenal, aortomesenteric, aortoiliac bypass)	-IV 3-dose perioperative repeat q 3h
Clean elective involving groin (Axillofemoral, aortofemoral, femoropopliteal, femorodistal)	-IV 3-dose perioperative repeat q 3h -topical antibiotics for groin wounds -consider in situ rifampin
Active distal infection	-IV therapeutic 7 to 10 days -topical antibiotics for all wounds -consider in situ rifampin
Aortic aneurysmorrhaphy	-IV 3-dose perioperative -extend to 2 weeks for positive aortic culture -consider in situ rifampin

(Courtesy of Bunt TJ: *Compl Surg* 46–52, 1991.)

Long-Term Prognosis of Myocardial Ischemia Detected by Holter Monitoring in Peripheral Vascular Disease

Raby KE, Goldman L, Cook EF, Rumerman J, Barry J, Creager MA, Selwyn AP (Brigham and Women's Hosp, Boston; Harvard Med School)
Am J Cardiol 66:1309–1313, 1990   6–12

Background.—There is a strong correlation between ST depression detected during ambulatory monitoring and other markers of myocardial ischemia in patients with coronary artery disease. This method has been used to predict in-hospital postoperative events in patients undergoing peripheral arterial surgery. A large group of these patients was followed to determine if preoperative ischemia can predict late adverse cardiac events.

Patients.—Prospective studies were made in 124 men and 52 women (mean age, 66 years) who were scheduled for elective peripheral arterial surgery. Before surgery the patients were monitored and had no alterations to their baseline medications. Prospective follow-up was done in the course of routine medical care that was provided by blinded, independent cardiologists and by subsequent telephone interviews with the patients. Myocardial ischemia was detected in 75 episodes in 32 patients; 73 episodes were asymptomatic. Mean follow-up time was 615 days.

Findings.—During follow-up there were 9 cardiac deaths, including 1 postoperative in-hospital death. There were 13 nonfatal myocardial infarctions, 4 of which occurred in the hospital. Twelve of the 32 patients with ischemia had some cardiac event, including 6 deaths, for a rate of 38%. There were 10 cardiac events in 144 patients without ischemia, including 3 deaths for a rate of 7%. The sensitivity of ischemia was 55%; specificity, 87%; positive predictive value, 38%; and negative predictive value, 93%. A multivariate Cox proportional hazards model was calculated for the variables of age, sex, coronary risk factors, history of angina, myocardial infarction, coronary artery disease, and antianginal medications. The only independent predictor of outcome was the presence of ischemia.

Conclusions.—Ambulatory monitoring for myocardial ischemia is a significant independent predictor of 1- to 2-year prognosis in patients with peripheral vascular disease. The technique is particularly helpful in patients who cannot perform adequate exercise tests. Patients without ischemia appear to be at low risk for future cardiac events.

▶ In the original article abstracted here, the authors' previously published study was summarized for reemphasis. The method of monitoring that was described in this study was able to predict postoperative cardiac events, but a limitation of the study was that few patients experienced cardiac death or myocardial infarction during the postoperative period. The events referred to were largely unstable angina or ischemic pulmonary edema. Preoperative monitoring appears to be a predictor of cardiac death and myocardial infarction in the late postoperative period. This is, of course, an important finding.

Selective Evaluation and Management of Coronary Artery Disease in Patients Undergoing Repair of Abdominal Aortic Aneurysms: A 16-Year Experience
Golden MA, Whittemore AD, Donaldson MC, Mannick JA (Harvard Med School)
Ann Surg 212:415–423, 1990   6–13

Introduction.—Patients with an abdominal aortic aneurysm (AAA) often have coexisting coronary artery disease (CAD) that increases the risk of perioperative cardiac mortality after AAA repair. A preoperative patient classification of cardiovascular risk status was evaluated in subsequent management of patients with AAA.

Patients.—During a 16-year period, 94 women and 406 men aged 42–94 years underwent urgent or elective operation for infrarenal nonruptured AAA. The patients were divided into 3 groups. The first group consisted of 260 patients (52%) with no clinical or ECG evidence of CAD. These patients underwent AAA repair without further cardiac evaluation. The second group consisted of 212 patients (42.4%) with clinical or ECG evidence of CAD. These patients underwent further cardiac evaluation, their CAD was found to be stable, and they underwent AAA repair. The third group consisted of 28 patients (5.6%) with clinical or ECG evidence of CAD. These patients underwent further cardiac evaluation, their CAD was found to be unstable, and they underwent repair of their cardiac disease before or during AAA repair.

Outcome.—Eight patients (1.6%) died within 30 days of operation. One patient was in the group with no CAD (mortality, .4%) and 7 were in the group with stable CAD before AAA repair (mortality, 3.3%). Five of the 7 patients with stable CAD before operation died of myocardial infarction. None of the patients with unstable CAD who underwent repair of cardiac disease before or during AAA repair died within 30 days of operation.

Conclusion.—Myocardial infarction is the leading cause of perioperative mortality in AAA repair. Repair of severe or unstable CAD before or during AAA repair seems to prevent operative mortality. Patients with known CAD should undergo further cardiac evaluation before being operated on for AAA. Those patients with no clinical or ECG evidence of CAD rarely have significant perioperative cardiac complications.

▶ Data from other studies corroborate the facts in this study. Those patients without clinical or ECG evidence of coronary artery occlusive disease do not require further investigations before aortic surgery. In contrast, patients with clinical or ECG evidence of coronary artery disease should have further investigations. Among these patients are those who should have preliminary coronary artery bypass grafting. In answering questions from the floor about the most cost-effective predictive screening tests in patients with coronary artery disease, the authors referred to the patients who had undergone ambulatory Holter monitoring. They suggested that it might ultimately prove to be the most sensitive test.

Which Deaths in Vascular Surgery are Avoidable? A Review of 150 Consecutive Deaths Occurring on the Oxford Regional Vascular Service
O'Kelly TJ, Collin J, Murie JA, Morris PJ (Univ of Oxford, England)
Eur J Vasc Surg 4:395–399, 1990   6–14

Objective.—The identification and prevention of avoidable deaths can improve the quality of surgical care. Deaths occurring between October 1984 and July 1988 at the Oxford regional vascular service were evaluated to determine which surgical deaths were avoidable.

Setting.—During this period, 2,449 patients were admitted to the vascular service and 1,796 operations were performed. A total of 150 consecutive deaths were reviewed. The primary vascular diagnosis was aneurysmal disease in 71 of the 150 patients who died and occlusive arterial disease in 76. Most of the deaths occurred in the elderly, 89% in patients older than 65 years of age, and 32% in patients older than 80 years. Most of the deaths were caused by the presenting disorder or associated conditions.

Results.—Thirty-four (23%) deaths were considered avoidable. Twenty-seven of these occurred in patients with aneurysms, including 21 with rupture. Eleven deaths involved delay in the management of the presenting condition. Delays included a wrong diagnosis in 7 cases and interhospital transfer of 4 patients with leaking aneurysm. The remaining 21 deaths involved 3 anesthetic errors and 18 technical mistakes made by surgeons. The latter included incorrect use of arterial clamps, prolonged arterial clamping, anastomotic disruption, graft sepsis, and 7 deaths that occurred as a direct consequence of hemorrhage from the anastomotic suture line, a single bleeding vessel, or generalized oozing from disrupted tissue. These were compounded by failure to recognize the continuing hemorrhage early.

Summary.—Although early diagnosis of abdominal aortic aneurysms and rapid transport to a vascular service are essential, technical management errors remain a major cause of avoidable deaths in vascular surgery.

▶ In this study, technical management errors are stressed as a cause of death after vascular surgery. Please note that in elective cases such as those reported in Abstract 6–13, there were no technical deaths. All of the causes of death were in the categories of myocardial infarction or pulmonary embolization.

7 Thoracic Aorta

Alterations of Elastic Architecture in Human Aortic Dissecting Aneurysm
Nakashima Y, Shiokawa Y, Sueishi K (Kyushu Univ, Fukuoka, Japan)
Lab Invest 62:751–760, 1990   7–1

Background.—The pathogenesis of human dissecting aneurysm is not clear. Some studies suggested that elastic alterations in the aorta may play a role in the pathogenesis of dissecting aneurysm.

Method.—The 3-dimensional architecture of elastin in the ascending aorta media was examined by scanning electron microscopy after treatment of the aortas with hot formic acid. The samples of aorta were obtained from 10 patients with type A dissecting aneurysm, 14 hypertensive patients, and 30 control subjects without cardiovascular diseases.

Findings.—In control subjects the elastin formed a honeycomb or framework-like continuous structure consisting of elastic laminae and interlaminar fibers that interconnected the laminae. In dissecting aneurysms, 6 cases showed similar alterations in the elastic architecture of the outer media. The alterations consisted of irregular arrangement and shape of interlaminar fibers, as well as a reduced number of interlaminar fibers. In 3 cases of dissecting aneurysm, cystic medial necrosis (CMN) was evident, but only 1 case showed a slight decrease of interlaminar elastic fibers in the area outside of the CMN. This suggested that the initiation of CMN did not relate directly to the decrease in interlaminar fibers. In hypertensives, the aortic media generally showed an increase of interlaminar fibers, particularly in the inner media. However, 3 cases showed focal decreases in the outer media that resembled those seen in the dissecting aneurysm. This finding suggests that hypertension relates to the etiology of the dissecting aneurysm through the architectural alterations in the media.

Discussion.—Human aortic dissecting aneurysm is associated with a decrease and a disarrangement of interlaminar elastic fibers, particularly in the outer media. This architectural alteration may relate to the medial weakness, causing a rarefaction of interconnection of each elastic lamina. Subsequently, the aortic wall becomes weak against the dissecting force of the laminae. This medial weakness may be related to the mechanism of initiation and progression of the dissecting aneurysm.

▶ Alteration of the elastic architecture suggests that the affected media allow progression of the dissection in a rapid and widespread fashion. A decrease in elastic fibers has not been demonstrated in dissecting aneurysms of non-Marfan's etiology.

Aortic Dissection With the Entrance Tear in the Descending Thoracic Aorta: Analysis of 40 Necropsy Patients

Roberts CS, Roberts WC (Natl Heart, Lung, and Blood Inst, Bethesda, Md)
Ann Surg 213:356–368, 1991   7–2

Background.—During the past 30 years, the National Heart, Lung, and Blood Institute has been studying patients with spontaneous aortic dissection. The entrance tear was in the ascending aorta in 70% of the patients, the transverse aorta in 7%, the descending thoracic aorta in 22%, and the abdominal aorta in 1%. The clinical and necropsy findings in patients in whom the entrance tear was in the descending thoracic aorta were examined.

Patients.—Forty patients, aged 39–91 years at death, were studied. Sixty percent were men. A total of 83% had a history of systemic hypertension, and the heart weights were increased in 78%. Of the 40 patients, 31 had no surgery, and 9 underwent operation for aortic dissection.

Outcomes.—The diagnosis of aortic dissection was established in life in 9 patients and at necropsy in 22 of the 31 patients who were not treated surgically. In 42%, the interval from aortic dissection to death was 30 days or less. Death was caused by rupture of the false channel in 69% and by renal failure in 15%; the cause was unclear in 15%. The time from aortic dissection to death was more than 30 days in 58% of the 31 patients who were not treated surgically. In these 18 patients, the cause of death was related to dissection in 61%. In the remaining 39%, death was unrelated to the dissection; however, a nonfatal complication—stenosis of the true channel from compression by a thrombus-filled false channel—occurred in 4 of these 7 patients. Therefore, only 3 of the 31 patients who were not treated surgically had no complications of aortic dissection. All 9 patients who had surgery did so because of a major complication of the dissection. In all cases, the aortic dissection occurred within 30 days. Four of these patients survived 8–84 months postoperatively.

Conclusions.—early operative intervention before complications occur appears to be justified in patients with aortic dissection with the entrance tear in the descending thoracic aorta. Such surgery may be done to prevent rupture of the false channel acutely or after initial healing, renal failure from compression of renal arteries by an aneurysmal false channel, true channel stenosis from compression by a thrombus-filled false channel, and possibly the recurrence of acute dissection.

▶ Elegant, classic, artistic renditions of the pathological process accompany the original publication of this study and are commended to the readers of this volume. This study confirms the clinical impression that dissections with the entrance tear in the descending thoracic aorta have the highest frequency of spontaneous healing. This is in contrast to the dissections in which the entrance tear is in the ascending aorta or in the transverse arch. Note that aneurysm formation of the false channel occurred in all 18 of the patients with healed dissections in this series. Rupture of this false channel aneurysm occurred in the largest of the aneurysms.

Ruptured Aneurysm of the Descending Thoracic and Thoracoabdominal Aorta: Analysis According to Size and Treatment

Crawford ES, Hess KR, Cohen ES, Coselli JS, Safi HJ (Baylor College of Medicine; Methodist Hosp, Houston)
Ann Surg 213:417–426, 1991   7–3

Introduction.—Several studies have concluded that rupture of a descending thoracic aortic aneurysm (DES) rarely occurs when the aneurysmal diameter is less than 10 cm. Some authors recommend that a DES less than 10 cm in diameter should be treated conservatively and that surgical treatment should be reserved for aneurysms greater than 10 cm in diameter. The records of 117 patients who were operated on for acute rupture of a DES or a thoracoabdominal aortic aneurysm (TAA) were reviewed.

Methods.—The study population consisted of 73 men and 44 women aged 16 to 87 years (median age, 69 years). Of the 117 patients, 80 had DES rupture and 37 had TAA rupture. Rupture of a DES occurred into either the lung or the esophagus in 8 patients, into the pleural cavity in 49, and into the mediastinum in 23. Rupture of a TAA occurred into the peritoneal cavity in 3 patients and into the retroperitoneal tissues in 34. Aneurysm size was recorded for 59 DESs and 27 TAAs.

Findings.—Of the 59 DESs 8 (14%) were 5–6 cm in diameter, 21 (36%) were 6–8 cm, 23 (39%) were 8–10 cm, and 7 (12%) were greater than 10 cm in diameter. Thus, in 52 (88%) patients the size of the DES was less than 10 cm at the time of rupture. Similarly, 22 (81%) of the 27 TAAs were less than 10 cm in diameter at the time of rupture (table). The overall 30-day mortality rate was 24%. In contrast, elective operation has an early mortality of 8%. The 5-year survival rate was 28%, whereas elective operation is generally associated with a 92% survival rate.

Conclusion.—Rupture of a DES or a TAA is usually a terminal disorder because most patients die before appropriate treatment can be instituted. The survival rate of patients who reach the hospital alive after aneurysmal rupture is significantly lower than that of patients who undergo elective operation. Elective operation should be considered when an aneurysm is 5 cm or larger or if a patient is symptomatic.

Estimated Aortic Diameter at Site of Rupture (86 Patients With Available Data)

Size Range (cm)	Abdomen	Thorax	Total
5.0–6.0	3 (11%)	8 (14%)	11 (13%)
6.1–8.0	13 (48%)	21 (36%)	34 (40%)
8.1–10.0	6 (22%)	23 (39%)	29 (34%)
10.1–17.0	5 (19%)	7 (12%)	12 (14%)
Total	27 (100%)	59 (100%)	86 (100%)

(Courtesy of Crawford ES, Hess KR, Cohen ES, et al: *Ann Surg* 213:417–426, 1991.)

▶ We will all miss Stanley Crawford's instructive and overwhelming reports to the American Surgical Association and to the Southern Surgical Association (such as this study).

Prevention of Paraplegia During Aortic Operations

Wadouh F, Wadouh R, Hartmann M, Crisp-Lindgren N (Heidehaus, Hannover, Germany)
Ann Thorac Surg 50:543–552, 1990   7–4

Background.—Paraplegia may result from spinal cord injury after cross clamping of the descending aorta whether or not there is aortic disease present. An early explanation for spinal cord injury in this circumstance held that the damage was caused by a proximal-to-distal reduction in the flow of the anterior spinal artery. Based on experimental evidence, it is suggested that a pressure gradient between vessels serving the spinal cord and the clamped aorta causes blood to flow back towards the hypotonic aorta, and that spinal cord injury results from a steal effect thus produced. This hypothesis was tested by measuring the oxygen tension (PO_2) in the spinal cord after simple or segmental clamping of the abdominal and thoracic aorta.

Methods.—A group of 20 pigs (weight, 25–30 kg) were anesthetized, ventilated, and cannulated for aortic pressure monitoring. In 1 group, the thoracic artery was occluded at T3 to T4; in the second group, the abdominal aorta was clamped at L1. Via laminectomies at T7 to T8 in the first group, and L3 to L5 in the second group, PO_2 was measured with an electrode on the surface of the spinal cord after simple aortic cross-clamping, double aortic cross clamping, occlusion of spinal cord blood supply, and resumption of aortic blood flow.

Results.—Regardless of where a simple clamp was applied, it resulted in a significant decrease in PO_2 distal to the clamp; however, if the thoracic aorta was excluded by an additional clamp at T13, PO_2 was restored to 30.8 mm Hg, near the normal level of 36 mm Hg. In contrast, PO_2 in the artery of Adamkiewicz was relatively unaffected by segmentation of the abdominal aorta as far as S-1.

Discussion.—Rather than supplying the spinal cord longitudinally, blood appears to dissipate away from it after aortic cross-clamping, aggravating spinal ischemia. A dramatic decline in PO_2 occurred distal to the clamp despite a relative perfusion pressure of 20 mm Hg between the aorta and the spinal cavity. Two techniques may reduce the risk of paraplegia in humans. To repair the aorta with the counterocclusion technique after injury or bursting, an additional clamp should be placed at T12 or distal to the arteria radicularis magna anterior (ARMA). An alternate, the bypass fractionated approach, requires perfusion pressure of at least 50 mm Hg and a volume of at least 2 L/min, with proximal-to-distal staged clamping of the aorta, blood flow restored at the previous stage as each new stage is clamped, thus reducing ischemic time. The location of the ARMA should first be localized by angiography.

▶ Whether or not a steal phenomenon occurs, as is claimed in this study, will be proven eventually. It is depressing that focused research on this subject has not uncovered a method of preventing paraplegia during thoracoabdominal surgery.

Traumatic Disruptions of the Thoracic Aorta: Treatment and Outcome
DelRossi AJ, Cernaianu AC, Madden LD, Cilley JH Jr, Spence RK, Alexander JB, Ross SE, Camishion RC (Cooper Hosp/Univ Med Ctr, Camden, NJ; Univ of Medicine and Dentistry of New Jersey)
Surgery 108:864–870, 1990   7–5

Introduction.—The overall mortality for traumatic transection of the thoracic aorta remains very high. During the past 3 years 27 patients were treated for acute disruption of the thoracic aorta.

Patients-Management.—All of the patients had associated major injuries, although 5 of the patients had no symptoms. Diagnostic aortography showed a definitive disruption of the aorta at the level of the isthmus, but failed to show multiple tears in 3 patients. On admission 3 patients were in profound shock, and 2 died of exsanguination before aortic repair. One patient had massive leakage from the aneurysm after aortography and died during surgery. The other 24 patients were hemodynamically stable on admission, and treatment was based on the extent of their injuries (table). Emergency thoracotomy was performed on patients with exsanguinating hemorrhage and signs of widened mediastinum, whereas orthopedic or abdominal injuries, or both, were considered after aortic repair. Eighteen patients, including 2 with multiple tears, underwent aortic repair with the "clamp and sew" technique and with intercalation of a woven Dacron prosthesis. The mean aortic cross-clamp (AXC) time was 26 minutes, but it was prolonged to 67 minutes in the 2 patients with multiple tears. Five patients had aortic repair with heparin-bonded Gott shunts, and mean AXC time was 38 minutes. One patient with multiple tears underwent a total cardiopulmonary bypass with a mean AXC time of 43 minutes.

Operative Procedures and Outcome

Operation	Survivors	Nonsurvivors
Thoracotomy	1	3*
Thoracotomy/orthopedic procedure	14	1
Thoracotomy/laparotomy	2	1
Laparotomy/thoracotomy	4	1
TOTALS	21	6

*Includes 2 patients admitted in shock and operated on an emergency basis.
(Courtesy of DelRossi AJ, Cernaianu AC, Madden LD, et al: *Surgery* 108:864–870, 1990.)

Outcome.—Six of the patients died, for an overall mortality of 22.2%. Of these 6 patients, 3 died of massive exsanguination before or during surgery; the 3 postoperative deaths were related to polytrauma, cardiogenic shock, and sepsis. Although the other 21 patients recovered, 3 had paraplegia, including 2 who required longer AXC time during repair. Follow-up at 1 year showed 100% survival, with only 1 patient having a significant neurologic deficit.

Conclusion.—The clamp and sew technique for the repair of traumatic dissections of the thoracic aorta is relatively safe and simple to perform and may allow for a more favorable outcome. Complicated lesions, however, may require the use of temporary shunts or cardiopulmonary bypass.

▶ This study emphasizes both the paraplegia caused by prolonged thoracic aortic cross-clamping and the lack of paraplegia observed during short clamp times. However, other observations do not support these findings. The problem remains vexing.

Rupture of Thoracic Aorta Caused by Blunt Trauma: A Fifteen-Year Experience

Cowley RA, Turney SZ, Hankins JR, Rodriguez A, Attar S, Shankar BS (Univ of Maryland)

J Thorac Cardiovasc Surg 100:652–661, 1990   7–6

Introduction.—Acute rupture of the thoracic aorta from blunt trauma is associated with a high rate of lethal exsanguination and a high incidence of postoperative paraplegia in survivors. There is still controversy concerning the protective effect of shunting during aortic crossclamping. The possible advantage of using a shunt during the bypass repair of a ruptured thoracic aorta was retrospectively assessed in 114 patients, aged 15–80 years, who were admitted with acute rupture of the descending thoracic aorta caused by blunt trauma. The study took place during a 15-year period.

Methods.—During the first 5 years, aortic repair was performed without shunt/bypass in 6 patients, all of whom survived, and with shunt/bypass in 25 patients, 19 of whom survived. Postoperative paraplegia was diagnosed in 1 survivor operated on with shunting. During the next 10 years, 25 of 83 admitted patients died of exsanguination during resuscitation, 7 died during operation, and 12 died within 30 days of operation. Of the 51 patients who initially survived operation, 34 were operated on with shunt/bypass (6 of whom had paraplegia) and 17 were operated on without shunt (4 of whom had paraplegia). All 10 patients with paraplegia had aortic crossclamp times exceeding 30 minutes. Of the 51 initial survivors, 21 had other major complications including adult respiratory distress syndrome, severe renal failure, severe sepsis, and pseudoaneurysm at the graft-aorta anastomosis.

Conclusion.—Blunt traumatic rupture of the thoracic aorta continues to be associated with high mortality and morbidity rates. There was no advantage to using or not using a shunt in preventing paraplegia.

▶ This enormous experience with blunt-induced traumatic aortic rupture presents a gloomy point of view on the whole subject and emphasizes our need in vascular surgery to effect the repair of this lesion promptly without producing paraplegia. There is very little hope that the epidemic of motor vehicle trauma will abate in any way.

8 Abdominal Aortic Aneurysms

The Epidemiologic Necropsy for Abdominal Aortic Aneurysm
McFarlane MJ (Case Western Reserve Univ; Univ of Kansas)
JAMA 265:2085–2088, 1991   8–1

Purpose.—The validity of epidemiological necropsy as a tool to measure the incidence of abdominal aortic aneurysm (AAA) in the general population was tested and compared with the occurrence of AAA as determined in screening surveys. When this research tool is used, bias initiated by selection for autopsy must be controlled. Adjustments were made for demographical differences between the necropsy and the general population, and the outside fatalities referred to the study hospital for autopsy were excluded, as were all patients in whom AAA was suspected or proven in life. Therefore, the meaning population was not selected for necropsy because of possible AAA.

Study Design.—Autopsy records from 1950 to 1984 for the University of Kansas Medical Center were evaluated; 56% of the patients who died in the hospital between 1962 and 1981 underwent necropsy. Patients younger than 20 years of age and those involved with medicolegal cases were excluded. Occurrences of AAA as a necropsy surprise or incidental observation were noted. The results were compared with those of 5 English language screening surveys for AAA; the surveys were made on varied populations and each used slightly different exclusion criteria. In preference to standardizing the studies, comparable demographic subgroups in each study were directly compared.

Outcome.—After exclusions, the epidemiological necropsy population of patients in whom AAA was not suspected or demonstrated in life comprised 7,297 patients, 4,155 males and 3,142 females. The detection rate differed significantly in men and women. The rates were .019 and .0009, respectively. In men and women between 20 and 49 years of age, AAA was infrequent. In the period from 1970 to 1984, the necropsy detection rates were comparable in men (.041) and women (.031) 70 years or older. After adjustment for demographic variations, there were no statistically significant differences between AAA incidence rates in this study, compared with those in the 5 screening surveys.

Discussion.—Because the incidence of AAA determined by live screening did not differ from that resolved by epidemiological necropsy, the latter may indeed be a valid tool for determining AAA rates in the general population. Confirmation would require replication of these results at different hospitals and comparison of screening surveys and epidemiological necropsy in the same population. Nevertheless, this study identified a higher incidence of AAA in older women, similar to that found in older men.

▶ Although the importance of autopsy in studying the natural history of disease is undeniable, the autopsy study detailed here teaches us much less than the screening studies on patients that were reported in previous editions of the YEAR BOOK OF VASCULAR SURGERY (1). Those studies indicated that first-order relatives, hypertensive men (especially those in cardiovascular clinics), and men and women older than 70 years of age are the best candidates for ultrasound screening for AAA.

Reference

1. Collin J: *Eur J Vasc Surg* 4:113, 1990.

Abdominal Aortic Aneurysm: Results of a Family Study
Webster MW, St Jean PL, Steed DL, Ferrell RE, Majumder PP (Univ of Pittsburgh; Indian Statistical Inst, Calcutta)
J Vasc Surg 13:366–372, 1991   8–2

Background.—Early detection and elective resection of asymptomatic abdominal aortic aneurysms (AAAs) can almost completely prevent death caused by rupture of the aneurysm. The risk factors implicated in the development of AAAs include hypertension, smoking, and atherosclerosis. Family clustering of AAAs has also been noted. Data on the families of 91 patients who had undergone elective or emergency AAA repair were collected and analyzed.

Patients.—The patient group consisted of 79 men (age range, 50–86 years) and 12 women (age range, 61–75 years)—a male:female sex ratio reflecting that of other studies. Information was obtained on each patient's spouse, parents, siblings, and children. The families were classified as simplex (with no affected first-degree relative) or multiplex (at least 1 affected first-degree relative of the proband).

Findings.—Seventeen first-degree relatives had AAAs. These relatives included 2 fathers, 1 mother, 8 brothers, and 6 sisters. No children were affected, but the majority (90%) of the probands' children were younger than 50 years of age and were thus unlikely to have AAA. There were 14 multiplex families (15.4%), 11 ascertained through male and 3 through female probands (table). In 11 of these families AAAs were observed in siblings; the remaining 3 families showed parent-offspring transmission. When both affected and unaffected siblings were considered, there was no statistically significant difference between the proportion of male and female siblings.

Conclusion.—The relative risk of having AAA was 3.97 for fathers, 4.03 for mothers, 9.92 for brothers, and 22.93 for sisters. The findings confirm that familial factors are important in the origin of AAA.

Proportions of Different Types of Families Observed in the Present and in 3
Previous Studies

Type of family	Present study*	Cole et al. (1989)	Tilson and Seashore † (1984)	Norrgård et al ‡ (1983)
Simplex (no affected first-degree relative of proband)	77 (84.6) §	271 (88.9)	Not given	75 (86.2)
Multiplex (At least one affected first-degree relative of proband)	14 (15.4)	34 (11.1)	49	12 (13.8)
Total	91 (100.0)	305 (100.0)	Not given	87 (100.0)
Among multiplex families:				
Affected siblings only	11 (78.6)	18 (52.9)	28 (57.1)	11 (91.7)
Affected parent(s) and offspring	3 (21.4)	16 (47.1)	21 (42.9)	1 (8.3)
Among multiplex families with affected siblings only:				
Affected brothers only	3 (27.3)	7 (38.9)	22 (78.6)	6 (54.5)
Affected sisters only	1 (9.1)	1 (5.6)	3 (10.7)	2 (18.2)
Both affected brothers and sisters	7 (63.6)	10 (55.6)	3 (10.7)	3 (27.3)

*Because data of the present study include only first-degree relatives of probands, data of other studies were recompiled to include first-degree relatives only.
  †Data on multiplex families have been reported in this study.
  ‡Data on intracranial aneurysms were excluded.
  §*Figures in parentheses* indicate percentages.
  (Courtesy of Webster MW, St Jean PL, Steed DL: *J Vasc Surg* 13:366–372, 1991.)

▶ In this study of 91 probands, the 15% incidence of individuals with AAAs must be taken as a baseline figure. No doubt, following these individuals over a longer period of time would have revealed an additional number with AAAs. Perhaps the incidence would range as high as 30% to 50%.

On the Inheritance of Abdominal Aortic Aneurysm
Majumder PP, St Jean PL, Ferrell RE, Webster MW, Steed DL (Univ of Pittsburgh; Indian Statistical Inst, Calcutta)
Am J Hum Genet 48:164–170, 1991   8–3

Background.—The 13th major cause of death in the United States is aortic aneurysm. The most common cause of aortic aneurysm mortality is rupture of an infrarenal abdominal aortic aneurysm (AAA); patients usually die before they can reach a hospital. Although AAA is frequently asymptomatic, it can be diagnosed accurately with ultrasound and CT scans. If individuals at risk for AAA could be identified and screened, they could take advantage of the relatively safe option of elective aneurysm repair. In view of multiple reports of familial clustering of AAA, a formal genetic study was undertaken to assess the familial risk of having an AAA.

Methods.—The 91 initial subjects, or probands, were 79 men and 12 women, all white individuals, who were identified from hospital records as having undergone elective or emergency AAA repair between 1985 and 1989. Telephone interviews were used to collect data on diagnoses, surgery and death of parents, siblings and children, all first-degree relatives of the proband, and on the spouse if the proband had children. Of the 91 families, 86 extended over 3 generations, with the initial subject in the middle generation. Statistical segregation analyses were done using several different genetic models of inheritance to find the simplest model that would explain the family data.

Results.— In 13 of the 91 families, at least 1 first-degree relative of the initial individual also had an AAA. The age of onset was in the late 60's in both probands and their affected relatives. The significant risk of having an AAA was calculated to be 3.97 for the father of the proband, 4.03 for the mother, 9.92 for the brother, and 22.93 for the sister. The segregation analysis showed that vulnerability to AAA was best explained by a major recessive gene at an autosomal diallelic locus, and that adding a multifactorial component to the major locus did not improve the predictive value of the model.

Discussion.— Many of the known risk factors for AAA (such as smoking, atherosclerosis, and hypertension) act in a nonspecific way in the age group in which AAA usually happens; many AAA patients are normotensive nonsmokers. Although asymptomatic AAAs were not included in the final analysis, their inclusion would be unlikely to alter conclusions. The present genetic analysis shows a significant single-factor recessive genetic risk for AAA.

▶ Sharp-eyed readers will recognize this statistical presentation as a companion piece to Abstract 8–2. Read on for further commentary.

▶ Elective repair of an AAA is one of the most successful operations performed by vascular surgeons. Several reports during the past few years have emphasized the familial tendency for AAA and have aroused our curiosity about the reasons for this tendency. The recent contribution by Majumder et al. (1) does not make easy reading. The authors conclude that the susceptibility to AAA is determined by a single recessive gene, a situation that is akin to the recessive mutations of the LDL-receptor causing familial hypercholesterolemia.

Ninety-one families were selected for detailed study, but the authors did not advise readers of the selection criteria (other than Caucasian) or of what bias this could have introduced to their statistical analysis (1). This is a major criticism, because we all know that if we selected groups of patients carefully enough we could demonstrate results of our choosing.

Majumder et al. took considerable trouble to screen with ultrasound many of the members of their chosen 91 families for silent AAAs. Of the 104 relatives scanned, only 6/104 (6%) were "positive." "Positive" was an infrarenal aortic diameter (transverse or anterior-posterior not specified) of > 2 cm. Would you accept the referral of a 2.2-cm AAA in a tall, well-built 62-year-old man? Even with this remarkable definition of an aneurysm, the number of AAAs found among the relatives was very low compared with the studies of Collin and Walton (2) and Bengtsson et al. (3) who found 25% or more of the brothers of patients with AAA had a dilated (> 3 cm) or aneurysmal aorta.

The central point of the paper by Majumder et al. is that susceptibility to AAA arises from a single recessive gene. The recent association of a mutation in the type III collagen gene with AAAs in a single family is an exciting pointer in this direction (4). However, this family was unusual because its members had aneurysms and a mild bleeding tendency at a young age (4). This same mutation was not found in 50 consecutive patients seen at Charing Cross for elective AAA repair (5). Furthermore, Majumder et al. have neglected the strong epidemiological evidence between smoking and AAA. This paper by Majumder et al. provides a hypothesis to prove or disprove, a challenge that is being taken up by several groups on both sides of the Atlantic.—Jane T. Powell M.D., and Roger M. Greenlaugh M.D.

References

1. Majumder PP, et al: *Am J Hum Genet* 48:164, 1991.
2. Collin J, Walton J: *Br Med J* 299:493, 1989.
3. Bengtsson M, et al: *Br J Surg* 76:789, 1989.
4. Kontusaari S, et al: *J Clin Invest* 86:1465, 1990.
5. Powell JT, et al: *Eur J Vasc Surg* 5:145, 1991.

A Mutation in the Gene for Type III Procollagen (COL3A1) in a Family With Aortic Aneurysms
Kontusaari S, Tromp G, Kuivaniemi H, Romanic AM, Prockop DJ (Thomas Jefferson Univ)
J Clin Invest 86:1465–1473, 1990   8–4

Background.—Aortic aneurysms are common, often fatal, and in many cases familial. In a rare genetic disorder, Ehlers-Danlos syndrome (EDS) type IV, mutations in the gene for type III collagen have disastrous consequences, including rupture of the aorta. Whether mutations in the same gene might be responsible for familial aortic aneurysms was assessed.

Case Report.—Woman, 37, in excellent health and physical condition, was found to have an extensive family history of sudden death by rupture of aortic or thoracic aneurysms. Although the patient did not meet the diagnostic criteria for either EDS or Marfan's syndrome, during a prior appendectomy the surgeon had noted excessive bleeding and friability of the tissues. At least 5 direct blood relatives had died of vascular catastrophes at early ages (15–55 years). Sample DNA was extracted from pathology slides available from the patient's late mother and maternal aunt. Saliva samples provided DNA from surviving family members. All of the DNA samples were analyzed by the sequencing of polymerase chain reaction (PCR) products for mutations in the type III procollagen gene. In addition, the effects of mutations on the thermal unfolding of procollagen extracted from cultured fibroblasts of the patient were evaluated.

Results.—The DNA of the patient, her late mother and aunt, and her living son, daughter, brother and aunt showed the same single-base genetic mutation: conversion of a codon for glycine to a codon for arginine in the α1 chain for type III procollagen. The mutated procollagen produced by the patient's fibroblasts was less thermally stable than normal procollagen.

Discussion.—The presence of the mutated gene in the patient's late mother and aunt suggested that the genetic defect caused the aortic aneurysms. The patient and her family members with the mutation were thus considered at risk for the same problem, and the diagnosis was made of familial aortic aneurysm. Because mortality caused by presurgical rupture of abdominal aortic aneurysms (AAAs) is 85% to 95%, but is less than 10% with elective surgery, there are important practical implications of these results. The time and skill required to initially detect a procollagen III gene mutation are considerable, but once it is detected family members can be screened for the same mutation with a simple PCR test. Careful monitoring and timely elective surgery become options for affected family members.

▶ Although this is undoubtedly an important study, the results obtained apply to a particular type of aortic aneurysm rather than the garden variety, fusiform aneurysms that are seen in clinical practice.

Elastase-Induced Experimental Aneurysms in Rats
Anidjar S, Salzmann J-L, Gentric D, Lagneau P, Camilleri J-P, Michel J-B (Hôpital Broussais-96, Paris; Hôpital Saint-Michel-33, Paris)
Circulation 82:973–981, 1990   8–5

Background.—In contrast to the pathophysiology of stenosis, which primarily involves the intimal layer of the arterial wall, the formation of aneurysms mainly results from changes in the medial layer. Recent human clinical investigations indicate that elastase may play a significant role in the early development of an aneurysm by contributing to the elastolysis of the aortic media. An in vivo experimental model was established to illuminate the function of elastase in the formation of aneurysms.

Methods.—The abdominal aortas of anesthetized rats were clamped and ligated around a femoral arterial catheter inserted to 1 cm downstream of the clamp. Two milliliters of a test solution slowly perfused from lumen to adventitia to media in the isolated segment. After perfusion, the femoral artery was ligated and aortic permeability was verified. The animals were killed 3 weeks later, some after angiography. Ten control rats were perfused with saline. Perfusion with pancreatic elastase and 4 other proteases was tested in 10 rats for each protease. In addition, groups of 3 rats each were perfused with 1, 3, 6, 10, or 15 units of elastase (1 unit equalled 1 mg hydrolyzed in 2 mL saline). Also, in situ macrophage secretion of elastase was induced by perfusion with thioglycollate (TGC) in 10 rats, and 10 more rats were perfused with TGC-activated macrophages. Plasmin alone (1 or 2 units) or in addition to 1 or 2 units of elastase or thioglycollate was also used for perfusion.

Results.—As increasing amounts of elastase were perfused, more damage occurred; 1 to 2 units did not produce lesions, 3 to 6 units produced microscopic damage of elastic tissue, and more than 6 units produced an

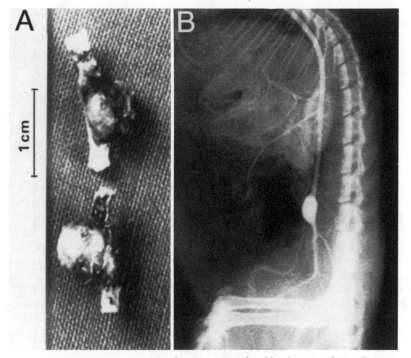

Fig 8–1.—**A**, macroscopic appearance of an aneurysm induced by elastase perfusion; **B**, aortogram of a typical aneurysmal dilation in a rat aorta perfused with 15 units of hog pancreatic elastase. (Courtesy of Anidjar S, Salzmann J-L, Gentric D, et al: *Circulation* 82:973–981, 1990.)

aneurysm (Fig 8–1). Perfusion with TGC or TGC-activated macrophages resulted in a complete loss of elastic tissue in the media near the activated macrophages. The media was completely invaded by activated macrophages after 9 days, but the aortas were more dystrophic than aneurysmal. Although plasmin alone had no effect, its addition to either thioglycollate or elastase always produced a sizable aneurysm.

Discussion.—The results suggest that elastase destroys the elastin network of the media and can induce the formation of aneurysms in a dose-dependent manner. Other proteases that were tested had a similar, though less dramatic, effect. Plasmin may facilitate the breakdown of elastin by breaking down matrix proteins or by activating a pro-elastase. The macrophages in the aortic media may be the source of elastase, causing destruction of elastic tissue and aneurysm formation.

▶ Although inheritance may influence the development of abdominal aortic aneurysms (AAAs) and predispose patients to the elongation and dilation of the arteries that accompany aneurysmosis, other factors are important. Among these is the balance between elastin and elastase. Clinical investigations suggest that there is an increase in elastase activity in human AAAs. This study notes that the destruction of the elastin network of the media is a necessary step in the genesis of aneurysmal dilation. Continuing investigations such as this one supplement clinical studies and will be rewarding in the future.

Aneurysmal Form of Aortoarteritis (Takayasu's Disease): Analysis of Thirty Cases

Kumar S, Subramanyan R, Ravi Mandalam K, Rao VRK, Gupta AK, Joseph S, Madhavan Unni N, Sreenivasa Rao A (Sree Chitra Tirunal Inst for Med Sciences and Technology, Kerala, India)

Clin Radiol 42:342–347, 1990   8–6

Background.—The aneurysmal form of the inflammatory disease aortoarteritis is less frequent and less well characterized than the nonaneurysmal form. The clinical and radiological characteristics of aneurysmal aortoarteritis, and the prognosis for a group of patients with the disease, are reported.

Patients.—Of 135 patients diagnosed with aortoarteritis during a 12-year period at this facility, 22% were determined to have the aneurysmal form; the latter group comprised 22 females and 8 males (average age, 27.4 years). The aneurysm patients satisfied Ishikawa's criteria for aortoarteritis and also met 1 or more of these criteria: the presence of aneurysms in the aorta or in its fusiform, saccular or dissecting branches not related to a constrictive lesion; large aneurysms including those distal to a stenosis; and substantial, diffuse widening of long stretches of aorta. Patients with an erythrocyte sedimentation rate (ESR) of 40 mm or more in the first hour received a diagnosis of aortoarteritis in the active inflammatory phase; diagnosis was confirmed by aortography. The patients were followed an average of 59.7 months; they were compared with a control group of 70 patients in whom nonaneurysmal aortoarteritis was diagnosed.

Results.—Equally distributed between the descending thoracic and abdominal aorta were 41 fusiform and 18 saccular aneurysms; 63.3% were type III aneurysms that combined involvement of the aortic arch and branches and the descending abdominal and thoracic aorta. Also, 24 diffuse dilatations were found, mainly in the ascending aorta. Half of the patients had multiple aneurysms (Fig 8–2), 47% had aortic regurgitations, and 77% had steno-occlusive lesions. There was no significant difference between the control and aneurysmal groups in symptoms, age at onset, sex, hypertension, or incidence of survival or events after 5 years; however, the aneurysm patients had significantly more aortic regurgitation and more frequently elevated ESR.

Discussion.—This type of aneurysm that occurs in young people should be distinguished from types that appear in older populations and are caused by syphilis, giant cell aortitis, or atherosclerosis. Multiple aneurysms, especially if saccular, are an important diagnostic attribute indicating aortoarteritic disease, as are aortic branch aneurysms. Aortoarteritic aneurysms can be differentially diagnosed in patients on the basis of female sex, youth, negative serological tests, location and multiplicity of aneurysms, and frequency of steno-occlusive lesions.

▶ This form of aortoarteritis is seldom seen in North America, yet the inflammatory infiltrate that is characteristic of the condition may be an important eti-

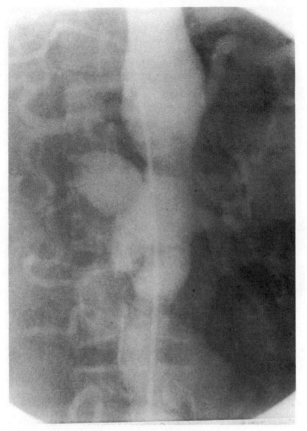

Fig 8–2.—Abdominal aortogram shows multiple aneurysms. (Courtesy of Kumar S, Subramanyan R, Ravi Mandalam K, et al: *Clin Radiol* 42:342–347, 1990.)

ological factor in the production of dilating disease. This is suggested in later abstracts in this chapter.

Incidence of Aneurysms in Takayasu's Arteritis

Matsumura K, Hirano T, Takeda K, Matsuda A, Nakagawa T, Yamaguchi N, Yuasa H, Kusakawa M, Nakano T (Mie Univ School of Medicine, Mie, Japan)
Angiology 42:308–315, 1991   8–7

Background.—Takayasu's arteritis was first described in 1908. It is an ophthalmic disease comprising unusual wreathlike arteriovenous anastomoses in the optic fundi. Aneurysmal lesions appeared as complications or secondary alterations of stenotic lesions in previous reports and were thus considered comparatively less-significant problems. The present evaluation reviews the angiographic findings and clinical significance of aneurysms in patients with this disorder.

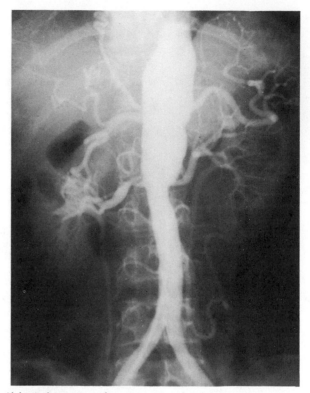

Fig 8—3.—Abdominal aortogram of a woman, 27, with Takayasu's arteritis showing a fusiform aneurysm of the abdominal aorta and stenosis of the right renal artery. (Courtesy of Matsumura K, Hirano T, Takeda K, et al: *Angiology* 42:308—315, 1991.)

Methods.—A series of 113 patients (93 females and 20 males) ranging in age from 10 to 68 years underwent angiography. The procedure was performed by introducing a catheter through the femoral artery by Seldinger's method under local anesthesia, and then injecting contrast medium (76% sodium and meglumine diatrizoate).

Outcome.—Stenotic or occlusive changes, chiefly in the major branches of the aortic arch, were the most common findings. Fusiform or saccular aneurysms were observed in 36 patients (31.9%) (30 females, 6 males). The average patient age was 43.5 years. A total of 26 patients had systolic blood pressure higher than 160 mm Hg, and 15 patients had multiple aneurysms. The aneurysms occurred in various locations of the aorta; 7 patients had aneurysms of the abdominal aorta (AAAs) (Fig 8—3). Eight patients had aneurysms in the pulmonary arteries, of which were fusiform aneurysms in the main pulmonary artery. Aneurysms in the ascending aorta that were complicated by aortic regurgitations were diagnosed in 7 patients.

Implications.—Angiography remains the best and most practical diagnostic procedure for Takayasu's arteritis. In this series of 113 patients, stenotic or occlusive alterations were the major problem, but fusiform or saccular aneurysms were observed in various sites in 36 patients (31.9%). Even younger patients experienced aneurysms. These aneurysms are considered a significant problem in younger patients with Takayasu's arteritis because the lesions can cause aortic regurgitation, coronary insufficiency, or rupture.

▶ Dilating disease is clearly frequent in aortoarteritis. The aneurysms can appear at an extremely young age, suggesting that the inflammation or the products of inflammation may be of importance in aneurysm genesis.

Human Abdominal Aortic Aneurysms: Immunophenotypic Analysis Suggesting an Immune-Mediated Response
Koch AE, Haines GK, Rizzo RJ, Radosevich JA, Pope RM, Robinson PG, Pearce WH (Northwestern Univ)
Am J Pathol 137:1199–1213, 1990   8–8

Purpose.—Because atherosclerosis is the most common cause of abdominal aortic aneurysm (AAA), the inflammatory cells may also be involved in the immunopathogenesis of AAA. The potential role of inflammatory cells in the development of AAA was investigated.

Methods.—Tissue samples were obtained from the infrarenal abdominal aortas of 32 patients. Four normal aortas were obtained at autopsy, 6 aortas were obtained during surgery for occlusive aortic disease, and 23 aortas were obtained from patients operated on for AAA, 5 of whom had inflammatory aneurysms. The 5 monoclonal antibodies used for the study were anti-CD3, anti-CD19, anti-CD11c, anti-CD4, and anti-CD8.

Findings.—The tissue samples from normal aortas contained few or no inflammatory cells. In contrast, 67% to 80% of the cells in the aortic tissue taken from the 3 disease groups were CD3-positive T lymphocytes. The locations of the T lymphocytes varied by disease. In occlusive aortas, only 25% of the CD3-positive T lymphocytes were found in the adventitia; the remainder was found in the media. However, in AAA and inflammatory aneurysm tissue, CD3-positive T lymphocytes were found predominantly in the adventitia (Fig 8–4). In all 3 groups of pathologic tissue, CD19-positive B lymphocytes were found mainly in the adventitia. The CD4-positive:CD8-positive ratio was greater in AAAs than in the other groups, both in the adventitia and in the media of the aortas; CD11c-positive macrophages were found throughout the diseased tissues.

Conclusion.—Aneurysmal disease may progress from occlusive disease, and it is characterized by an increase in chronic inflammatory cells, as well as by a redistribution of these cell types. Whereas it is likely that aortic aneurysmal disease represents an immune-mediated response, it is also possible that the inflammation seen in aneurysmal tissue is an epiphenomenon.

▶ Normal aortic tissue contains few inflammatory cells. Aneurysms with occlusive disease show a mild inflammatory change and AAAs show a more severe

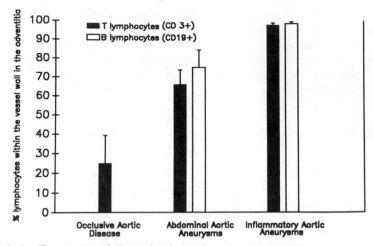

Fig 8–4.—The percentage of CD3+ T lymphocytes located in the adventitia (compared with the media) is shown *(filled bar)*. The percentage of CD19+ B lymphocytes in the adventitia (compared with the media) is also shown *(open bar)*. Because the number of CD19+ B cells within the occlusive aortas was so small, no percentage of cells located in the adventitia is shown for this group. (Courtesy of Koch AE, Haines GK, Rizzo RJ, et al: *Am J Pathol* 137:1199–1213, 1990.)

change. The so-called inflammatory aneurysm represents the far end of the spectrum of inflammation. The findings of this study suggest that AAAs and inflammatory aneurysms can be considered variants within the spectrum of aneurysmal disease rather than distinct pathological entities. Further studies are needed to establish the relationship between inflammatory cells and the progression of aneurysmal degeneration.

Survival in Patients With Abdominal Aortic Aneurysms: Comparison Between Operative and Nonoperative Management
Johansson G, Nydahl S, Olofsson P, Swedenborg J (Karolinska Hosp, Stockholm)
Eur J Vasc Surg 4:497–502, 1990   8–9

Background.—Elective repair of an asymptomatic abdominal aortic aneurysm (AAA) is beneficial when the risk of death from rupture exceeds the expected mortality associated with surgery. A study was undertaken to evaluate the risk benefit relationship of surgical treatment of AAA and the relevance of selective management of patients with AAA on the basis of whether the diameter of the aneurysm was larger or smaller than 5 cm.

Patients.—Among the 213 patients with AAAs confirmed by CT, patients with aneurysms > 5 cm were generally operated on if no serious contraindications were present and if those with AAAs < 5 cm were followed by repeated CT examinations and operated on when an increase in size occurred. Mean follow-up time was 5 years, 4 months.

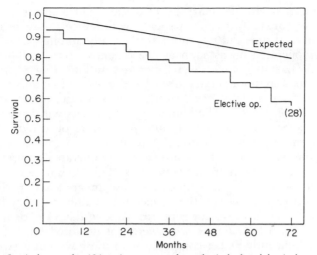

Fig 8–5.—Survival curve for 134 patients operated on electively for abdominal aortic aneurysm compared with an age- and sex-matched normal population. The *number within parentheses* represents the number of patients still alive at the end of the observation period. (Courtesy of Johansson G, Nydahl S, Olofsson P, et al: *Eur J Vasc Surg* 4:497–502, 1990.)

Results.—Among the 134 patients operated on electively, the operative mortality rate was 7.5%. Another 7 patients died later of causes related to surgery, for an overall mortality rate of 13%. Life table analysis showed that survival in patients operated on electively was 68% at 5 years (Fig 8–5). The mean survival time was 45 months. Surgically

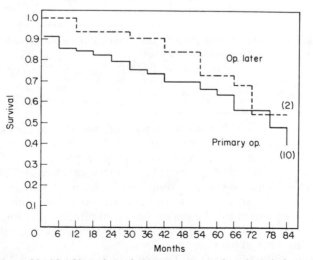

Fig 8–6.—Survival by life table analysis of 102 patients operated on electively for AAA as soon as possible after diagnosis was established, compared with 32 patients who were operated on at a later date. There is no significant difference between the 2 curves. The *numbers within parentheses* represent the number of patients at the end of follow-up. (Courtesy of Johansson G, Nydahl S, Olofsson P, et al: *Eur J Vasc Surg* 4:497–502, 1990.)

treated patients with coronary heart disease had a lower survival rate (48%) than surgically treated patients without coronary heart disease (68%). Survival time did not differ significantly among the 102 patients who were operated on as soon as the diagnosis was established, compared with 32 patients who were operated on later (Fig 8–6). Seventy-nine patients were not operated on. Of those, 42 had an aneurysm with a diameter < 5 cm initially, but 3 of the aneurysms ruptured and all 3 had grown to a size > 5 cm. The remaining 39 patients with aneurysms < 5 cm in diameter were followed up and no rupture occurred. The risk of rupture in those patients whose AAA remained < 5 cm was significantly less than the risk of death from surgery in the operated group with aneurysms > 5 cm. The mortality rate was slightly, but not significantly higher in patients with aneurysms < 5 cm compared with patients operated on electively. However, the former was mainly attributed to deaths caused by cardiac disease, not ruptures. Among the 34 patients with aneurysms > 5 cm in diameter who were not operated on, the mortality rate was significantly higher compared with those who underwent operation; only 14% of the former patients survived.

Summary.— In conclusion, patients with AAAs < 5 cm in diameter can be followed up with repeated CT examinations and operated on only when the size of the aneurysm approaches or exceeds 5 cm. Unless serious contraindications are present, patients with an AAA > 5 cm in diameter should undergo surgery.

▶ A number of good studies now show that it is possible to observe patients with 3 cm and 4 cm aortic dilation. Among the criteria for surgery is expansion of the lesion by 1 cm or the development of symptomatology.

Utility of Computed Tomography for Surveillance of Small Abdominal Aortic Aneurysms: Preliminary Report
Krupski WC, Bass A, Thurston DW, Dilley RB, Bernstein EF (Scripps Clinic and Research Found, La Jolla, Calif)
Arch Surg 125:1345–1350, 1990   8–10

Background.— The decision to repair an abdominal aortic aneurysm (AAA) is commonly based on aneurysmal diameter as monitored by serial B-mode ultrasound. The accepted average expansion rate for AAAs is .5 cm/year, but actual AAA expansion rates vary widely between patients. The influence of various clinical variables on AAA expansion rates have been examined, but most studies have been inconclusive. Because CT has proven useful for the diagnosis and treatment planning of AAAs, CT scans were used to identify the AAA characteristics that might be predictive of an AAA expansion.

Methods.— The CT scans of 25 men and 5 women, aged 34–95 years, who had 2 or more scans at least 6 months apart during a 26-month follow-up period were analyzed. The initial AAA diameters ranged from 3 cm–6.4 cm. All of the patients were initially managed conservatively.

Eighteen of the patients (60%) were hypertensive, 17 (57%) had coronary artery disease, 5 (17%) were diabetic, and 27 (90%) had a history of cigarette smoking; 16 (53%) of the 27 smokers quit smoking after the AAA was discovered. Twenty-eight AAAs were discovered during routine physical examinations.

Findings.—Nineteen patients had an increase of 3 mm or more in AAA diameter on CT scans during follow-up, confirming that the AAAs were expanding. The average expansion rate for the enlarging AAAs was 4 mm/year. The other 11 patients showed little or no AAA expansion on CT scans and had an average expansion rate of only .02 mm/year. A comparison of the clinical features in patients with and without AAA expansion revealed that only serum cholesterol levels correlated with an increased risk of AAA expansion. There was no difference in AAA size at initial diagnosis between the 2 groups. Two (18%) of the 11 patients with stable AAAs and 6 (31%) of the 19 patients with expanding AAAs underwent surgical repair of the AAA. There were no operative deaths. Three patients died during the follow-up period of causes other than AAA.

Conclusion.—Serial CT scanning is an effective technique for monitoring AAA size in patients who have received a diagnosis of small AAAs and who are initially being treated conservatively.

▶ This study is valuable because it shows no relationship between calcification, lumen location, thrombus-lumen ratio, or diameter of the arterial lumen and the expansion of the aneurysm wall. Only the perhaps chance observation that thrombus area was measured in cm² was related to aneurysm enlargement.

Selective Use of Arteriography in the Assessment of Aortic Aneurysm Repair
Campbell JJ, Bell DD, Gaspar MR (Long Beach Surgical Group, Long Beach, Calif)
Ann Vasc Surg 4:419–423, 1990   8–11

Background.—Despite the fact that arteriography is potentially dangerous and costly in terms of both time and resources, it is frequently a routine procedure before aortic aneurysm repair. The predictive validity of specific indications for arteriography was judged retrospectively based on how frequently an operative modification was based on arteriography.

Methods.—The arteriograms and medical and operative records were analyzed for 100 patients who had undergone elective aortic aneurysm repair; preoperative arteriography was carried out in 41 cases. All of the cases were reviewed for specific indications proposed as criteria for preoperative arteriography, including claudication, decreased lower extremity pulses, hypertension in patients younger than 60 years of age, thoracic aneurysm, serious coronary artery disease, cerebrovascular disease, mesenteric angina, renal abnormalities, previous vascular surgery, peripheral

Cases Modified by Arteriography

Case	Arteriogram finding	Modification
#15	Delineated blood supply to ectopic fused kidney	Allowed safer preservation of ectopic blood supply
#27	Multiple iliac occlusions and stenosis; occluded SFAs*	Aortobifemoral bypass; bilateral profundoplasty added
#29	Multiple iliac stenosis with occluded left hypogastric artery	Aortobifemoral bypass; right hypogastric endarterectomy added to improve pelvic flow
#45	Right SFA occlusion	Right SFA endarterectomy added
#50	Occlusion of left proximal popliteal suggestive of aneurysm	Excision and repair of popliteal aneurysm
#68	Occluded left renal artery	Left nephrectomy added
#84	Multiple iliac stenoses; occlusion of right hypogastric artery	Reimplant, left hypogastric
#88	Stenosis, left renal artery	Graft to left renal artery
#89	Bilateral renal artery stenosis	Bilateral renal artery TEA
#94	Bilateral renal artery stenosis	Bilateral renal artery TEA

Abbreviations: SFA, superficial femoral artery; *TEA,* thromboendarterectomy.
(Courtesy of Campbell JJ, Bell DD, Gaspar MR: *Ann Vasc Surg* 4:419–423, 1990.)

aneurysm, and blue toe syndrome. Significant arteriographic abnormalities were defined as those that resulted in modification of the operative procedure and that would not have been detected during surgery. The 59 surgeries performed without arteriogram were analyzed to determine which intraoperative modifications might have been averted had that information been available.

Results.—In 10 of 41 cases with arteriography, the operative plan was changed because of the findings (table). Intraoperative modifications that might have been predicted by arteriography were necessary in only 3 of the 59 cases without the procedure. An index of the predictive validity of the various indications for arteriography showed that significant hypertension in relatively young patients was the best predictor of finding significant anomalies in an arteriogram (.6 index), followed by claudication (.35), decreased lower extremity pulse (.33), and coronary artery or cerebrovascular disease (.28 each). Multiple indications only increased the probability of operative modification when there were 4 or more.

Discussion.—Arteriography is justified, not by how frequently it detects an anomaly, but by how often the information results in a modification of operative procedure. Although the proponents of routine arteriography claim this outcome in 20% to 75% of cases, many of these modifications could have been planned based on thorough clinical observation. The relatively high rate of modification resulting from arteriograms in the current study (24%) validates the accuracy of the clinical selection process that was used by this group before ordering the procedure. These results support the conclusion that routine arteriography before aneurysm surgery is not warranted; it should be done only when there are specific clinical indications.

▶ As it happens, economical considerations coincide with non-aortographic imaging developments to suggest that routine aortography can be eliminated in patients with aortic aneurysm. therefore, this review by an experienced group that has previously analyzed their own practice in this regard is especially timely.

The Role of the Aortic Aneurysm Diameter Aortic Diameter Ratio in Predicting the Risk of Rupture
Louridas G, Reilly K, Perry MO (Univ of the Witwatersrand, Johannesburg, South Africa; Vanderbilt Univ)
S Afr Med J 78:642–643, 1990   8–12

Introduction.—It is well established that the diameter of an aneurysm predicts the risk of aneurysmal rupture reliably. In an attempt to define those aneurysms that are at the greatest risk of rupture, the ratio between the size of an infrarenal aortic aneurysm and the proximal normal aorta was studied.

Methods.—All 130 patients with infrarenal abdominal aortic aneurysms underwent a CT scan of the abdomen. The ratio was calculated by dividing the diameter of the normal aorta at the level of the superior mesenteric artery (cm) into the diameter of the aneurysm at its widest diameter (cm).

Findings.—For the 100 asymptomatic patients the mean aneurysm-aortic ratio was 2 (range, 1.1–4.2) (table). For the 17 symptomatic patients with no evidence of rupture, the mean ratio was 2.7 (range, 2–4.5) and for the 13 with a contained rupture, the mean ratio was 3.4 (range, 2.2–9). The differences in mean ratio between the asymptomatic and symptomatic patients was significant. None of the patients with a ratio of less than 2.2 had a ruptured aneurysm.

Conclusions.—These findings suggest that the aneurysm-aortic ratio may be helpful in identifying the high-risk aneurysm. Abdominal aortic aneurysms with a ratio of 2.7 or greater are likely to become symptomatic, whereas those with a ratio of 3.4 or greater are at risk of rupture.

▶ A simple but informative study that confirms that surgery can be recommended for patients whose aneurysms are 2 to 3 times the size of the native artery.

Ratios and Diameters of Aortas in Different Groups of Patients

	Asymptomatic	Symptomatic without contained rupture	Symptomatic with contained rupture
No. of patients	100	17	13
Aorta (cm)			
Range	1,5 - 4,2	2,3 - 3,5	2,0 - 3,6
Mean	2,8	2,8	2,8
Aneurysm (cm)			
Range	2,9 - 13,3	4,6 - 13,5	6,5 - 20,0
Mean	5,8	7,8	9,5
Ratio			
Range	1,1 - 4,2	2,0 - 4,5	2,2 - 9,0
Mean	2,0	2,7	3,4

(Courtesy of Louridas G, Reilly K, Perry MO: *S Afr Med J* 78:642–643, 1990.)

Ultrafast Computed Tomography in the Diagnosis of Aortic Aneurysms and Dissections

Stanford W, Rooholamini SA, Galvin JR (Univ of Iowa)
J Thorac Imag 5:32–39, 1990   8–13

Background.—Because of its excellent (.75 mm–1.5 mm) spatial resolution, rapid (50 msec–400 msec) scan times, and excellent vascular opacification, ultrafast CT (UFCT) is an ideal imaging technique for assessing aortic aneurysms and dissections.

Patients.—Using the Imatron C-100 UFCT scanner, 50 patients with suspected aortic aneurysms and/or dissections were studied. Of the patients, 18 had thoracic or thoracoabdominal aneurysms, 17 had thoracic or thoracoabdominal dissections, and 7 had abdominal aneurysms; no aneurysms were found in the other 8 patients. In 30 patients the UFCT images were correlated with findings on angiography, surgery or autopsy. The criteria for the diagnosis of aneurysms were similar to those of conventional CT; dissection was considered when intimal calcification was displaced 5 mm or more inward from the aortic wall on unenhanced images or when a dissection flap was visualized on contrast-enhanced images (Fig 8–7).

Findings.—Of the 35 patients with thoracic or thoracoabdominal aneurysms or dissections, UFCT confirmed the diagnosis in 23 (95.8%) of 24 patients with angiographic, surgical, or autopsy findings. There was 1 false positive UFCT finding. Of the 7 patients with abdominal aneurysms, 4 were confirmed by UFCT and the other 3 were examined clinically. Of the 8 patients without aneurysms or dissections, UFCT confirmed the negative findings in 2 patients who subsequently underwent angiography and/or surgery, whereas clinical follow-up for a mean 14.8 months in the other 6 patients failed to show findings suggestive of aortic abnormality.

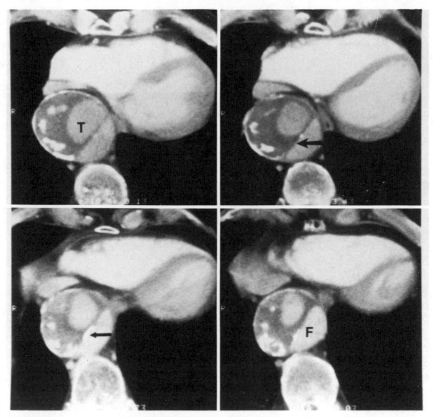

Fig 8–7.—Large thoracoabdominal dissecting aortic aneurysm in a 73-year-old hypertensive man. The UFCT sequential images show a large dissecting thoracoabdominal aortic aneurysm. Note the intimal flap *(large arrow)*, true *(T)* and false *(F)* lumina, and medial displacement of the intimal calcification *(small arrow)*. (Courtesy of Stanford W, Rooholamini SA, Galvin JR: *J Thorac Imag* 5:32–39, 1990.)

Conclusion.—Ultrafast CT is a rapid, minimally invasive imaging technique for the screening and follow-up of patients with aortic aneurysms or dissections.

▶ Computed tomography scanning has a proven role in the evaluation of aortic aneurysms. Ultrafast CT that can obtain 40 slices in 76 seconds or less merely extends the utility further.

Distal Embolization as a Presenting Symptom of Aortic Aneurysms
Baxter BT, McGee GS, Flinn WR, McCarthy WJ, Pearce WH, Yao JST (Northwestern Univ)
Am J Surg 160:197–201, 1990   8–14

Background.—The operative risks for patients with initial symptoms of distal embolization from an abdominal aortic aneurysm (AAA) have not been well defined. Data on 302 patients who underwent AAA repair during a 5-year period were reviewed.

Patients.—Of the 302 patients, 248 (82%) were asymptomatic, 32 (11%) had ruptured AAAs, and 15 (5%) had distal embolization as the first evidence of AAA. In 13 of the latter 15 patients, embolization was spontaneous, but in 3 patients the release of emboli to distal sites was provoked by the aortographic or angiographic procedures. Microembolic events evidenced by focal digital ischemia occurred in 11 patients. During surgery, care was taken to avoid manipulations that could release more emboli.

Results.—The AAAs in these patients were small, ranging from 3.2 to 6.3 cm (mean, 4.3 cm). The special features of the aortic thrombus with the AAA were well-demonstrated by contrast-enhanced CT; the thrombus was heterogeneous and had fissures and calcifications. Although aortography performed in all 15 patients demonstrated an irregular luminal surface. Suggestive of atheromatous occlusive disease, it failed to detect the AAA in 7 patients. Complications included 3 major and 5 minor amputations, developing or worsening renal failure in 5 (33%) patients, and death in 2 (13%).

Discussion.—The 20% incidence of related embolization in this series, combined with failure to diagnose AAA in 47% of the patients, suggest that it should be used very selectively, especially when CT scans or symptoms indicate an unstable thrombus. A contrast-enhanced CT scan provides substantial diagnostic accuracy and detail, enables the prescreening of patients for angiography, and should be considered the safe diagnostic tool of choice for patients with a suspected AAA. The risk of embolization did not correlate with decreasing aneurysm size, indicating the potentially dangerous nature of smaller aneurysms.

▶ Many patients with ruptured AAAs are not being seen at university centers. This study reemphasizes the importance of the distal atheromatous complications of AAAs. Furthermore, it emphasizes the occult nature of the aneurysm itself and the importance of its detection by CT scanning.

Repair of Abdominal Aortic Aneurysms: A Statewide Experience
Richardson JD, Main KA (Univ of Louisville; Kentucky Legislative Research Commission, Frankfort)
Arch Surg 126:614–616, 1991   8–15

Background.—Many hospitals have had excellent results with the elective treatment of abdominal aortic aneurysms (AAAs). However, no one has compared the results of this type of surgery in a large geographic region in which patients were treated by different surgeons at different hospitals. Therefore, a statewide experience with abdominal aortic aneurysm repair was reviewed.

Methods.—The results of AAA repair for all Medicare recipients during 1 year in Kentucky were analyzed. A group of 52 surgeons in 31 hospitals performed 136 operations.

Results.—The overall operative mortality was 18%. The mortality rates for elective and emergency surgery were 6% and 49%, respectively. Advancing age did not influence the treatment outcome; however, deaths caused by ruptured aneurysms were more frequent in smaller hospitals than in larger ones.

Conclusions.—An overall operative mortality of 18% and an elective operative mortality of 6% were found among patients undergoing AAA repair. Because the death rate associated with elective procedures is so much lower than that accompanying the treatment of ruptured aneurysms, the liberal use of AAA repair is indicated, even in elderly populations.

▶ Who should operate on AAAs will be debated increasingly during the years to come. the abundant documentation that appears in this study and others points out that a trend exists showing that surgeons with a higher operative volume encounter fewer complications. Furthermore, the mortality cited in association with an elective aneurysm exceeds 5% and contrasts with some reports of clinical series from vascular centers. This suggests an actual higher mortality from operation than is usually quoted.

Abdominal Aortic Aneurysms: Is There an Association Between Surgical Volume, Surgical Experience, Hospital Type and Operative Mortality?
Amundsen S, Skjærven R, Trippestad A, Søreide O, Members of the Norwegian Abdominal Aortic Aneurysm Trial (Univ of Bergen, Norway)
Acta Chir Scand 156:323–328, 1990   8–16

Introduction.—A previous study found that postoperative mortality after vascular surgery decreased when the number of operations performed increased, suggesting that patients would benefit from undergoing vascular surgery in specialized surgical centers. A prospective multicenter study further examined the effects of surgical experience, surgical volume, and type of hospital on the operative mortality in patients operated on for abdominal aortic aneurysm (AAA). Surgical experience was expressed as the number of vascular operations performed per year in the unit.

Study Design.—Seven university hospitals, 9 county hospitals, and 10 local hospitals participated in the study. There were 444 patients with AAAs, including 279 (63%) admitted electively and 165 (37%) admitted emergently. Twenty-four elective patients were not operated on. Of the 165 emergency patients, 114 had a ruptured AAA and 51 had an impending rupture. Eleven patients with a ruptured AAA died after admission but before reaching the operating room and 29 died during operation. Two patients with impending rupture also died before operation.

Findings.—For the patients admitted electively, there was a significant difference in mortality between the hospitals in which more than 10 AAA repairs were performed during the study period and the hospitals in which less than 10 such procedures were performed. The operative mortality for elective patients treated in units with vascular surgical experience was 4.8%, compared with 11.3% in the other units. There was no statistically significant difference with respect to surgical experience for emergency patients. Operative mortality by university, county, and local hospitals did not differ significantly.

Conclusion.—The outcome after operation for AAA is related to the number of vascular operations performed and to the vascular surgical experience of the unit. The type of hospital in which the operation is performed does not seem to be important.

▶ Vascular surgery requires little extra equipment. The facilities for advanced general surgery suffice for the performance of major vascular surgery. Once again, the results of treatment are in the hands of the operating surgeon—not in the policies or facilities of the institution.

Elective Resection of 332 Abdominal Aortic Aneurysms in a Southern West Virginia Community During a Recent Five-Year Period
AbuRahma AF, Robinson PA, Boland JP, Lucente FC, Stuart SP, Neuman SS, Hall MD, Hoak BA (West Virginia Univ Health Sciences Ctr-Charleston Area Med Ctr, Charleston; Pfizer Central Research, Groton, Conn)
Surgery 109:244–251, 1991   8–17

Objective.—More than half of the elective aneurysm repairs performed in the United States are done in hospitals with less than 400 beds. The average number of such surgeries performed at these hospitals is 2.2 per year. The variables that might have affected the outcome of elective abdominal aortic aneurysm (AAA) resections performed by variably experienced surgeons in 4 different hospitals in 1 community were assessed.

Methods.—Using univariate and multivariate statistics, 33 variables pertaining to demographics, pulmonary status, cardiac complications, colon ischemia, acute renal failure, surgery concomitant to aneurysm repair, angiography and CT results, early death (before 30 days), and other complications were analyzed for each of 332 patients who underwent elective AAA repair during a 5-year period. The group comprised 256 men and 76 women aged 39–89 years (average age, 69 years). Of these patients, 68% were smokers, 54% were hypertensive, and 8% were diabetic.

Results.—In similarity to comparable series, early mortality was 2.1%. There was at least 1 postoperative complication in 32.2% of the patients. Five independent factors had significant positive correlations with postoperative complications: the number of blood transfusions, a history of prior cardiac catheterization, more than 50% renal artery constriction, left renal vein ligation, and a relative lack of experience in the procedure by the surgeon. An increasing number of postoperative complications correlated positively and significantly with increased mortality; both of these factors appeared to vary independently of the other clinical, surgical, and demographic factors analyzed, including age of the patient and

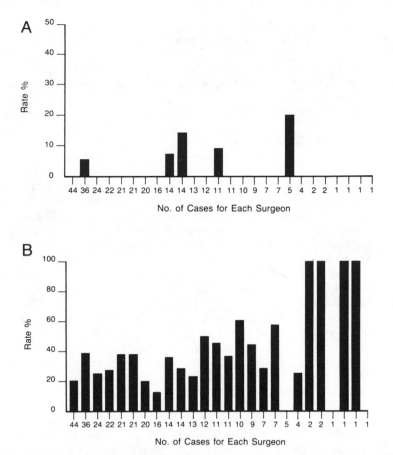

Fig 8–8.—**A,** graph showing mortality for individual surgeons. **B,** graph showing surgical morbidity (complications) for each surgeon and proportion of patients with 1 or more events. (Courtesy of AbuRahma AF, Robinson PA, Boland JP, et al: *Surgery* 109:244–251, 1991.)

size of the aneurysm. The mortality and morbidity rates for individual surgeons are shown in Figure 8–8.

Discussion.—These results strongly suggest that the patients of surgeons who perform a particular procedure more often have fewer complications and lower mortality. In the present study, the mortality varied from 1% with more experienced surgeons to 4% with those who were less practiced. Preoperative angiography did not increase risk; therefore, it seems prudent for less experienced surgeons to order this test and to refer especially those patients with marked renal artery constriction or coronary artery disease to practitioners with more experience in abdominal aortic aneurysm repair.

▶ This study suggests that many AAA repairs are performed in community hospitals. The mortality of aneurysm resection is quite acceptable in these hospitals but the overall postoperative complication rate is alarmingly high. The less experienced surgeons have a greater number of complications, and the mortality and morbidity are not related to institution size.

Long-Term Survival in Patients Undergoing Resection of Abdominal Aortic Aneurysm

Vohra R, Reid D, Groome J, Abdool-Carrim ATO, Pollock JG (Glasgow Royal Infirmary, Scotland)
Ann Vasc Surg 4:460–465, 1990   8–18

Background.—Rupture of an abdominal aortic aneurysm (AAA) is uniformly fatal unless it is surgically treated. For elective cases the operative mortality is less than 5%, but it increases to between 21% and 78% with rupture. Long-term survival was examined in 338 patients who had elective, emergency, or urgent repair of abdominal aortic aneurysms.

Patients.—Of the 185 patients included in the elective group, 153 had surgery. Of the 153 patients, 50 were in the urgent group, 41 underwent excision, and 37 had graft replacement. Eleven of 103 patients with ruptured AAAs died before surgery could be performed. Seventy-one patients had aortic bifurcation grafts and 20 received straight tube grafts. Intermittent claudication was the most common symptom of aneurysm in the elective group. In 23% of the cases aneurysm was an accidental finding. In the urgent and ruptured groups, most patients had abdominal pain and backache, and 25% of the patients with rupture presented with vomiting. In all of the groups the most common presenting sign was a pulsatile mass. Nearly a third of the elective cases had signs of peripheral ischemia. Patients were followed up for 5 years.

Results.—The 30-day hospital mortality in surgical patients was 39% in the ruptured group and 24% in the urgent group, but it was only 8.5% in the elective group. Survival in patients who had surgery was 68.9% compared with 29.6% in those not receiving surgery. However, the latter group contained severely unfit patients. Long-term survival in patients who had successful surgery did not differ significantly whether surgery had been elective, urgent, or emergency. Age older than 70 years did not significantly affect long-term survival, but after 1,000 days the survival was poor in these patients. Neither myocardial infarction nor hypertension significantly reduced long-term survival. Fifty percent of late deaths in the surgical group were caused by atherosclerosis that involved coronary, cerebral, and renal arteries, and 3 patients in the unoperated group died of ruptured aortic aneurysms.

Conclusions.—All aneurysms should be considered for surgery. Although there are initial differences in operative mortality, long-term survival is similar in patients having elective, urgent, and emergency repair. In this series patients with 2 or more risk factors had 44% operative mortality, but long-term survival in patients with myocardial infarction and hypertension did not differ from that in patients who were disease free.

▶ Vascular surgery is gradually being credited with preventing stroke, decreasing the incidence of amputation, and, in the case of aortic aneurysm, extending life expectancy. Late deaths are caused by cardiac and cerebrovascular disease and malignancy.

The Results of Surgery in 114 Cases of Aneurysms of the Infrarenal Abdominal Aorta in Patients Aged Over 75 Years
Chaillou P, Patra P, Chapillion M, Meresse S, Lescalie F, Enon B, Chevalier JM, Bourseau JC, Dupon H (Hôpital G et R Laënnec, Nantes, France; CHU d'Angers, Angers, France)
J Chir (Paris) 127:319–324, 1990   8–19

Introduction.—The discovery of an infrarenal abdominal aneurysm in an elderly patient raises the question whether there is an age limit beyond which the patient should not be operated on. It also questions whether operation in elderly patients is associated with prohibitive postoperative morbidity and mortality when compared to the risk associated with spontaneous disease progression.

Patients.—During a 10-year period, 80 men and 34 women (age range, 75–94 years; mean age, 79 years) underwent repair of an infrarenal abdominal aneurysm. Of these patients, 62 underwent elective operation and 52 underwent urgent operation; 27 were classified as extremely urgent, 15 as moderately urgent, and 10 as semi-urgent (Fig 8–9). Only 6 patients had no preoperative risk factors, 21 had 1 risk factor, and 22 had 2 risk factors. Forty-seven patients had arterial hypertension, 35 of whom also had coronary insufficiency; 24 had cardiac insufficiency and 22 had respiratory insufficiency. The other patients were operated on "cold" (without previous assessment of risk factors) because they could not be questioned.

Results.—Thirty-five patients (31%) had no medical or surgical complications during the first 30 postoperative days. The other 79 patients

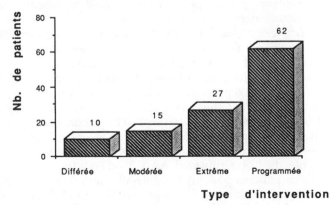

Type d'intervention

Fig 8–9.—Classification according to the degree of urgency for operation. (Courtesy of Chaillou P, Patra P, Chapillion M, et al: *J Chir (Paris)* 127:319–324, 1990.)

experienced a total of 26 surgical complications and 104 medical complications. Four of the 9 patients who had ischemia of the colon required operation. Twenty patients had renal insufficiency, whereas 19 had respiratory complications. Thirty-six patients (31%) died either during operation or within the first month after operation; 32 of these had undergone urgent operation. The other 4 patients died after undergoing elective operation. An additional 14 patients died during an average follow-up of 32 months. Of the patients who survived the first postoperative month, 96% were living independently at the end of the study or at the time of death. There was no statistically significant difference in the actuarial survival between patients who underwent elective aneurysmal repair and an age- and gender-matched control population.

Conclusion.—Repair of an infrarenal abdominal aneurysm in elderly patients has an acceptable morbidity and mortality. Age in itself is not a surgical contraindication. It is not even a risk factor in elderly patients who have a reasonable life expectancy and no obvious contraindications for operation. Therefore, surgical intervention in these patients appears to be justified.

▶ Previous reports from Canada (1986), Texas (1982), and Cleveland (1982) have shown the value of offering aneurysm resection to octogenarians, but this report underscores those observations.

Probability of Rupture of an Abdominal Aortic Aneurysm After an Unrelated Operative Procedure: A Prospective Study

Durham SJ, Steed DL, Moosa HH, Makaroun MS, Webster MW (Univ of Pittsburgh)
J Vasc Surg 13:248–252, 1991   8–20

Background.—Some physicians assume that patients with abdominal aortic aneurysms (AAAs) are at a greater risk of rupture after unrelated surgery. The incidence of postoperative aneurysmal rupture in 1 series of patients was documented.

Patients.—Between 1986 and 1989, 33 patients with known AAAs underwent 45 operations. Twenty-eight patients had an infrarenal AAA; 5 had a thoracoabdominal aneurysm. The AAAs varied in transverse diameter from 3 cm to 8.5 cm (average, 5.6 cm). A total of 27 patients had only 1 operation, and 6 had 1–6 procedures. The Operations were abdominal in 13 cases, cardiothoracic in 9, head and neck in 2, other vascular in 11, urologic in 7, amputation in 2, and breast in 1. The anesthesia used was general in 29 cases, spinal/epidural in 6, and regional/local in 10.

Findings.—One patient died of cardiopulmonary failure after surgery, whereas another died of a ruptured AAA 20 days after coronary artery bypass. Fourteen patients had AAA repair an average of 18 weeks after their other surgery. During the 40-month study period, 2 other patients with unknown AAAs died of ruptures at 21 and 77 days after another surgical procedure.

Conclusions.—These findings cast doubt on the assumption that an unrelated operative intervention hastens the rupture of an AAA. However, such a relationship is still possible. The study of biochemical changes in the aneurysm wall induced by surgical trauma should shed more light on this question.

▶ What was formerly an accepted truth is rapidly becoming an acknowledged myth.

Experience in Managing 70 Patients With Ruptured Abdominal Aortic Aneurysms

Cohen JR, Birnbaum E, Kassan M, Wise L (Long Island Jewish Med Ctr; Albert Einstein College of Medicine, New York)
N Y State J Med 91:97–100, 1991   8–21

Objective.—Ruptured abdominal aortic aneurysms (RAAAs) present diagnostic and operative urgency to hospitals and physicians. Mortality rates are still high (25% to 80%), even with improved technology. Preoperative, operative, and postoperative factors were examined in 70 patients treated for RAAA during a 14-year period from January 1975 to January 1989. For the first 10 years, 11 different surgeons repaired the RAAAs; after 1985, only 6 surgeons did the repairs with 1 surgeon performing most of them (20/28).

Results.—Factors such as history of heart disease, chronic obstructive pulmonary disease, hypertension, diabetes, cerebral vascular accident, peptic ulcer, and carcinoma did not correlate with mortality. Significant correlations (Fig 8–10) existed between mortality and admitting systolic blood pressure, blood pressure at the time of skin incision, the number of

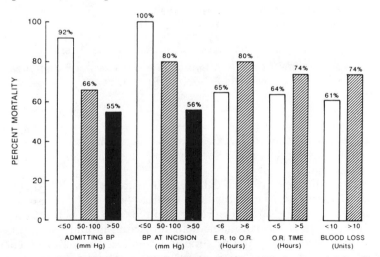

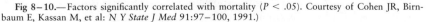

Fig 8–10.—Factors significantly correlated with mortality ($P < .05$). Courtesy of Cohen JR, Birnbaum E, Kassan M, et al: *N Y State J Med* 91:97–100, 1991.)

hours between transfer emergency room to operating room, time in operating room of less than 5 hours compared with more than 5 hours, and blood loss. It was also noted that a smaller number of surgeons operating on a majority of the RAAAs improved survival.

Discussion.—Prompt action in cases of RAAA is important. The stable patient with a systolic blood pressure of 100 mm Hg or more has a better chance of survival. Chance of survival will be even greater if the patient is transferred within 6 hours of admission to a facility experienced in RAAA repair.

▶ Important lessons can be derived from reports of the experience in dealing with RAAAs. In this study, we again see emphasis on the status of the patient at the time of presentation.

▶ An RAAA is a catastrophic complication of a condition that is entirely curable when discovered and treated electively. Cohen et al. found that mortality rates after RAAA correlate with hypotension at admission, and that the correlation is even stronger when hypotension persists. Excessive blood loss and prolonged time in the operating room (frequently associated with technical complications such as inadvertent venous injury) were also predictive of a poor outcome. In addition, technical expertise—or at least experience—probably matters. Mortality decreased when a smaller number of surgeons with more extensive vascular expertise managed critically ill and technically challenging patients. Ouriel and colleagues made a similar observation (1). Excessive mortality rates after RAAA, as reported in this study and in other recent series (2), will persist until routine ultrasonographic screening of populations at high risk for AAA becomes the norm.—K. Johansen, M.D., Ph.D.

References

1. Ouriel K, et al: *J Vasc Surg* 11:493, 1990.
2. Johansen K, et al: *J Vasc Surg:* 13:240, 1991.

Ruptured Abdominal Aortic Aneurysm: The Harborview Experience
Johansen K, Kohler TR, Nicholls SC, Zierler RE, Clowes AW, Kazmers A (Univ of Washington)
J Vasc Surg 13:240–247, 1991   8–22

Background.—Ruptured abdominal aortic aneurysm (RAAA), which is treatable and curable, is the 15th leading cause of death among men in the United States.

Patients.—Between 1980 and 1989, 186 patients with RAAA were admitted to the Harborview Medical Center, Seattle. Of these patients, 96% had a systolic blood pressure less than 90 mm Hg before admission. Management involved paramedic field resuscitation and transport, a diagnostic protocol completed in a mean 12 minutes in the emergency department, rapid transport to an emergency operating room, aneurysmorrhaphy, and skilled postoperative care in the intensive care unit.

Findings.—Despite these steps, 130 patients (70%) died within 30 days of surgery. Three percent died in the emergency department, 13% died in the operating room, 51% died in the intensive care unit, and 3% died in the ward or after discharge. A greater than 90% likelihood of dying was associated with age older than 80 years, the female sex, persistent preoperative hypotension despite aggressive crystalloid and blood replacement, an admission hematocrit level of less than 25, and transfusion requirements above 15 units. None of the patients with preoperative cardiac arrest survived for more than 24 hours.

Conclusions.—Although optimal prehospital, emergency department, operating room, and postoperative care can improve the outcomes of patients with RAAAs in shock, most of these patients will still die. Certain clinical features predict excessive death rates after RAAAs, suggesting that withholding surgery may be justified. Screening patients who are at high risk for AAA and elective aneurysmorrhaphy is warranted.

▶ In this terribly important report from the Harborview Medical Center, it has been proven that efficiency in evaluation and swiftness in transport to the operating room does not contribute to decreased mortality. The obvious conclusion is that AAAs must be discovered in patients before symptomatology occurs.

Factors Affecting Survival After Rupture of Abdominal Aortic Aneurysm: Effect of Size on Management and Outcome
Murphy JL, Barber GG, McPhail NV, Scobie TK (Ottawa Civic Hosp, Ont)
Can J Surg 33:201–205, 1990   8–23

Background.—Survival rates after rupture of abdominal aortic aneurysms (AAAs) remain low. To determine factors that may influence outcome after rupture of an AAA, 172 consecutive patients who underwent surgery for a ruptured AAA between 1970 and 1985 were studied.

Findings.—The mean age of the patients was 69.8 years. The correct diagnosis was made promptly by the emergency department physician in 77% of the cases, and the average time from arrival to transfer to the operating room was 2.37 hours. The overall mortality rate was 49.4%. The factors that were significantly predictive of mortality included intraoperative urine output less than 100 mL, systolic blood pressure less than 90 mm Hg on admission or in the operating room, cardiac arrest, and a history of collapse. Information gathered in the emergency department combined with intraoperative variables correctly classified 90% of survivors and 84% of nonsurvivors, but the false positive rate was 10% and the false negative rate was 16%. The average diameter for 133 aneurysms with documented size was 8.78 cm. Thirteen aneurysms had a diameter less than 6 cm. Compared with the overall data, patients with these small aneurysms were more likely to receive a correct diagnosis (46% vs. 77%), had a longer time from arrival to transfer to the operating room (6.71 hours vs. 2.37 hours) and were more likely to die (77% vs. 45% in larger aneurysms).

Summary.—The mortality rate after rupture of AAAs remains high. The major contributing factors to mortality include the degree of shock and renal insufficiency. The ability to predict outcome is very limited, and aggressive diagnosis and surgical treatment remains the preferred approach in the subset of patients with aneurysms less than 6 cm in diameter.

▶ In this third abstract on the experience with ruptured AAAs, the lessons of Abstracts 8–21 and 8–22 are underscored in the last line of the abstract.

Aortocaval Fistulas and the Use of Transvenous Balloon Tamponade
Ingoldby CJH, Case WG, Primrose JN (St James's Univ Hosp, Leeds; Clayton Hosp, Wakefield, England)
Ann R Coll Surg Engl 72:335–339, 1990   8–24

Introduction.—Aortocaval fistulas are rare, and their diagnosis and management remain a challenge. Data on 6 patients with acute aortocaval rupture were reviewed.

Patients.—Aortocaval fistula was caused by a spontaneous rupture of aortic aneurysms in 5 patients and by trauma in 1 patient. The diagnosis was suspected before surgery in 4 patients. Diagnosis was made after the aneurysm sac was opened in the other 2 patients; both of these patients died. The useful diagnostic features included inappropriate venous pulsation in the neck with distended jugular veins despite hypotension and shock in 5 patients, lower abdominal and trunk cyanosis in 3, and a palpable thrill in 3 patients. Preoperative diagnosis allowed preliminary con-

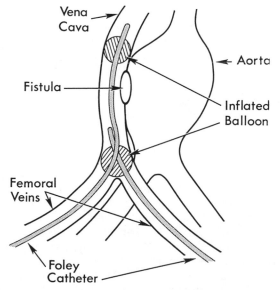

Fig 8–11.—The technique of control of caval bleeding by use of balloon catheters inserted from the groins. (Courtesy of Ingoldby CJH, Case WG, Primrose JN: *Ann R Coll Surg Engl* 72:335–339, 1990.)

trol of venous hemorrhage in 3 patients, including the use of balloons through the aortic sac in 1 and the transvenous positioning of balloon catheters in the vena cava before aortic opening in 2 (Fig 8–11). Venous bleeding was not a problem during surgery in the latter 2 patients. Four patients survived.

Conclusion.—Both preoperative recognition of the signs of an acute aortocaval rupture and preliminary balloon tamponade appear to be valuable in the management of acute aortocaval fistulas.

▶ Rupture of abdominal aortic aneurysms usually occurs into the retroperitoneum. When such rupture occurs into the peritoneal cavity, the patients rarely survive. At the opposite end of the spectrum is rupture into the vena cava, requiring the patient to receive an autotransfusion. This study details techniques of management that might or might not prove useful.

Recurrent and Fatal Haemoptysis caused By an Atheromatous Abdominal Aortic Aneurysm
Villar MTA, Wiggins J, Corrin B, Evans TW (Westminster Hosp, London; Brompton Hosp, London)
Thorax 45:568–569, 1990   8–25

Introduction.—Although hemoptysis is a rare but well-documented complication of thoracic aortic dissection, it is not a complication of abdominal aortic aneurysm (AAA).

Case Report.—Woman, 74, who was a smoker with chronic airflow limitation, had a 2-month history of recurrent hemoptysis. An initial chest radiograph showed an unfolded, dilated aorta and clear lung fields. Bronchoscopy revealed blood in the left main bronchus, and aspirated secretions gave no evidence of malignancy. A repeat chest radiograph taken 2 weeks later showed a rounded opacity in the right cardiophrenic angle and a small pleural effusion. Contrast-enhanced CT disclosed aneurysmal dilatation of the lower thoracic and upper abdominal aorta. Surgery was deemed inappropriate because of the patient's poor general medical condition, and the patient later died of massive hemoptysis. Postmortem examination showed a fusiform dilatation of the lower thoracic and upper abdominal aorta with an atheromatous saccular aneurysm arising just below the diaphragm. The aneurysm had ruptured into the liver and retroperitoneal tissues and through the diaphragm into the right lower lobe. There was no evidence of aortic dissection.

Conclusion.—Recurrent hemoptysis may result from an atheromatous AAA. Contrast-enhanced CT can be useful early in the assessment of a patient with recurrent hemoptysis.

▶ Indeed, an avis rara.

Ruptured Abdominal Aortic Aneurysm Presenting as an Obstruction of the Left Colon

Politoske EJ (Univ of Southern California; Corona Community Hosp, Corona, Calif)

Am J Gastroenterol 85:745–747, 1990

8–26

Introduction.—The clinical diagnosis of an expanding abdominal aortic aneurysm (AAA) may not always be obvious, because the typical triad of abdominal pain, pulsate mass, and hypotension may be absent. Delay in the treatment of a ruptured AAA is associated with a mortality in excess of 50%. Data were reviewed on a patient in whom a large bowel

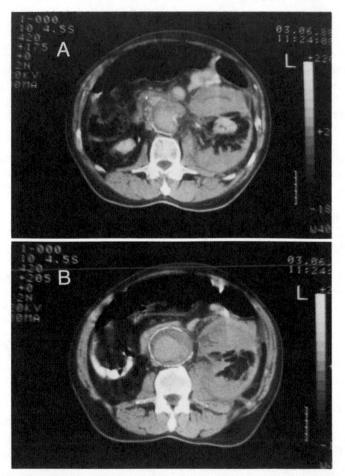

Fig 8–12.—These films (**A** and **B**) show the abdominal aortic aneurysm with thrombus present in the lumen. A defect is present along the left lateral wall of the aorta. Extravasation into the left renal bed is also noted. Marked colonic dilatation immediately overlying the aneurysm is seen. (Courtesy of Politoske EJ: *Am J Gastroenterol* 85:745–747, 1990.)

obstruction was diagnosed but who was found at operation to have a ruptured AAA.

Case Report.— Man, 72, was evaluated for progressive abdominal pain with distention of 1 week duration. After unsuccessful treatment at home with mild analgesics, antispasmodics, and antiemetics, the patient went to the emergency room because of intolerable pain. Abdominal examination revealed marked distention with tympany and increased bowel sounds, and no palpable masses or bruits were heard. The presumed admission diagnosis was peptic ulcer disease with gastrointestinal tract bleeding and a reactive ileus. Because of rapid deterioration, the patient was transferred 8 hours later to the intensive care unit. A CT scan revealed a 6 cm AAA at the level of the kidney containing a large thrombus (Fig 8–12). At emergency operation the colon was massively dilated, and the entire colon was pulled over to the left side overlying the aneurysm. There was no frank blood in the peritoneal cavity, but when the colon was removed there was immediate brisk bleeding in the retroperitoneal space. The patient had asystole and died on the operating table. Local tamponade involving both the retroperitoneal fascia and the left colon probably controlled the leakage from the aneurysm so that hemodynamic stability was maintained until very late.

Conclusion.— A partially ruptured AAA may be very difficult to diagnose. Timely diagnosis involves maintaining a high index of clinical suspicion, particularly in elderly men who smoke.

▶ As the legendary Murphy once said, "Anything that can happen, will happen."

Ringer's Lactate With or Without 3% Dextran-60 as Volume Expanders During Abdominal Aortic Surgery

Dawidson IJA, Willms CD, Sandor ZF, Coorpender LL, Reisch JS, Fry WJ (Univ of Texas, Dallas)
Crit Care Med 19:36–42, 1991   8–27

Introduction.— There is still controversy concerning the optimal replacement fluid during surgery. Experiments have suggested that a 3% colloid solution is optimal in fluid resuscitation necessary for shock and during surgery. Ringer's lactate (RL) was therefore compared with a solution of 3% dextran-60 (D60) in RL as a maintenance fluid during aortic reconstructive surgery.

Methods.— In a randomized control trial, 20 consecutive patients who underwent elective abdominal aortic reconstructive surgery received either D60 in RL or RL alone as maintenance fluids during surgery and for 24 hours postoperatively. The infusion rates were guided by a pulmonary artery occlusion pressure (PAOP) of at least 10 mm Hg and a urine output of > 30 mL/hr.

Results.— The infused volume of 3% D60 averaged 36 mL/kg, and that of RL alone was 104 mL/kg, for an infusion volume ratio of 1:2.9.

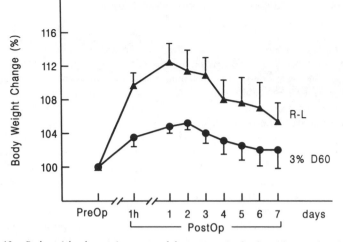

Fig 8–13.—Body weight changes in percent of the preoperative level at 1 hour and 24 hours after surgery in patients receiving either 3% D60 or RL (mean ± SEM). (Courtesy of Dawidson IJA, Willms CD, Sandor ZF, et al: *Crit Care Med* 19:36–42, 1991.)

The body weight gain at 24 hours was significantly greater with Rl alone (12.5%) than with D60 (4.8%) (Fig 8–13), despite a significantly greater intraoperative urine output with RL. In both groups, the total intravascular albumin decreased by .7 g/kg, closely matching the calculated plasma volume (PV) loss of 13 mL/kg to 15 mL/kg without fluid infusions. One hour after surgery, blood volume (BV) and PV increased to 102% and 115% of the preoperative level in the D60 group, respectively. In contrast, both BV and PV decreased significantly to about 83% of preoperative levels in the RL alone group. Furthermore, only 6% of the infused RL remained as PV at 1 hr after surgery, whereas 51% of the infused D60 remained as PV. Cardiac output, PAOP, central venous pressure, and mean arterial pressure were similar in the D60 and RL groups.

Conclusion.—A diluted colloid solution in RL is of significant value in maintaining intravascular volumes and hemodynamics both during and after major surgery.

▶ Neither this study nor the references cited in the original will answer the question implied by the title.

Infrarenal Abdominal Aortic Disease: A Review of the Retroperitoneal Approach
Grace PA, Bouchier-Hayes D (Beaumont Hosp, Dublin)
Br J Surg 78:6–9, 1991   8–28

Background.—the most widely used approach to the infrarenal aorta has been through transabdominal exposure. Over the past 30 years a number of surgeons have used a retroperitoneal approach.

Indications.—The retroperitoneal approach has been used for the elective repair of infrarenal AAAs and occasionally for the repair of ruptured AAAs. Use of the retroperitoneal route to gain access to juxtarenal and suprarenal aneurysms has also been reported. A further indication for using the retroperitoneal approach is aortoiliac occlusive disease in which the route has been used extensively in procedures such as aortoiliac obliteration, aortoiliac bypass, aortofemoral bypass, and celiac and renal artery angioplasty or bypass.

Discussion.—Many studies have found that the retroperitoneal approach yields better results in specific areas. It is associated with better perioperative oxygenation and preservation of lung volume and a lower incidence of pulmonary complications. Hospital stay and morbidity were reduced in most cases, and a shorter time to alimentation is often noted. Only a few drawbacks to using the retroperitoneal approach have been reported; these include the extended time used in positioning the patient on the table (which may not occur when the Lisberg incision is used), inability to fully explore the abdomen before repair of the aneurysm, and extreme technical demands.

▶ History repeats itself. Recent vascular surgery has seen a return to the retroperitoneal approach to AAAs despite a lack of concrete proof that the approach is less morbid. However, the observations of many experienced clinical surgeons who favor the retroperitoneal operation cannot be discarded.

Is Tube Repair of Aortic Aneurysm Followed by Aneurysmal Change in the Common Iliac Arteries?
Provan JL, Fialkov J, Ameli FM, St Louis EL (Univ of Toronto; Wellesley Hosp, Toronto)
Can J Surg 33:394–397, 1990   8–29

Introduction.—There are concerns that aneurysmal changes in the common iliac arteries may occur after repair of an abdominal aortic aneurysm (AAA) with a tube prosthesis. Computed tomography scans were used to assess the maximum intraluminal diameters of the common iliac arteries before and 3–5 years after tube repair of AAAs in 23 patients.

Findings.—Before operation, 9 patients had minimal ectasia of the common iliac arteries (defined as a generalized dilatation to more than 1.5 cm but less than 3 cm in diameter). At follow-up none of the 23 patients had aneurysmal changes that were greater than 3 cm. There were no significant changes between the preoperative and follow-up maximum diameters (Fig 8–14), regardless of whether follow-up was at 3, 4, or 5 years. None of the patients had symptoms that have been associated with common iliac artery aneurysms.

Conclusion.—The repair of AAAs with tube prostheses is not followed by marked aneurysmal changes in the common iliac arteries for up to 5

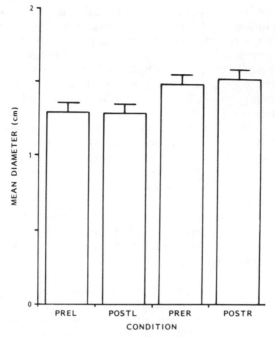

Fig 8–14.—Mean common iliac artery diameters for 23 right and 23 left arteries measured before and after operation show no significant change. *Abbreviations: PREL*, preoperative, left; *POSTL*, postoperative, left; *PRER*, preoperative, right; *POSTR*, postoperative, right. (Courtesy of Provan JL, Fialkov J, Ameli FM, et al: *Can J Surg* 33:394–397, 1990.)

years after operation, even if there is previous minimal dilatation of the common iliac arteries.

▶ Thirty years of experience with tube repair of AAAs has revealed the astounding fact that when AAAs recur, they do so in the aorta proximal to the previous AAA repair, not in iliac arteries.

Does Division of the Left Renal Vein During Aortic Surgery Adversely Affect Renal Function?

Huber D, Harris JP, Walker PJ, May J, Tyrer P (Royal Prince Alfred Hosp, Sydney, Australia)
Ann Vasc Surg 5:74–79, 1991   8–30

Introduction.—The effect of left renal vein division on renal function remains controversial. Although the division of this vein improves exposure of the juxtarenal aorta during aortic surgery, adverse effects have been demonstrated. The differing approaches and attempts to show the effect on renal function were investigated in 355 patients who had elective aneurysm resection and 123 who had emergency surgery for ruptured aortic aneurysm.

Methods.—The left renal vein was divided during surgery in 28 of the 355 elective patients and 17 of the 123 emergency surgery patients. Serum creatinine levels were measured to assess renal function. Cardiac, respiratory, and cerebral events; distal ischemia; postoperative bleeding; graft infections; and any other complications that may have compromised renal function were recorded.

Results.—In both the elective surgery and the emergency surgery groups, the immediately postoperative creatinine values were significantly greater in patients with division of the left renal vein. At 1-month follow-up, the creatinine levels decreased, but the values were significantly higher than the values in those patients whose renal vein was left intact. Suprarenal cross-clamping appeared to cause a significant increase in creatinine levels.

Discussion.—The high venous pressures associated with division of the left renal vein can impair renal function. Although there was no increase in the need for permanent dialysis, nor any difference in 5-year survival after division of the renal vein, the significant increases in creatinine levels can cause an adverse effect on renal function. This complication should be considered in surgical procedures involving the division of the left renal vein.

▶ The 1969 report from Detroit that suggested transsection of the left renal vein as a technical aid in aortic surgery influenced aortic surgery for the next 20 years (1). It has been understood gradually that such renal vein division is associated with the hazard of decreased renal function in the affected kidney. A review of the original article reveals that the authors suggested reanastomosis of the renal vein after temporary division.

Reference

1. Szilagyi DE, et al: *Surgery* 65:32, 1969.

Combined Myocardial Revascularization and Abdominal Aortic Aneurysm Repair

Hinkamp TJ, Pifarre R, Bakhos M, Blakeman B (Loyola Univ Med Ctr, Maywood, Ill)
Ann Thorac Surg 51:470–472, 1991
8–31

Background.—Late survival after repair of an abdominal aortic aneurysm (AAA) appears to be affected directly by coronary artery disease. The stress on the myocardium resulting from AAA repair may be heightened by coronary artery disease. Myocardial revascularization and AAA repair were combined in 17 in hemodynamically stable patients during a 5-year period.

Methods.—Of 128 patients who underwent either elective or urgent AAA repair, 17 had a combined procedure after undergoing coronary angiography for coronary artery disease. There were 15 men and 2 women (average age, 66 years). Fourteen patients who underwent elective AAA repair had evidence of coronary artery disease at catheterization, and 3 had increasing angina. Cardiopulmonary bypass with myocardial revascularization was performed through a median sternotomy that was then extended for AAA repair. All of the patients were hemodynamically stable before abdominal surgery began.

Results.—The operations were uneventful. Complications included mediastinal bleeding, tension pneumothorax, and a small subendocardial myocardial infarction. One patient died within 30 days; the rest were alive and well at follow-up. The average transfusion requirements were 4 units of packed red blood cells and 1.7 units of fresh frozen plasma; however, routine use of the Cell Saver significantly reduced the need for blood in the later patients in the series.

Conclusions.—In patients with serious coronary artery disease and AAA, both conditions can be safely treated in a single operation. The mortality of this procedure is low, and the cost and length of hospitalization are decreased.

▶ One wonders why a single center would find so many patients who required combined coronary artery bypass grafting and AAA resection.

Perigraft Pseudocyst Complicating Repair of Ruptured Aortic Aneurysm: Successful Treatment by Percutaneous Aspiration
Wynn JJ, Bates WB III, Teeslink CR, Nesbit RR Jr (VA Med Ctr, Augusta; Med College of Georgia, Augusta)
South Med J 83:1102–1103, 1990   8–32

Introduction.—Pancreatitis is usually associated with biliary tract disease or alcoholism rather than with surgery. A patient with a pancreatic pseudocyst was successfully treated by repeated percutaneous aspiration.

Case Report.—Man, 64, underwent repair of a ruptured infrarenal abdominal aortic aneurysm (AAA) that was complicated by shock. Computerized tomography demonstrated a large cystic mass enveloping the polytef prosthesis. The patient's serum amylase level postsurgery measured 205 units per L (normal, 20 units to 110 units per L). On the 71st postoperative day, more than 2,500 mL of sterile cloudy fluid was aspirated from the cyst, which had an amylase concentration of 6,216 units per L. A CT scan after aspiration showed partial decrease in pseudocyst size. A second aspiration 4 weeks later produced 460 mL of fluid with an amylase level of 1,800 units per L. Examination over 12 months after surgery demonstrated the continuing decrease of fluid around the graft. The most recent CT scan showed no signs of the pseudocyst.

Conclusions.—The medical literature had no previous reports of pancreatic pseudocysts after aortic surgery. Successful treatment of this patient suggests that percutaneous aspiration offers a means of therapy for patients who cannot tolerate the stresses of surgery.

▶ Pancreatitis after AAA resection is seen occasionally. A resulting pseudocyst is rare, and the authors of this study could find no previous case.

Prognostic Factors in Acute Renal Failure Following Aortic Aneurysm Surgery
Berisa F, Beaman M, Adu D, McGonigle RJS, Michael J, Downing R, Fielding JWL, Dunn J (Queen Elizabeth Hosp; Univ of Birmingham, England)
Q J Med New Series 76:689–698, 1990   8–33

Background.—Acute renal failure is a serious complication of aortic aneurysm surgery after elective or emergency operation for rupture. Because the reasons for the high mortalities (range, 47%–100%) associated with such failure are unclear, the prognostic factors affecting the survival of 70 patients who had acute renal failure after aortic aneurysm surgery were studied.

	Prognostic Factors				
	Total no of patients	Survived	Died	χ^2	p
Age					
> 65 yrs	43	12	31	5.351	0.02
< 65 yrs	27	15	12		
Aneurysm surgery					
rupture	49	15	34	4.367	0.04
elective	21	12	9		
Mechanical ventilation					
> 3 days	44	11	33	9.209	0.002
< 3 days	26	16	10		
Time in ITU					
> 7 days	46	11	35	12.167	0.0005
< 7 days	24	16	8		
Inotropic support	38	6	32	18.209	< 0.0001
No inotropic support	32	21	11		
Evidence of sepsis					
Yes	45	14	31	2.960	0.09
No	25	13	12		
Pre-existing cardiovascular disease					
Yes	28	10	18	0.161	0.69
No	42	17	25		
Further operations					
Yes	36	13	23	0.189	0.66
No	34	14	20		

(Courtesy of Berisa F, Beaman M, Adu D, et al: *Q J Med New Series* 76:689–698, 1990.)

Patients.—Of the 70 patients investigated, 49 had undergone surgery for a ruptured aneurysm and 21 had undergone an elective procedure; 59 received hemodialysis. Although 33 patients (47%) survived an episode of acute renal failure, 6 of these patients died within 3 months of recovery. Therefore, the overall survival rate was 39%.

Results.—A stepwise logistic regression analysis identified 3 factors that had an adverse affect on survival: a need for inotropic support, ventilation lasting longer than 3 days, and age greater than 65 years (table). Using these factors, a model was developed that provided a basis for predicting outcome.

Conclusions.—The high mortality rate associated with acute renal failure remains a major problem. Although the model for predicting outcome correctly predicted 72% of the patients who survived and 80% of the patients who died, it must be validated by a prospective study of patients with acute renal failure after aortic aneurysm surgery.

▶ Early studies of dialysis after AAA resection suggested that few patients survived. During the 1980s, an increasing incidence of survivors was noted gradually until, at present, one would expect a minimum of 30% to 50% of patients to leave the hospital.

The Role of Inflammation in Nonspecific Abdominal Aortic Aneurysm Disease

Brophy CM, Reilly JM, Walker Smith GJ, Tilson MD (Harvard Surgical Service, Boston: Yale Univ; Roosevelt/St Luke's Hosp, New York)
Ann Vasc Surg 5:229–233, 1991   8–34

Introduction.—Elastin degradation is a predominant pathologic feature of abdominal aortic aneurysm (AAA). The potential role of inflammation in nonspecific AAA was investigated.

Methods.—In 10 patients who underwent aortic reconstruction for aneurysm disease, specimens were taken from the anterior wall of the infrarenal aorta. Control specimens were taken from the aortic tissues of individuals with atherosclerotic disease who underwent vascular reconstruction and also from a normal organ donor. The specimens were examined for type and distribution of inflammatory cells, and the soluble extracts were examined for immunoglobulins.

Results.—In 8 of the 10 AAA specimens, a mononuclear inflammatory infiltrate was present. There were areas of undetectable elastin with no inflammation, and areas of marked inflammation with normal elastin amounts. In contrast to the atherosclerotic and normal control extracts, the inflammatory component in AAA was associated with immunoglobulins in soluble extracts from aneurysmal tissue.

Conclusions.—The inflammatory infiltrate is common in AAA, but it does not appear to contribute to loss of elastin. In addition, immunoglobulins are more likely to be present in the aneurysmal aorta than in the control aorta. Release of antigens, recruitment of inflammatory cells, and immunoglobulin production may be associated with aneurysmal degradation.

▶ As suggested by experience with aortoarteritis, an inflammatory infiltrate may play a role in the genesis of AAAs. This study suggests that proteolytic enzymes are not the active agent, and that other factors play a much more important role.

The Cellular Component in the Parietal Infiltrate of Inflammatory Abdominal Aortic Aneurysms (IAAA)
Stella A, Gargiulo M, Pasquinelli G, Preda P, Faggioli GL, Cenacchi G, D'Addato M (Bologna Univ, Italy; S Orsola Hosp, Bologna, Italy)
Eur J Vasc Surg 5:65–70, 1991   8–35

Introduction.—Inflammatory abdominal aortic aneurysms (IAAAs) are a subgroup of abdominal aortic aneurysms (AAA) with clearly defined anatomical and pathological characteristics; however, their cause remains unknown.

Study Design.—By using light microscopy, transmission electron microscopy, and immunohistochemistry, 8 IAAAs and 10 atherosclerotic AAAs were studied to define both the parietal inflammatory process and the degree of cell activation and alteration of connective tissue.

Results.—In IAAAs the parietal infiltrate consisted mainly of B lymphocytes with an accessory cell-mediated process in which the T4/T8 ratio was preserved. All of the cells appeared to be activated, as was evidenced by the widespread presence of interleukin-2 (IL-2) receptors and HLA-DR antigen. In follicular lesions part of the cell populations were in the proliferative phase, as was shown by positiveness for ki-67. The interstitial matrix contained deposits of IgG, IgM, and C3c together with an increase in type III collagen and a reduction in elastin that appeared fragmented and swollen. The same inflammatory cell population was observed in 1 case of AAA, but fibrosis was absent.

Summary.—When there is inflammation of the arterial wall, a cell population consisting mainly of B lymphocytes with an accessory cell-mediated process is activated. The degree of activation of these cell components and the activation of complement suggest that the relevant antigen may have been localized in the aneurysm wall at the time of observation.

▶ Further study of the inflammatory infiltrate in AAAs suggests that an antigen antibody reaction is important to the formation of the aneurysm. This factor may be most important in the future in the prevention or treatment of patients with aneurysm disease.

Inflammatory Abdominal Aortic Aneurysms
Boontje AH, van den Dungen JJAM, Blanksma C (Univ Hosp, Groningen C, The Netherlands)
J Cardiovasc Surg 31:611–616, 1990   8–36

Background.—The inflammatory abdominal aortic aneurysm (IAAA) is a variant of atherosclerotic AAA that may be considered a separate clinical entity. Without treatment the aneurysm may rupture or the patient may become uremic. The operative management of an IAAA has some special features.

Methods.—Forty-five of the 517 patients treated for abdominal aortic aneurysm were diagnosed as having an IAAA. At surgery, all of the patients had a thick, white, glistening perianeurysmal fibrous layer that usually adhered to adjacent structures. Of the patients, 38% were symptom free, 38% had chronic pain, and 24% had acute severe or progressive pain in the abdomen, flank, or back. Only 1 patient had a ruptured IAAA. In 9 patients hydronephrosis was the initial diagnosis. Aneurysm was an accidental finding in 4 patients, and IAAA was diagnosed before operation in only 10 of 45 patients. All 45 patients underwent surgery (6 on an emergency basis). All IAAAs were infrarenal. Ureterolysis was performed in 8 of the 9 patients with hydronephrosis. The preoperative diagnostic procedures included excretory urography, ultrasonography, and CT scans of the abdominal aorta.

Results.—All of the patients with preoperative pain had complete relief. Apart from the usual complications of aortic surgery, there was a slightly increased incidence of secondary retroperitoneal hemorrhage. Two patients died within 1 month of surgery from myocardial infarction. All 8 patients who underwent unilateral or bilateral ureterolysis had complete resolution of hydronephrosis and complete recovery of renal function. At follow-up 1 patient had recurrent ureteral obstruction that resolved with a second operation.

Conclusions.—All patients with an IAAA should undergo aortic replacement to achieve pain relief and to prevent rupture. When hydronephrosis is present, ureterolysis is strongly recommended. It may be performed safely with excellent results.

▶ Inflammatory infiltrate in AAAs may or may not be related to the inflammatory process seen anterior to some 4% to 10% of infrarenal aneurysms. This latter condition spreads laterally to entrap ureters and presents certain technical problems. As yet, it does not throw any light on the obscure problems of the genesis of aneurysms.

Abdominal Aortic Aneurysm With Perianeurysmal Fibrosis: Experience From 11 Swedish Vascular Centers

Lindblad B, Almgren B, Bergqvist D, Eriksson I, Forsberg O, Glimåker H, Jivegård L, Karlström L, Lundqvist B, Olofsson P, Plate G, Thörne J, Troëng T (Hospitals in Malmö, Uppsala, Västerås, Falun, Göteborg, Varberg, Karlstad, Stockholm, Helsingborg, Lund, and Karlskrona, Sweden)
J Vasc Surg 13:231–239, 1991   8–37

Background.—Between 3% and 10% of all abdominal aortic aneurysms (AAAs) are associated with retroperitoneal fibrosis. Therefore, patients with AAAs (without perianeurysmal fibrosis) who underwent treatment at 11 vascular centers in Sweden were analyzed in a case-control study.

Patients.—Of the 2,026 patients who underwent surgery for AAAs at the 11 centers, 98 patients (4.8%) had inflammatory AAAs. Eighty-two patients from the same centers who had noninflammatory AAAs were also studied for comparison.

Findings.—Four aneurysms in the inflammatory group and 16 in the noninflammatory group were ruptured. More patients with inflammatory AAAs had symptoms that indicated radiographic assessment. The median erythrocyte sedimentation rate was 39 mm in the inflammatory group and 19 mm in the noninflammatory group; serum creatinine levels increased in 27 and 8 patients, respectively. Preoperative examination showed ureteral obstruction in 19 patients with inflammatory AAAs. Twelve of these patients had preoperative nephrostomy or ureteral catheter placement. An additional 20 patients had fibrosis around 1 or both ureters at surgery. Although 19 patients underwent ureterolysis, the preoperative and postoperative creatinine levels were comparable in these patients and in the conservatively treated patients. The length of surgery, intraoperative blood loss, and complications were also similar in the 2 groups. The overall 30-day operative mortality was also comparable (11% and 12%, respectively), but it was higher for patients who had elective surgery for inflammatory AAAs.

Conclusions.—In sum, the inflammatory AAAs were more often symptomatic and less likely to have ruptured. They also increased erythrocyte sedimentation rates or creatinine levels frequently. The surgical techniques used against the ureter did not affect the renal function abnormalities of patients with inflammatory AAAs.

▶ Although the summary of Swedish experience expressed in this study presents little new information, some of the observations made are pertinent. Among these is the lack of progression of the process after surgical decompression. Also, the process does not progress as far distally as the external iliac artery, and concomitant ureterolysis is unnecessary when the aneurysm is excluded from the circulation. After operation, regression of the inflammatory process is to be expected. My personal bias is to implant ureteral catheters before operating on patients with inflammatory aneurysms.

Inflammatory Abdominal Aortic Aneurysms: A Disease Entity? Histological Analysis of 60 Cases of Inflammatory Aortic Aneurysms of Unknown Aetiology
Leu HJ (Univ of Zürich, Switzerland)
Virchows Arch [A] 417:427–433, 1990   8–38

Background.—Takayasu's disease and nonspecific aortitis can currently be distinguished from inflammatory abdominal aortic aneurysms (IAAA) by their affected populations and clinical course only. The latter disease usually affects older male patients and has a benign clinical course after surgical intervention. The affected tissue need not be removed, nor is further medication required. In contrast, Takayasu's disease affects young women primarily, and the prognosis is poor. Histology of the affected tissue is, however, identical in the 2 syndromes. The histological specimens from 60 cases of IAAs of unkonwn etiology were re-examined in the hope of discovering a distinctive histology to identify IAAA.

Methods.—Serial tissue sections from 51 men (mean age, 61 years) and 8 women (mean age, 43.8 years) were differentiated with a variety of histological stains. The marked adventitial fibrosis considered indicative of Takayasu's disease, the derivation of tissue (thoracic or aortic), and the presence of granulomas giant cells, fibrinoid necrosis, plasma cells, and eosinophils were all assessed. Accompanying demographic data were extracted from medical records.

Results.—The histopathological characteristics of the 39 abdominal and 21 thoracic aneurysms were identical. In all of the specimens, the thickened adventitia contained inflammatory cells in a diffuse or follicle-like arrangement. There were also focal lymphatic infiltrates with germinal centers. Takayasu's disease and IAAA could not be distinguished on a morphological basis in subgroups divided on the basis of age, sex, site of aneurysm, or racial origin.

Discussion.—The morphological changes that occur in IAAA do not warrant its designation as a distinct disease entity. A sufficient descriptor at this time is "abdominal (or thoracic) aortic aneurysm of apparently inflammatory origin." The presence of lymph follicles with germinal centers is common in many autoimmune diseases. Thus, the histopathology observed in the aneurysms could have an autoimmune etiology.

▶ One would expect that experienced pathologists looking at the IAAA would be able to relate the condition to garden variety retroperitoneal fibrosis or non-specific aortoarteritis. It is disappointing that this study fails to do so.

Abdominal Aortic Aneurysms Infected With *Salmonella:* Problems of Treatment
Trairatvorakul P, Sriphojanart S, Sathapatayavongs B (Ramathibodi Hosp, Bangkok, Thailand)
J Vasc Surg 12:16–19, 1990   8–39

Introduction.—*Salmonella* infection of abdominal aortic aneurysms (AAAs) creates a range of problems for the treating physician. The best alternatives of treatment for patients with infected aneurysms were examined.

Methods.—Seven patients with *Salmonella*-infected AAAs were studied. Cultures from the aneurysm wall confirmed the presence of *Salmonella* in all of the patients. Treatment with broad-spectrum antibiotics was started immediately after the diagnosis was made. Three patients underwent resection and axillofemoral bypass reconstruction; 2 patients had total removal of the aneurysmal wall and infected periaortic tissue. The aneurysmal wall of 1 patient was left intact to cover the in situ graft (*Salmonella infection* had not yet been diagnosed); 1 patient died during emergency laparotomy.

Results.—Two of the patients with an axillofemoral bypass graft died, and a third patient had a difficult postoperative course. All of the patients with in situ graft survived.

Discussion.—In situ graft placement with extensive débridement of the infected tissue and aneurysmal wall had the most successful results when combined with effectively monitored antibiotic therapy for a minimum of 6 weeks. Early diagnosis and treatment are essential for recovery and survival.

▶ Aneurysms infected with *Salmonella* organisms and other bacteria continue to be an important problem. Management by extra-anatomical techniques or by in situ repair have their advocates, however, as yet, no best method of management has been determined.

Salmonella choleraesuis Aortitis and Abdominal Abscess
VanRoy VL, Smith PW (Univ of Nebraska)
Infect Surg 10:21–24, 1991   8–40

Background.—*Salmonella choleraesuis* can cause bacteremia and vascular infection. A patient had an infected aortic graft and abdominal abscess caused by *S. choleraesuis.*

Case Report.—Man, 60, had intermittent pain in his right buttock and lower back. The patient's past history included a ruptured abdominal aortic aneurysm and placement of a subcutaneous axillofemoral bypass graft. Blood culture grew *S. choleraesuis* and a pathological report revealed acute and chronic inflammatory infiltrates of the vascular tissues. Since then, recurrent soft tissue abscesses occurred in the flank and groin area; the patient also had a fever. During the present admission, purulent material was draining from a lesion at the right buttock. An abdominal CT scan revealed a large left psoas abscess. At surgery, the abscess communicated with a right buttock sinus tract. Cultures grew *Salmonella* species group C1, and a stool culture was negative for *Salmonella*. Intravenous ampicillin was started, followed by oral ciprofloxacin for 6 months. The patient improved.

Discussion.—*Salmonella choleraesuis* can cause aortitis with rupture of an abdominal aneurysm. Of the 9 reported patients with *S. choleraesuis,* 8 had sustained a rupture by the time of diagnosis. Four underwent bypass graft surgery and only 1 survived. Axillofemoral bypass surgery for *Salmonella* abdominal aortic infection avoids the contaminated field and is probably the procedure of choice. There have been no controlled trials to determine the optimum antibiotic therapy, but ampicillin is recommended traditionally and ciprofloxacin has also been shown to be effective.

▶ The extra-anatomical repair of a ruptured *Salmonella*-infected AAA is certainly not free of complications.

Primary Aorto-Enteric Fistula: A Practicable Curable Condition? Pathogenetic and Clinical Aspects
Nohr M, Juul-Jensen KE, Balslev IB, Jelnes R (Aalborg, Denmark)
Int Angiol 9:278–281, 1990   8–41

Background.—Aorto-enteric fistulas occur most often after reconstructive vascular surgery on the abdominal aorta, and they can be lifethreatening. To illustrate the etiology, pathogenesis, and diagnostic possibilities of primary aorto-enteric fisultas, 3 cases were evaluated.

Case Reports.—Three men, 41, 51, and 61, were admitted to the hospital with upper gastrointestinal hemorrhage or abdominal pain. Two of the 3 patients had a typical bleeding pattern: small repeated attacks of gastrointestinal bleeding ("herald" or "sentinel" bleeds) followed by a massive hemorrhage resulting in hemodynamic changes and requiring immediate laparotomy. The third patient had no herald bleeding, only a massive and lethal hemorrhage. The diagnosis of a fistula was not established in any of the patients before laparotomy. Each patient had only 1 fistula, the 3 fistulas were caused by atherosclerotic aneurysm, mycotic aneurysm, and radiation-induced ulcer of the duodenum, respectively. One of the patients underwent an aortic graft and a duodenal suture, whereas a second patient underwent a direct suture of the aortic defect and a duodenal resection. The third patient died before surgery could be performed, and only 1 of the 2 patients operated on survived.

Conclusions.—Clinicians should maintain a heightened index of suspicion when a patient has gastrointestinal bleeding of obscure origin, abdominal or back pain, and an abdominal mass. Although endoscopy and diagnostic imaging may identify a fistula, there is a high rate of false negative results. Laparotomy is the safest diagnostic method and may save the patient's life.

▶ Vascular surgeons will encounter primary aortoduodenal fistula in association with aortic aneurysms. This is a situation in which an in situ repair can be accomplished with expectation of success.

9 Aortoiliac Occlusions

Aorto-Iliac Arteriosclerotic Disease in Young Human Adults
Jensen BV, Egeblad K (Aalborg Sygehus, Aalborg, Denmark)
Eur J Vasc Surg 4:583–586, 1990   9–1

Background.—Although peripheral arteriosclerotic arterial disease of the lower extremities is found most often in common men, some studies have found a higher incidence of the disease in women in the younger age groups, particularly when the lesion is located in the aortoiliac segment. A group of younger patients with a predominance of women was assessed.

Patient Selection.—During a 7-year period, 404 patients underwent primary operations for an obliterative lesion in the aortoiliac segment; 96 of these patients were younger than 50 years of age. An arteriogram demonstrated stenosis/occlusion of the aortoiliac segment with normal distal arteries in 45 patients. The arteriograms of an additional 11 patients showed the same lesion, but with insufficient contrast in the peripheral arteries to allow proper evaluation. The case notes of these 56 patients, (18 men and 38 women) were reviewed.

Symptoms and Treatment.—Of the patients, 35 had bilateral symptoms and 21 had only 1 affected limb. Intermittent claudication was reported in 73 limbs and rest pain and gangrene noted in 18. Few patients had an associated disease; most were judged to be otherwise healthy. A variety of surgical procedures were performed in 102 lower limbs. Although 12 patients had postoperative complications, no patients died postoperatively or during follow-up ranging from 21–96 months. The overall cumulative patency rate at 4 years was 89%. A total of 48 patients were completely free of symptoms at follow-up.

Implications.—The outcome was better for women than for men. In addition, more women were free of symptoms and had normal pulses after surgery. In this highly selected group of younger patients, particularly the women, an isolated aortoiliac arteriosclerotic lesion appeared to be a separate disease entity that was both benign and curable.

▶ One type of aortoiliac occlusive disease occurs in patients approximately 50 years of age. This group of individuals was first described by Leriche, and it represents the most favorable class for hemodynamic reconstruction. This study emphasizes female dominance; however, of greater importance is the fact that these individuals have a great capacity for life expectancy. In addition, reconstruction allows complete rehabilitation. This group of patients can be reconstructed for claudication alone, not for distal gangrene.

Aortofemoral Dacron Reconstruction for Aorto-Iliac Occlusive Disease: A 25-Year Survey

Nevelsteen A, Wouters L, Suy R (Univ Clin, Gasthuisberg, Leuven; Janssen Research Found, Belgium)

Eur J Vasc Surg 5:179–186, 1991   9–2

Background.—The aortofemoral Dacron reconstruction has been used for aortoiliac occlusive disease during the past 4 decades. Most reports on the procedure usually focus on the patency after operation. The results of a review of medical experience with 869 patients who received an aorto(bi)femoral Dacron graft for occlusive disease during a 25-year period were evaluated.

Methods.—The medical and surgical records of all patients referred to the Department of Cardiovascular Surgery for elective aortofemoral (AF) reconstruction between 1963 and 1987 were reviewed. The follow-up data were collected between October 1987 and February 1988. Angiography or noninvasive examinations were performed if deterioration was noted. A total of 869 patients (820 men and 49 women) with a mean age of 61 years were assessed. Cardiac status was judged normal by history, ECG, and clinical examination in 547 patients.

Results.—The early results showed an operative mortality of 4.5% (39 patients died 1 month after surgery). Myocardial infarction was the leading cause of death. The operative mortality remained somewhat steady throughout the study. Early morbidity occurred in 162 patients (20%), with the incidence of morbidity significantly increasing in patients who were older, who had advanced ischemia, and who had combined surgeries. Systemic complications were found in 39 patients (4.5%), whereas local, nonvascular complications were observed in 99 patients (12%). The median survival time was 8.2 years (Fig 9–1). Late events were observed in 216 patients (26% of the total population). Graft-related problems were the most frequent late event, occurring in 78.5% of the 216 patients. Late occlusion was the most frequent functional problem. The primary patency rate decreased from 99% at discharge to 74% after 10 years and to 70% after 15 years. Further surgery improved patency (Fig 9–2). Anastomotic aneurysms were found in 47 patients and recurrent stenoses occurred in 23 patients. The primary event-free rate decreased to 51% and 40% after 10 years and 15 years, respectively, but it increased to 70% and 61% after reoperation.

Conclusion.—These results indicate that atherosclerotic events cause most perioperative and late deaths after surgery. The long-term functional results of AF Dacron reconstruction depended primarily on the smoking habits of the patients after surgery, the operation date, and the presence of concomitant femoropopliteal occlusive disease.

▶ It is discouraging to note a decrease in the late patency of aortofemoral reconstructions. The deterioration of graft patency appears to be dependent upon the progression of distal occlusive disease and the occurrence of false aneu-

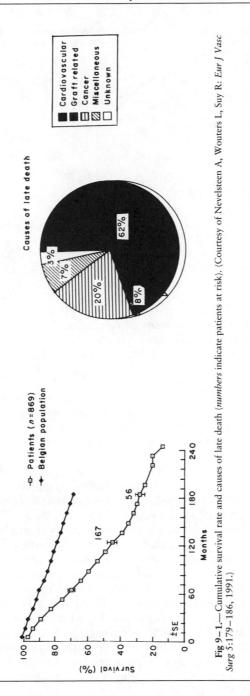

Fig 9–1.—Cumulative survival rate and causes of late death (*numbers* indicate patients at risk). (Courtesy of Nevelsteen A, Wouters L, Suy R: *Eur J Vasc Surg* 5:179–186, 1991.)

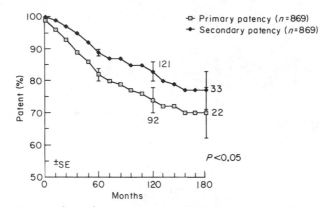

Fig 9–2.—Primary and secondary patency rate (*numbers* indicate patients at risk). (Courtesy of Nevelsteen A, Wouters L, Suy R: *Eur J Vasc Surg* 5:179–186, 1991.)

rysms with thrombosis. This study points out that smoking has a deleterious influence.

Recent Changes in the Treatment of Aortoiliac Occlusive Disease by the Oxford Regional Vascular Service

Davies AH, Ramarakha P, Collin J, Morris PJ (Univ of Oxford; John Radcliffe Hosp, Oxford, England)
Br J Surg 77:1129–1131, 1990   9–3

Purpose.—Percutaneous transluminal angioplasty has been used increasingly in the treatment of occlusive arterial disease. The impact of this technique on the surgical treatment of patients with aortoiliac disease was evaluated.

Data Analysis.—Between 1985 and 1988, 192 patients were treated for aortoiliac occlusive disease by the Oxford Regional Vascular Service. The number of patients treated by percutaneous transluminal angioplasties increased from 2 in 1985 to 34 in 1987 (Fig 9–3). This increase coincided with a decrease in the number of patients treated by aortobifemoral bypass, although the number of patients treated by extraanatomical bypass remained constant. There were twice as many patients in the fourth year as in the first year, and the number of surgical operations increased despite the fact that many patients were treated exclusively with percutaneous transluminal angioplasty. There was a 109% increase overall in the number of patients treated for mandatory indications (rest pain or critical ischemia) and an 85% increase in patients treated for optional indications (intermittent claudication). Percutaneous transluminal angioplasty was initially used only in patients with optional indications for treatment. However, it was later used just as frequently for patients in whom treatment was mandatory.

Conclusion.—The introduction of percutaneous transluminal angioplasty for the treatment of aortoiliac occlusive disease has caused a sub-

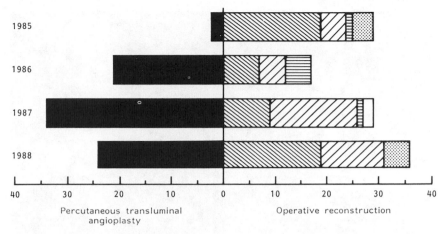

Fig 9–3.—Number of patients treated per year by the various techniques. *Narrow hatched bars,* aortobifemoral bypass; *wide hatched bars,* femorofemoral bypass; *filled bars,* percutaneous transluminal angioplasty; *open bars,* endarterectomy; *dotted bars,* axillobifemoral bypass; *horizontally striped bars,* femorofemoral and percutaneous transluminal angioplasty. (Courtesy of Davies AH, Ramarakha P, Collin J, et al: *Br J Surg* 77:1129–1131, 1990.)

stantial reduction in the number of surgical operations performed; however, this effect is shortlived. The availability of percutaneous transluminal angioplasty appears to stimulate increased referral of patients who are otherwise candidates for major arterial surgery only. Therefore, there is a doubling of the workload for the vascular service with an increased demand for surgical reconstruction.

▶ It could have been predicted that percutaneous transluminal angioplasty of the aortoiliac segment would increase both the number of patients studied and the number of those referred for treatment by surgical intervention. One advantage of this procedure is that it allows intervention before occlusion takes place, thereby obviating the need for an immediate bypass.

Obstruction of the Infrarenal Portion of the Abdominal Aorta: Results of Treatment With Balloon Angioplasty
Ravimandalam K, Rao VRK, Kumar S, Gupta AK, Joseph S, Unni M, Rao AS
(Sree Chitra Tirunal Inst for Med Sciences and Technology, Kerala, India)
AJR 156:1257–1260, 1991   9–4

Background.—Some patients with vascular disease have stenoses of the lower abdominal aorta and its bifurcation. These lesions are usually treated surgically with endarterectomy for focal stenoses or with a bypass for more extensive conditions. Balloon angioplasty of the lower abdominal aorta was used in 27 patients with obstruction of the infrarenal section of the abdominal aorta.

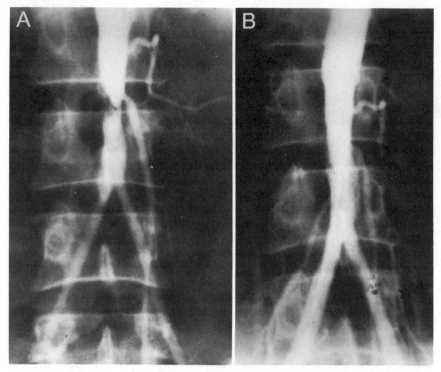

Fig 9–4.—Radiographs of a man, 40, with a history of claudication and impotence. **A,** transaxillary aortogram showing stenosis of abdominal aorta at the level of the inferior mesenteric artery; **B,** angiogram obtained after dilatation with a single 12mm balloon. The lumen of the inferior mesenteric artery was preserved. The patient was asymptomatic with normal sexual function 27 months later. (Courtesy of Ravimandalam K, Rao VRK, Kumar S, et al: *AJR* 156:1257–1260, 1991.)

Methods.—A total of 27 patients, 2 women and 25 men between the ages of 22 and 70 years, had disabling claudication of the lower limbs. The condition was ascribed to atherosclerosis in 24 of the patients and to nonspecific aortoarteritis in 3. Angiography was conducted through the transaxillary brachial artery route in 12 patients, transfemorally in 11, and by intravenous digital subtraction angiography in 4. All of the balloon dilatations were performed transfemorally, employing the 2-balloon technique in 22 patients and the single-balloon method in 5.

Findings.—Guidewires and balloon catheters successfully crossed the lesions from both femoral arteries in 22 patients and from 1 femoral artery in 5. The single-balloon technique was used in the latter group of patients because of failure to puncture the opposite femoral artery or to cross an eccentric stenosis. Nine of the 10 patients observed for 10–38 months (mean, 22 months) showed no symptoms at the last follow-up visit. The 7 patients who were followed for 3–8 months (mean, 4.4 months) were also symptom free. Six of the 8 males with sexual dysfunction experienced a significant improvement in erectile function after the procedure (Fig 9–4). Emboli occurred in the left common iliac artery in

1 patient and in the left superficial femoral artery in another patient. The first patient refused further intervention despite symptoms. The second patient, with blue-toe syndrome and rapidly progressive ischemia of both legs, required above-the-knee amputations 3 months after angiography. The patient later died of renal failure and bowel ischemia. Bleeding at the puncture site occurred in 2 patients, and 1 patient had infection at this site.

Implications.—Angioplasty has general advantages over surgery, including reduced morbidity, mortality, hospital stay, and cost. One added advantage of balloon angioplasty is the improvement in sexual function in males.

▶ Because percutaneous transluminal angioplasty can be used before occlusion occurs, it is heartening to know that these techniques are applicable to the aorta as well as to the iliac vessels. The expected results are quite good.

Multilevel Occlusive Vascular Disease Presenting With Gangrene
Scher KS, McFall T, Steele FJ (Wright State Univ, Dayton, Ohio)
Am Surg 57:96–100, 1991   9–5

Background.—The presence of multilevel occlusive disease must be identified before beginning treatment for atherosclerotic occlusion. A study determined the incidence of multiple segment occlusive disease in patients who undergo major amputations of the lower extremity and defined the need for distal reconstruction in multilevel occlusion patients who present with tissue loss.

Methods.—Records of all patients who underwent lower-limb amputation during a 3-year period were reviewed. The vascular status of the affected limb was noted, including the presence of multiple-level vascular disease and previous arterial reconstructive surgery. In a follow-up study, 41 consecutive patients with multilevel occlusive disease and tissue loss during the next year were investigated. A total of 18 patients were treated with proximal revascularization or inflow procedures only, and 23 had distal bypass simultaneously or within 3 months of the more proximal reconstruction. The patients were followed up every 3 months for 1 year.

Results.—According to review, neither advanced age nor the presence of multiple medical problems predisposed to higher amputation levels. Diabetes did not increase the likelihood of above-knee (AK) amputations, but diabetic patients were more likely to undergo amputation because of sepsis than nondiabetic patients. The patients who had previous arterial surgery were no more likely to undergo AK amputation; however, despite patent proximal inflow revascularization procedures, limb salvage was achieved in few of these patients. Amputation level could not be predicted by several presumed risk factors. Combined segment (aorto-iliac and femoropopliteal) occlusive disease was more common in patients who had AK amputations than in those who had more distal amputations. In the follow-up study, 56% of the patients in the inflow procedures only group required amputation, compared with 13% of those who underwent distal revascularization.

Conclusions.—Distal bypass should be added to inflow procedures for patients who have tissue loss resulting from multilevel arterial occlusion. Even with profundoplasty, proximal revascularization only is frequently insufficient to salvage the limb. No test or factor on its own can predict which patients need distal bypass grafting.

▶ When ischemic necrosis is present, the pulsatile blood flow should be delivered as distally as possible. Aortofemoral bypass alone should not be expected to provide sufficient revascularization to prevent amputation. On the other hand, proximal and distal reconstruction performed as staged procedures should decrease the need for amputation in patients with multisegment occlusive disease.

Evaluation of Hematoma by MRI in Follow-Up of Aorto-Femoral Bypass
Di Cesare E, Di Renzi P, Pavone P, Marsili L, Ventura M, Spartera C, Passariello R (Univ of L'Aquila, Italy)
Magn Reson Imaging 9:247–253, 1991   9–6

Introduction.—Many reports suggest the use of MRI in differentiating the blood flow from the vascular wall. The presence of periprosthetic hematoma and its complications using MRI were assessed.

Methods.—A total of 20 patients who underwent graft implantations for infrarenal aortic aneurysm (11 patients) and aortoiliac obstructive arteriopathy (9 patients) were evaluated. The 20 individuals (2 women and 18 men) had a mean age of 63.2 years. In the 11 patients who had surgical repair of an aortic aneurysm, the graft was placed end-to-end at the level of the proximal and distal anastomosis; the natural aorta was wrapped around the graft. In the 9 patients who underwent repair of an aortoiliac obstructive arteriopathy, the graft was placed end-to-side for the proximal and distal ends and was positioned ventral to the patient's aorta. The MRI studies were done using a superconductive magnet operating at .5 T. A total of 61 examinations were performed.

Findings.—Of the 20 patients, 18 had minimal to moderate periprosthetic fluid collection at 1 week after surgery. The signal intensity of perigraft collection, as related to the ileopsoas muscle, was medium-low in T1-weighted spin-echo sequences (w.s.) and high in the T2 w.s. in 9 patients with the aneurysmatic condition. In 6 of these 9 patients, small areas of high signal intensity in the T1 w.s. and low signal intensity in T2 w.s. were observed (Fig 9–5). At the 1-month control observation, a slight size reduction and persistent medium-low signal intensity in T1 and high signal intensity in T2 was found. The 3-month postsurgery results in patients with obstructive disease showed a disappearance of the residual areas in 5 and the minimal residual areas in 4. The patient who received end-to-end anastomosis repair experienced a size reduction in residual ar-

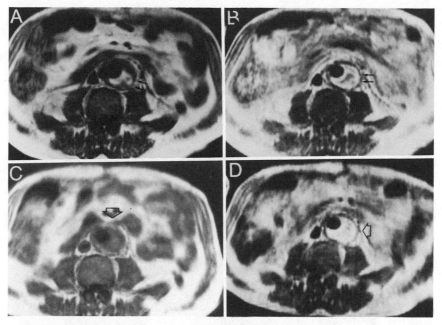

Fig 9–5.—Patient operated for aneurysmatic aortic condition. **A and B,** a large aneurysm around the graft is evident; inside the collection there is an area of high signal intensity in T_1 and T_2 w.s. *(arrows)* related to the presence of metahemoglobin compounds. **C and D,** after 1 month a slight size reduction, a disappearance of paramagnetic effects, and a persistence of medium-low signal intensity in T_1 w.s. and high intensity in T_2 w.s. *(open arrows)* were found. (Courtesy of Di Cesare E, Di Renzi P, Pavone P, et al: *Magn Reson Imaging* 9:247–253, 1991.)

eas; however, they had persistent low signal intensity in T1 w.s. and high signal intensity in T2 w.s.

Conclusion.—These findings indicate that perigraft collection and low signal intensity in both T1 w.s. and T2 w.s. disappear or are greatly reduced 3 months after surgery for aortoiliac stenosis. In patients with an abdominal aortic aneurysm, this progressive reduction did not occur until after 6 months. The high signal intensity of the perigraft collection on T2 w.s. may reflect infection after only 3 or 6 months, depending on the type of surgery. Infection can only be demonstrated by the inflammatory involvement of the surrounding tissues, which is observed through enhancement with gadolinium-diethylenetriaminepentaacetic acid.

▶ Complete healing of perigraft hematomas occurs over a long period of time and may take longer than 6 or more months after surgical intervention.

Left Atrial Myxoma Metastasizing to the Aorta, With Intraluminal Growth Causing Renovascular Hypertension

Kotani K, Matsuzawa Y, Funahashi T, Nozaki S, Tarui S, Matsuda H, Tokunaga K, Kasugai T, Sakurai M (Osaka Univ, Japan)
Cardiology 78:72–77, 1991

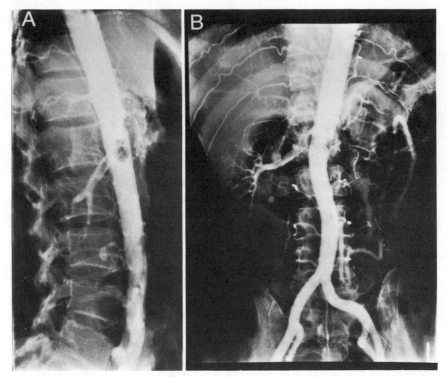

Fig 9–6.—Right lateral (**A**) and anterior (**B**) abdominal aortograms showing a globular filling defect at the takeoff of the renal arteries, with one branch extending into the right renal artery. The distal left renal artery, the celiac axis, and the superior mesenteric artery are occluded. (Courtesy of Kotani K, Matsuzawa Y, Funahashi T, et al: *Cardiology* 78:72–77, 1991.)

Background.—Myxomas, the most common cardiac tumors, have been thought to have a good prognosis after surgery. However, many local recurrences and rare metastases have been reported. A patient was seen in whom systemic metastases from a left atrial myxoma occurred.

Case Report.—Man, 48, had a left atrial tumor removed by local excision. Histological analysis showed the tumor to be a typical benign myxoma arising from the free left atrial wall. Three months after surgery, the patient had multiple subcutaneous nodules on his trunk and extremities that were shown to be myxomas on biopsy. One year later, an intracranial myxoma tumor was found. The patient's right calf became swollen, prohibiting ambulation. At hospitalization the patient's erythrocyte sedimentation rate was 27 mm/hour and the white blood cell count was 7,100/mm^3. Biopsy of his left leg on the seventh hospital day demonstrated a well-encapsulated tumor in the gastrocnemius muscle. Abdominal ultrasonography and CT suggested a tumor in the abdominal aorta, which was verified by aortography (Fig 9–6). Surgical removal revealed a tumor extending from the proximal aorta into the renal arteries. A left atrial tumor was detected and confirmed as a recurrent myxoma 6 months later. The patient underwent cardiotomy, but subacute hepatitis and multiple organ failure occurred and the patient died.

Literature Review.—A total of 10 patients with metastasizing left atrial myxomas have been reported in the medical literature. These few reports show that the metastases occur most often in the brain and frequently in bone and skin. This study is the first to describe a patient with metastasizing myxoma of the aorta. Because each tumor found in this patient extended flat branches to the orifice of the eighth intercostal artery, a fragment of the primary left atrial myxoma may have blocked the opening of the intercostal artery.

Conclusions.—Left atrial myxomas beginning at sites other than the interatrial septum appear more likely to metastasize. The metastasis may grow like a runner of ivy and block the branches of the aorta as it progresses.

▶ This is a curious case that may be a prelude to more curious cases.

Atherosclerotic Occlusive Disease After Radiation for Pelvic Malignancies
Pettersson F, Swedenborg J (Karolinska Hosp, Stockholm)
Acta Chir Scand 156:367–371, 1990   9–8

Introduction.—There have been several reports of radiation-induced atherosclerotic injury of the large arteries. Most of these reports involved radiation injury to the carotid and subclavian arteries; the iliac and femoral arteries were affected infrequently. The incidence of arterial occlusive disease in the iliac arteries or distal aorta was determined in women treated previously by irradiation for pelvic malignancies. In addition, the role of risk factors in the pathogenesis of arterial occlusive complications was assessed.

Study Design.—The patient population consisted of 15 women (aged 38–68 years) who had previously undergone radiation therapy for pelvic malignant disease and who had symptoms of arterial occlusive disease in the pelvic area. Each index patient was paired with 3 age-matched controls who were treated in the same year and who had the same initial diagnosis and stage. The risk factors that were assessed were smoking history and radiation dose. All of the index patients had intermittent claudication as the predominant symptom, and 3 had rest pain. The time of symptom onset varied from less than 1 year to 15 years after radiation therapy. A group of 12 patients underwent revascularization that relieved their symptoms (table).

Results.—The mean radiation dose was 36.3 Gy for the index patients and 25.8 Gy for the controls. The difference was statistically significant. Seven of the 15 index patients, but only 1 of the 45 control patients, had severe radiation reactions that affected other organs in the pelvis. The bladder or the rectosigmoid, or both, were most commonly

Clinical Data of Patients Developing Atherosclerotic Occlusive Disease After Radiation

Case no.	Site of malignant disease	Age at radiation treatment	Onset of arterial symptoms (years after radiation)	Symptoms	Operation
1	Cervix	40	6	Intermittent claudication	Aortobifemoral bypass
2	Cervix	54	6	Intermittent claudication	Left iliofemoral bypass
3	Cervix	49	3	Rest pain ulcers	Aortobifemoral bypass
4	Ovary	52	1	Intermittent claudication	Aortobifemoral bypass
5	Cervix	53	8	Intermittent claudication	Thromboendarterectomy
6	Ovary	63	1	Intermittent claudication	No operation
7	Cervix	56	6	Intermittent claudication	Aortobifemoral bypass
8	Cervix	39	15	Intermittent claudication	No operation
9	Body of uterus and ovary	47	5	Intermittent claudication	Iliofemoral bypass
10	Body of uterus	58	1	Rest pain	Aortoiliac bypass
11	Ovary	43	11	Intermittent claudication	Aortobifemoral bypass
12	Cervix	68	3	Intermittent claudication	No operation
13	Cervix	41	1	Rest pain	Iliofemoral bypass
14	Cervix	48	12	Intermittent claudication	Aortobifemoral bypass
15	Cervix	38	10	Intermittent claudication	Left iliofemoral bypass

(Courtesy of Pettersson F, Swedenborg J: *Acta Chir Scand* 156:367–371, 1990.)

affected. Smoking history data were available for all index patients and for 38 of the 45 controls. All 15 index patients smoked more than 10 cigarettes a day, whereas 18 of the (47%) controls were nonsmokers, 3 were ex-smokers, and 4 smoked fewer than 10 cigarettes a day. The remaining 13 controls smoked more than 10 cigarettes a day. One control who smoked more than 20 cigarettes a day also had a severe radiation reaction with a rectovaginal fistula.

Conclusion.—Atherosclerotic occlusive disease of the aorta or iliac arteries, or both, can occur as a late complication of irradiation for pelvic malignancy. Smoking appears to increase the risk. Radiation injury to other organs is more common in patients who have arterial disease after irradiation.

▶ A particular pattern of occlusive disease occurs after pelvic radiation. This pattern is more distal than the pattern that is usually associated with atherosclerotic aortoiliac disease, and Treatment is complicated by the intraperitoneal adhesions and retroperitoneal fibrosis. The principles of proximal inflow and the ensurance of distal outflow aid in planning effective reconstructions.

Femoro-Femoral or Ilio-Femoral Bypass for Unilateral Inflow Reconstruction?

Perler BA, Burdick JF, Williams GM (The Johns Hopkins Med Insts)
Am J Surg 161:426–430, 1991   9–9

Introduction.—The aortofemoral graft has been the optimal technique for bilateral inflow reconstruction during the past 2 decades. Femorofemoral and iliofemoral bypass are the 2 popular choices for unilateral inflow reconstruction. A comparison of these 2 techniques assessed their relative advantages and disadvantages.

Patients.—The records of 70 consecutive patients who underwent either femorofemoral or iliofemoral grafts for unilateral inflow reconstruction were analyzed. A total of 50 femorofemoral grafts were performed in 49 patients, whereas 22 iliofemoral grafts were done in 21 patients. Of the procedures, 92% were done for occlusive disease and 8% for aneurysmal conditions. The 70 patients included 24 women and 46 men with a mean age of 66 years. The femorofemoral grafts were performed through longitudinal groin incisions with the patient supine; the iliofemoral grafts were done through longitudinal groin and transverse lower quadrant retroperitoneal incisions with the patient supine and the operated side elevated 30°.

Outcome.—Hospital operative mortality was 10% for the femorofemoral grafts and 9% for the iliofemoral grafts. This reflects the increased risk inherent in performing these surgeries simultaneously with other procedures or as an emergency (3 of 6 patients died in the hospital after emergency femorofemoral grafts). No deaths occurred among the 30 femorofemoral grafts, and 1 death (6%) occurred among the 17 iliofemoral grafts that were performed as elective, solitary operations. The mean operative duration, blood loss, fluid and blood transfusions, time to oral

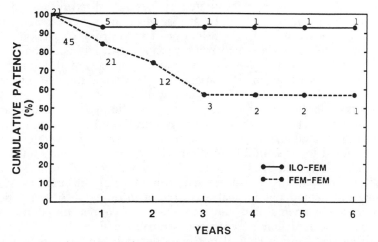

Fig 9–7.—Cumulative patency for all femorofemoral *(FEM-FEM) and iliofemoral (ILO-FEM)* grafts. (Courtesy of Perler BA, Burdick JF, Williams GM: *Am J Surg* 161:426–430, 1991.)

diet, and postoperative course duration were similar for both types of procedures. At 30 days after surgery, 96% of the iliofemoral grafts and 86% of the femorofemoral grafts were patent. At 3 and 5 years, primary patency was 93% for the iliofemoral procedure and 57% for the femorofemoral operation (Fig 9–7). Among the femorofemoral reconstructions, better overall patency occurred in grafts with Dacron than occurred in those with polytetrafluoroethylene.

Conclusion.—These findings suggest that, although the femorofemoral operation has been the popular choice for unilateral inflow reconstruction in many institutions, the iliofemoral bypass should be used more often, particularly because of the longer-lasting patency it confers on the graft.

▶ Unilateral iliofemoral reconstruction was abandoned in the 1960s, yet it has continued to be performed occasionally in all vascular centers. The disadvantages of unilateral reconstruction include progression of occlusive disease in the contralateral arterial tree. The retroperitoneal approach minimizes morbidity in the unilateral procedure. Therefore, it has its own indications that are separate from those for femorofemoral or aortofemoral reconstruction.

Donor Limb Vascular Events Following Femoro-Femoral Bypass Surgery
Veterans Affairs Cooperative Study
Arch Surg 126:681–686, 1991   9–10

Background.—There have been few studies of the early and late changes in the donor leg in patients who undergo femorofemoral bypass surgery for unilateral iliac arterial disease. The patency of various types of vein grafts was compared. Postoperative vascular changes were examined in the donor limbs of 317 femorofemoral bypass surgery patients.

Methods.—Patients were evaluated by a standardized history of claudication, rest pain, or necrosis (Fig 9–8). Mean age was 62 years. Diabetes was diagnosed in 19%, 31% had prior myocardial infarctions, 18% had prior stroke, and 4% had prior vascular procedures. Tobacco was used by 98%. Percutaneous transluminal angioplasty of the donor iliac vessel had been done in 45 patients. The average follow-up was 38 months, and 35% of patients were followed for more than 4 years.

Results.—Seven percent of the patients had "unmasked" claudication. There was new claudication related to a "steal" in 3.5%, progression of preoperative claudication in 1%, and new rest pain in 1.7%. New necrosis was noted in .7%. In 3% of the patients, the donor limb ankle-brachial index decreased by .3 or more. This index decreased from .15 to .29 in 6% of the patients and decreased from .1 to .14 in another 6%. A clinical and hemodynamic steal was present in only 3% of the patients. Only a few patients had late vascular procedures for donor iliac stenosis—3% had iliac percutaneous transluminal angioplasty and inflow bypasses. Neither clinical nor hemodynamic steal events were predicted by angiography. In most cases, the symptoms of claudication in

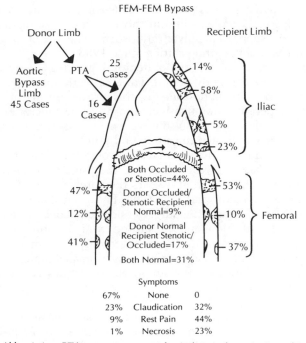

FEM-FEM Bypass

Symptoms

67%	None	0
23%	Claudication	32%
9%	Rest Pain	44%
1%	Necrosis	23%

Fig 9–8.—*Abbreviation: PTA,* percutaneous transluminal angioplasty. Angiographic profile in 317 patients having a femorofemoral (FEM-FEM) bypass, (Courtesy of Veterans Affairs Cooperative Study: *Arch Surg* 126:681–686, 1991.)

the donor limb represented previous arterial insufficiency that had become apparent on improvement of the recipient limb.

Conclusions.—In femorofemoral bypass surgery patients, both early and late morbidity in the donor limb are rare, suggesting that steal phenomenon and progressive donor iliac occlusive disease are rare. Both limbs must be watched postoperatively to assess these changes when they occur. The use of femorofemoral vascular reconstruction for patients with minimal donor iliac occlusive disease should be continued.

▶ This large Veteran's Administration study shows few deleterious effects on the donor limb when femorofemoral reconstructions are used.

Clinical Results of Axillobifemoral Bypass Using Externally Supported Polytetrafluoroethylene
Harris EJ Jr, Taylor LM Jr, McConnell DB, Moneta GL, Yeager RA, Porter JM
(Portland VA Hosp, Portland, Ore; Oregon Health Sciences Univ)
J Vasc Surg 12:416–421, 1990   9–11

Background.—Axillobifemoral grafting has been used selectively in those patients with clear contraindications to aortobifemoral bypass grafting. Low patency rates were noted when axillobifemoral grafting was used in high-risk patients and in those with coexisting systemic disease. Externally supported polytetrafluoroethylene (xPTFE) grafts have been used for axillobifemoral grafting since 1983.

Methods.—A total of 76 axillobifemoral graftings were done with xPTFE during a 6-year study period. Patients were not chosen, but they included the entire population having this procedure at the designated hospitals. Postoperative, noninvasive, laboratory peripheral arterial measurements and evaluations of pulse were used to assess patency. Any loss of primary patency indicated the study end point.

Results.—Operative indications were absolute in 26% of the patients and relative in 74%. At 1-year follow-up, the primary patency was 93% for the axillobifemoral grafts; at 4 years the patency was 85%. The limb salvage rate was 92% at 4-year follow-up. Five graft failures occurred between 2 weeks and 3 years after surgery and included 2 caused by thrombosis, 1 caused by infection, and 2 resulting from anastomotic disruption.

Conclusions.—Treatment of lower extremity ischemia with axillobifemoral grafting with xPTFE was successful in this patient population. It is not known if the externally supported prosthesis is needed to support improved patency.

▶ Although this is an optimistic report and may indeed herald the greater use of reinforced grafts for axillofemoral reconstruction, it should be noted that mean follow-up extended to slightly more than 2 years and that 52 of the grafts were done in the 2 years immediately preceding the study. Time will tell whether this is a real or illusory advance.

10 Femorodistal Occlusions

The Value of Digital Subtraction Angiography in the Investigation of Severe Chronic Ischaemia of the Lower Limbs
Bartoli JM, Kuredjian S, Espinoza H, Ternier F, Di Stefano-Louineau D, Branchereau A, Kasbarian M (CHU Timone, Marseilles, France)
Ann Radiol 33:250–254, 1990   10–1

Introduction.—Severe chronic ischemia of the lower limbs requires amputation after less than 1 month when left untreated. Clinical evidence of gangrene with locally severe ischemia should always be investigated angiographically. A maximal arterial ankle pressure of less than 50 mm Hg with the patient at rest is a good criterion of severe ischemia. There has been much progress in the area of limb salvage surgery during the past few years; however, the planning of limb-saving bypass requires excellent preoperative documentation of the vascular tree. The vascular imaging quality of conventional angiography was compared with digital subtraction angiography (DSA).

Patients.—A group of 11 men and 12 women (median age, 71 years) with severe, chronic ischemia in 24 limbs was studied. One patient had bilateral involvement. The patients had conventional angiography under local anesthesia with a 6-French catheter inserted via a femoral or axillary artery, followed by DSA after a median interval of 11 days. The patients were placed in identical positions for both examinations. Only 2 limbs were amputated; 22 limbs were revascularized. A total of 2 bypass operations failed after 30 days to 4 months; both limbs were then amputated.

Results.—Comparison of the 2 imaging techniques revealed that all arterial segments seen on conventional angiography were also visualized by DSA. In 14 cases, the therapeutic approach was changed after looking at the DSA films. In 4 cases, the surgical approach was changed and in 10 cases, the decision to amputate after conventional angiography was changed to distal bypass after looking at the DSA films (Fig 10–1). In 6 cases, the therapeutic indications remained the same; however, the prognosis was upgraded after DSA showed an intact distal collateral vasculature that was not seen during conventional angiography. Both the therapeutic approach and the surgical prognosis were identical for conventional angiography and DSA in 4 cases.

Conclusions.—The use of DSA under local anesthesia is less traumatic and requires fewer films and less contrast medium than conventional an-

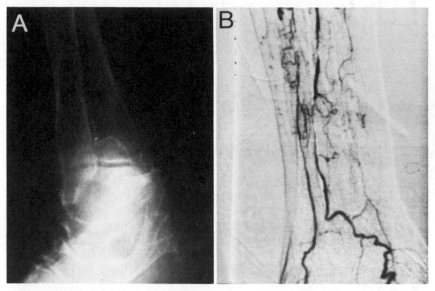

Fig 10–1.—Surgical indication: correlation between conventional angiography and digital subtraction angiography in the right lower limb of a woman, 89, who was diabetic. **A**, conventional angiography: amputation. **B**, digital subtraction angiography: satisfactory distal anterior tibial and peroneal arteries, therefore indication for right femorodorsalis pedis bypass graft. (Courtesy of Bartoli JM, Kuredjian S, Espinoza H, et al: *Ann Radiol* 33:250–254, 1990.)

giography. The results of this study clearly demonstrate the superiority of DSA to conventional angiography.

▶ This very experienced French group has emphasized the need for excellent arteriography when planning operations for correction of severe chronic ischemia. Similar studies have been done in this country. Clear arteriographic studies have used 4-second external iliac artery injections with volumes as low as 60 mL and have taken step films of the distal circulation after a 12-second delay.

Deterioration Following Delay in Performing Femoral Angioplasty
Spencer JA, Fletcher EWL (John Radcliffe Hosp, Oxford, England)
Brit J Radiol 63:919–921, 1990   10–2

Background and Methods.—Arteriographic deterioration may occur after diagnostic lower limb arteriography if there is a delay between assessment and attempted angioplasty. The frequency of early deterioration and its relationship to the site of arterial puncture and other variables were studied retrospectively. In 61 patients with peripheral vascular disease there was a wait of more than 24 hours after assessment before superficial femoral artery (SFA) angioplasty was attempted. The appearance of the SFA at initial arteriography was compared with the direct preangioplasty femoral arteriogram. These pairs were scored as no difference, or as a worsening of SFA appearance to the extent that angioplasty was difficult or impossible. The patients were classified according to whether initial arteriogram puncture was ipsilateral or contralateral to the angioplasty site.

Results.—Of the 61 patients, 6 had arteriographic deterioration. In 3 patients, the deterioration precluded angioplasty. In 33 patients the assessment arteriogram was ipsilateral to the SFA angioplasty site, and in 28 patients, it was contralateral. Four of the 6 patients who had deterioration had initial ipsilateral studies, but this finding was not statistically significant. In 5 of the 6 patients, there were no immediate complications to account for the findings. No features on assessment arteriograms suggested more severe lesions in the deteriorated group than in the group who did not have deterioration, and there were no differences in age or other specific risk factors, such as diabetes mellitus. There was a mean delay of 14.6 days between the arteriogram and the angioplasty attempt.

Conclusions.—Almost 10% of the patients had early and significant arteriographic deterioration after assessment. Although this series did not identify the exact cause of deterioration, surgeons should schedule angioplasty with a minimum of delay to prevent such deterioration.

▶ The reasons for the deterioration of distal outflow after arteriography are numerous. Among these reasons are procedure-associated acute thromboses secondary to hyperactive platelets. The recognition of contralateral and/or remote thrombotic events after any form of arteriography is important to the practice of vascular surgery.

Femoral-Distal Bypass With In Situ Greater Saphenous Vein: Long-Term Results Using the Mills Valvulotome
Donaldson MC, Mannick JA, Whittemore AD (Harvard Med School; Brigham and Women's Hosp, Boston)
Ann Surg 213:457–465, 1991   10–3

Introduction.—The autologous greater saphenous vein is widely used as a conduit for revascularization below the inguinal ligament. The saphenous vein was originally used in reversed fashion, but refinement of the valvulotome and of small-vessel surgical techniques has led to the widespread use of the in situ greater saphenous vein for infrainguinal arterial reconstruction. A large experience with in situ saphenous vein bypass was performed at a single institution.

Methods.—During a 7-year study period, 371 patients underwent 440 in situ greater saphenous vein bypass operations in the treatment of atherosclerotic occlusive disease. Saphenous vein bypass was the primary reconstruction in 406 (92%) procedures, and a previous infrainguinal revascularization had been performed in the remaining 34 cases. A modified Mills valvulotome was used for all operations. In all of the procedures, the proximal anastomosis was at the groin level. An infrapopliteal artery was the site of distal anastomosis in 200 (45%) procedures. The indications for arterial bypass were critical ischemia in 299 limbs and disabling claudication in 141 limbs.

Results.—Surgical complications occurred in 104 patients (24%), 33 of whom had major cardiopulmonary, renal, or cerebrovascular complications. Technical problems attributable to the in situ method occurred in 5 of 27 early occlusions. Nine of the patients (2%) died within the first 30 days of operation. The mean postoperative follow-up was 20.4 months. Of the 440 grafts, 352 (80%) were followed to known end points. Graft surveillance identified 18 stenotic grafts (4.1%) that were revised while patent, but that required a total of 30 revisions to maintain patency during follow-up. Of the grafts, 68 (15%) occluded during follow-up; 36 of these underwent initial disobliteration and required a total of 52 revisions during follow-up. A 5-year life-table analysis showed an overall primary patency rate of 72%, primary revised patency of 78%, secondary patency of 83%, limb salvage of 88%, and patient survival of 66%.

Conclusion.—In contrast to reversed vein grafts, long infrapopliteal in situ grafts have long-term secondary patency similar to that of shorter femoropopliteal bypass grafts. Therefore, in situ greater saphenous vein grafting is the procedure of choice for long infrapopliteal bypass.

▶ In the discussion after the presentation of this paper to the Southern Surgical Association meeting, the first author emphasized that femorodistal bypass is a "game of palliation." In addition, emphasis was placed on the hypercoagulable state that affects results adversely during the first 30 days after surgery. This may be linked to the hypercoagulability discussed in Abstract 10–2, which dealt with deterioration of the distal tree after arteriography. Searching for the cause of the hypercoagulability becomes very important in the postoperative period if graft thrombosis occurs. A 6-point screening profile, including lupus anticoagulant and anticardiolipin antibody, should be a part of such surveillance.

Femoro-Popliteal and Femoro-Distal Bypass: A Comparison Between In Situ and Reversed Technique
Bergmark C, Johansson G, Olofsson P, Swedenborg J (Karolinska Hosp, Stockholm)
J Cardiovasc Surg 32:117–1290, 1991   10–4

Background.—Conventionally, the excised autogenous saphenous vein is reversed before being placed as a femoropopliteal bypass reconstruction. An alternative is to leave the vein in its bed if the valves have been disrupted somehow. New instruments for valve ablation have revived the in situ approach that is presently the preferred method for below-knee bypass at many centers.

Study Design.—A group of 40 patients had bypass surgery using the in situ technique, and they were compared with an equal number of patients who underwent reversed bein grafts below the knee in previous years.

The 2 groups were similar in concomitant cardiovascular and pulmonary disorders. The preoperative ankle-brachial indices were .26 in the in situ group and .32 in the reversed vein group.

Results.—The 6-month patency rates were 84% in the patients given in situ bypasses and 49% in those who had reversed vein bypass surgery. The difference was especially marked for patients with the distal anastomosis at the infrapopliteal level. Four patients in the in situ group and 8 in the reversed vein group required re-operation for thrombosis within 30 days. Limb salvage was 75% in both groups at 6 months. Of the 10 patients in the in situ group who had amputation, 6 had patent grafts; none of the amputees in the reversed vein group had patent grafts.

Conclusion.—In situ saphenous vein grafting has yielded better results than reversed vein grafting, at least in infrapopliteal reconstructive operations.

▶ Students of vascular surgery will recognize that this study reflects one side of the continuing controversy about types of distal reconstruction. If 2 sides of an argument are espoused vigorously in medical science, then both sides are probably right.

Comparison of In-Situ and Reversed Saphenous Vein Grafts for Infrageniculate Bypass
Ricci MA, Graham AM, Symes JF (Royal Victoria Hosp Montreal; McGill Univ)
Can J Surg 33:216–220, 1990   10–5

Objective.—There is still controversy on the superiority of in situ bypass over the reversed vein technique for infrainguinal reconstruction in the ischemic limb. To investigate further, the records of 161 patients who had infrageniculate bypass with autogenous saphenous vein grafts between 1982 and 1987 were reviewed retrospectively.

Procedures.—Of the 92 in situ bypasses, 42 were to the popliteal artery below the knee, and 50 were to the tibial vessels. Of the 69 reversed vein grafts, 51 were performed on the popliteal artery below the knee, and 18 were performed on the tibial vessels. Sixty-seven in situ and 43 reversed grafts were performed for foot salvage. The patients were classified based on the objective criteria of the Society for Vascular Surgery/ International Society for Cardiovascular Surgery (SVS/ISCVS) Committee on Reporting Standards.

Results.—Patency rates did not differ significantly overall between the in situ and reversed saphenous vein bypasses. Patency rates for in situ grafts were 81.1% at 30 days, 77% at 1 year, and 59.8% at 5 years, with corresponding rates of 85.2%, 76.8%, and 42.3% for reversed vein grafts. The secondary patency rates did not differ significantly between procedures; they were 72.8% at 3 years for in situ and 67.2% for reversed vein bypasses. Although the trend favored in situ bypass at the tibial level as well as in terms of the SVS/ISCVS classification, the difference between procedures was not significant. The foot salvage rates at 3 years were 91% for in situ bypass and 78.9% for reversed vein.

Conclusion.—No significant differences were found in the primary, secondary, and limb-salvage rates between in situ and reversed saphenous vein bypasses, regardless of the distal anastomotic site or the severity of disease. Further studies with longer follow-up and perhaps a randomized evaluation are needed.

▶ As has been summarized eloquently and succinctly in the past, "vein is vein."

Semi-Closed, Ex-Situ, Non-Reversed or Reversed Autogenous Vein Grafting: A Technique for Femoro-Distal Arterial Bypass

Myers KA (Prince Henry's Hosp, Melbourne)
J Cardiovasc Surg 32:110–116, 1991   10–6

Introduction.—The best method of femorodistal vein bypass grafting may be that which assures good long-term results but takes relatively little time and causes the least possible trauma.

Technique.—Arteries are chosen by digital subtraction arteriography and duplex scanning. A spinal anesthetic block is best if the long saphenous vein is used. After this vein is divided, it is removed retrograde using a semi-closed method. A Mayo stripper is then passed to consecutive tributaries until sufficient length is gained; 4 to 6 small incisions are usually required. If 2 divisions of the vein below the knee are used for a double bypass, the distal end of each is exposed and stripped antegrade to its junction. The vein is not reversed if it tapers more than 1 mm and if its distal end is less than 4 mm in diameter. The valves are broken down using the Hall stripper. The distal anastomosis is done first, creating a deep tunnel that passes between the gastrocnemius heads. The proximal anastomosis is then made and followed by completion arteriography.

Results.—A total of 33 patients received 35 grafts, including 30 initial femorodistal bypasses of the ipsilateral long saphenous vein. Two primary occlusions occurred, and 4 later occlusions occurred by 6 months. All of the late occlusions were in patients with critical ischemia.

Conclusion.—This semi-closed, ex situ vein bypass technique appears to be as effective as conventional methods, and it causes less trauma to the patient.

▶ This third technique for the utilization of vein and distal reconstruction comes from the service of a very distinguished vascular surgeon who performed fundamental studies on vascular physiology and the effects of vascular interventions 30 years ago at St. Mary's Hospital in London.

Results of Vein Graft Reconstruction of the Lower Extremity in Diabetic and Nondiabetic Patients

Rosenblatt MS, Quist WC, Sidawy AN, Paniszyn CC, LoGerfo FW (New England Deaconess Hosp, Boston; Harvard Med School; VA Hosp, Washington, DC; George Washington Univ; VA Med Ctr, Providence, RI; et al)
Surg Gynecol Obstet 171:331–335, 1990   10–7

Objective.—Distal arterial reconstructions to the tibial, peroneal, and pedal arteries are becoming increasingly successful in patients with advanced distal occlusive disease. The influence of diabetes mellitus on the patency of vein grafts and on the salvage of the extremities was evaluated in 171 patients, including 89 with diabetes mellitus and 82 nondiabetics. All of the patients underwent vein graft reconstruction of the lower extremity. Patency was evaluated by using a life-table analysis.

Data Analysis.—The indications for operation included claudication in 21 patients; rest pain, ulceration or gangrene in 141; and aneurysm or trauma in 9. Significantly more diabetic patients had bypass grafting for extremity-threatening ischemia, whereas more nondiabetics underwent bypass grafting for claudication. Also, significantly more bypasses to the tibial, peroneal, and pedal arteries were necessary in diabetics, whereas more femoropopliteal grafts were performed in nondiabetics. Minor amputations, such as digital and transmetatarsal, were more common in the diabetic group, whereas major amputations were more frequent in nondiabetics. For all indications, 1-year and 4-year patency rates for patients with diabetes were 95% and 89%, respectively; for nondiabetics, the rates were 85% and 80%, respectively. The difference was not significant

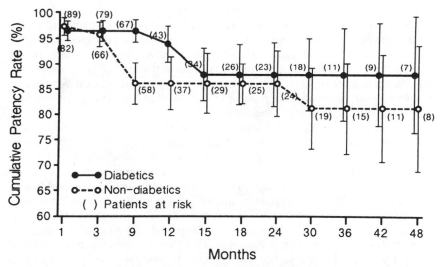

Fig 10–2.—The cumulative primary patency rate of vein grafts placed in diabetic and nondiabetic patients for all indications: claudication, salvage of extremity, aneurysm, and trauma (*P* indicates not significant). (Courtesy of Rosenblatt MS, Quist WC, Sidawy AN, et al: *Surg Gynecol Obstet* 171:331–335, 1990.)

(Fig 10–2). Among the patients who underwent bypass for extremity-threatening ischemia, the difference in patency rate approached statistical significance at 1 year, favoring the diabetic group (94% versus 79%).

Conclusion.—Arterial reconstruction of the lower extremity can be performed in patients with diabetes with the same high success rate as in the nondiabetic patient. When gangrene is managed by minor amputation, the patient with diabetes may be at an advantage for arterial reconstruction in the presence of extremity-threatening ischemia.

▶ The diabetic patient presents a paradoxical situation. Internists consider diabetes an end artery disease as seen in the glomulerus or retina. The conventional 1-segment occlusion, seen frequently in the proximal femoropopliteal artery, is often accompanied by gangrene caused by trauma or thermal injury to the toes. Such situations are eminently satisfactory for revascularization and contribute to the favorable 1-year results of vascular reconstruction seen in diabetes. Unfortunately, there is also a population of diabetics with multilevel distal occlusive disease in which severe ischemia is caused by multiple segmental occlusions. In this particular cohort, reconstructions are difficult and the results of surgery are not as favorable hemodynamically as they are in the former group.

The "All-Autogenous" Tissue Policy for Infrainguinal Reconstruction Questioned

Killewich LA, Bartlett ST (Univ of California, Davis)
Am J Surg 160:552–555, 1990   10–8

Background.—An "all-autogenous" policy has been proposed for infrainguinal reconstruction. Proponents of this policy suggest that the lesser saphenous vein, arm vein, endarterectomy, profundaplasty, or patch angioplasty can be used when the greater saphenous vein is unavailable. They contend that polytetrafluoroethylene (PTFE) grafts are significantly inferior and should be used only as a last resort. A series of patients who received either autogenous or PTFE grafting for infrainguinal reconstruction was investigated.

Methods.—A group of 84 patients underwent 92 infrainguinal vascular reconstructions. The patients ranged in age from 36 to 91 years; mean age was 56 years. Fifty-nine patients received translocated, nonreversed in situ saphenous vein; 3 received reverse saphenous vein; and 30 received PTFE grafts. The mean preoperative ankle-arm index (AAI) was .26. Intra-operative prebypass contrast arteriography was necessary to identify a graftable pedal or tibial artery in 40% of the cases. The results of autogenous and PTFE bypass were compared at 1 year and 3 years.

Results.—Patency after 1 year was 85% for autogenous bypasses and 67% for PTFE bypasses. For autogenous bypass, the limb salvage was 90% compared with 70% for PTFE bypass. At 3 years, the cumulative patency rates were 80% for autogenous grafts and 57% for PTFE grafts. Both AAI and duplex scanning were useful in detecting failing grafts. Secondary procedures were often required to maintain patency, regardless of the graft material used. A total of 9 patients required a reversed vein jump, and 3 required thrombectomy.

Conclusions.—In patients with combined superficial femoral and severe infrapopliteal occlusive disease, the PTFE bypass is an excellent alternative when suitable autogenous reconstruction is impossible. Long-term aspirin and warfarin therapy may contribute to a favorable prognosis. Regardless of the graft material used, most failures will occur during the first year.

▶ It should be noted that PTFE is an alternative in infrainguinal revascularization. However, even if patients are treated with anticoagulation and antiplatelet agents, the long-term patency is not favorable. Surgeons must be flexible in their approach to distal reconstructions. In addition, they must always remember that the autogenous vein (from whatever source) is the favored conduit and that prosthetic material is distinctly inferior.

A Flexible Approach to Infrapopliteal Vein Grafts in Patients With Diabetes Mellitus
Pomposelli FB Jr, Jepsen SJ, Gibbons GW, Campbell DR, Freeman DV, Gaughan BM, Miller A, LoGerfo FW (Harvard Med School)
Arch Surg 126:724–729, 1991   10–9

Background.—The pattern of infrapopliteal artery occlusion with sparing of the foot vessels is commonly seen in diabetic patients with ischemic foot lesions, and it requires bypass grafts to the distal tibial or pedal arteries. There is no consensus as to the best technique for handling the vein.

Methods.—In a period of nearly 4 years, 156 dorsalis pedis artery bypasses were performed in 146 patients, all for the purpose of limb salvage. There were 96 men and 50 women (mean age, 65.6 years); 95% had diabetes mellitus. For the purposes of shortening surgery, limiting the length of incisions, and obtaining the best possible size match between the vein grafts and the arteries, a variety of surgical techniques was used. The arterial inflow was from the common femoral artery in 58 cases and from the distal superficial femoral or popliteal artery in 88. The inflow was from a tibial artery in 3 cases and from a preexisting bypass in 7. The bypasses used were in situ in 75 cases, ex situ reversed or nonreversed vein in 62, composite vein in 9, and polytetrafluoroethylene in 1.

Results.—Four patients (2.7%) died within 30 days of surgery. During the same period, 4.5% of the grafts failed. At postoperative follow-up of 6–52 months, the actuarial patency was 87.1% and the limb salvage was 9.6%. For the in situ vein grafts, the patency was 93.2%. This was not significantly different from the 89.7% rate in ex situ vein grafts (Fig 10–3). Neither was there any difference in patency when the inflow site was the common femoral artery or the distal superficial femoral or popliteal artery; the rates were 89.3% and 88%, respectively.

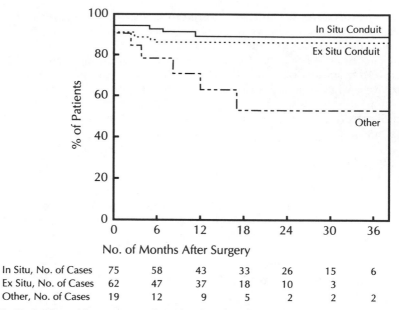

Fig 10–3.—Actuarial patency rates of 156 dorsalis pedis artery bypass grafts according to the type of conduit used. *Ex situ* includes reversed and nonreversed translocation vein grafts. *Other* includes arm vein grafts, composite vein grafts, and 1 polytetrafluoroethylene graft. (Courtesy of Pomposelli FB Jr, Jepsen SJ, Gibbons GW, et al: *Arch Surg* 126:724–729, 1991.)

Conclusions.—In performing infrapopliteal vein grafts, all of the available techniques can provide excellent results when the choice of technique is based on practical issues. The surgeon should be comfortable with all of the techniques and should follow a flexible approach toward devising the best procedure for the individual patient.

▶ Flexibility is the key to success in distal reconstruction operations, many of which are most difficult and extremely demanding.

Mechanism of Long-Term Degeneration of Arterialized Vein Grafts
Kohler TR, Kirkman TR, Gordon D, Clowes AW (Univ of Washington)
Am J Surg 160:257–261, 1990   10–10

Purpose.—Increasing constriction caused by atherosclerotic changes such as deposition of lipids and calcium, ulceration, and calcification results in the failure of more than 30% of femoropopliteal and aortocoronary saphenous vein grafts within 5 years of surgery. Increased production of smooth muscle, endothelial cells, and matrix thicken the intima, but these dynamic processes are essentially complete during the first 24 weeks. The evolution of atherosclerotic changes in vein grafts at 1 year was studied.

Methods.—A segment of the external jugular vein was interposed end-to-end in the common carotid artery in 6 anesthetized adult rabbits. After

1 year, the rabbits were anesthetized and injected intravenously with tritiated thymidine (to label dividing cells) and Evans blue dye. They were then killed by exsanguination by perfusion after a 1-hour radioisotope incorporation period. The graft samples were processed for standard histology and morphometry, autoradiography, and transmission electromicroscopy (TEM).

Results.—Although all of the grafts were appropriately thickened and cellular at 1 year, the abdominal staining of large areas of the graft surface by Evans blue indicated a breakdown of permeability barriers. No endothelial breakdown was evident in the TEM studies. A total of 3 grafts showed substantial deposition of subendothelial fibrin that was often associated with foam cells and signs of prior hemorrhage, but thymidine incorporation indicated that none of these changes altered the reproductively quiescent state of the smooth muscle cells.

Conclusions.—Intimal hyperplasia is responsible for the stenosis of vein grafts in the first year and the adaptive, necessary strengthening of the graft wall; subsequently, atherosclerotic changes occlude the graft without compensating benefits. The latter changes are more common in vein grafts into arterial circulation. The penetration of red blood cells and protein into the intima may result from increased tension on the graft wall or from flow separation peculiar to this particular experimental model. The loss of intimal integrity after 1 year may resemble the late course of progression of atherosclerosis in human vein grafts.

▶ In commenting on this study, the editor of the *American Journal of Surgery* said, "This work is exciting because of its possible broader bearing upon the fundamental cause of arteriosclerosis."

Use of Terminal T-Junctions for In Situ Bypass in the Lower Extremity
Sharp WJ, Shamma AR, Kresowik TF, Corson JD (Univ of Iowa Hosps and Clinics)
Surg Gynecol Obstet 172:151–152, 1991   10–11

Background.—In situ bypass using the saphenous vein has become a popular method for revascularization of a lower extremity. However, during construction of the distal anastomosis a kink or a buckle may occur at the heel of the anastomosis, particularly when the distal anastomosis is sewn into a popliteal segment at an abrupt angle below the knee (Fig 10–4). A new technique was devised to eliminate this problem.

Technique.—A branch point located strategically along the in situ vein was used in the anastomosis. The branch point was incised along its concavity, opening this as an in situ vein T-junction. This T-junction was then oriented in a heel-to-toe manner and sewn routinely to the outflow vessel.

Conclusion.—The use of terminal T-junctions allows the distal anastomosis of the arterialized in situ vein to be performed without kinking or buckling. It is particularly useful when the distal portion of the mobilized

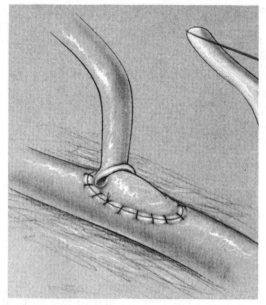

Fig 10–4.—Kink or buckle opposite the heel of the anastomosis. (Courtesy of Sharp WJ, Shamma AR, Kresowik TF, et al: *Surg Gynecol Obstet* 172:151–152, 1991.)

segment of an in situ vein is placed in a deeply located infragenicular popliteal segment.

▶ Although this technique has been in common use for more than 25 years, its reemphasis at this time—with the excellent illustration provided—may allow a wider application.

Lower Extremity Revascularization via the Lateral Plantar Artery
Friedman SG, Krishnasastry KV, Doscher W, Deckoff SL (North Shore Univ Hosp; Cornell Med College, Booth Memorial Med Ctr, Flushing, NY; Long Island Jewish Med Ctr, New Hyde Park, NY)
Am Surg 56:721–725, 1990   10–12

Background.—The use of a lateral plantar artery (LPA) for lower extremity revascularization in patients with atherosclerotic limb-threatening ischemia was first reported in 1970. However, the outcome with these grafts has not been well reported. Six patients underwent femoral artery to LPA bypass for gangrene of the forefoot.

Patients.—During a 19-month period, 6 insulin-dependent diabetics (age, 48–83 years) underwent arterial bypass of the LPA. Of the 6 patients, 4 did not have a suitable vessel for bypass on the preoperative angiogram. The posterior tibial artery was explored, and an acceptable LPA was chosen for reconstruction. A completely autogenous reconstruction was possible in 5 patients. An in situ vein bypass was used in 4 of these patients. The sixth patient had undergone 2 previous unsuccessful femoral-popliteal bypasses. A composite graft consisting of polytetrafluoroethylene and in situ vein was used in this patient.

Results.—The patient who received the composite graft had early graft failure on the first postoperative day. Visual inspection of the distal anastomosis and repeated completion angiography revealed no explanation for the failure. The patient subsequently underwent a below-knee amputation. After a follow-up period ranging from 3 to 22 months, all 5 completely autogenous reconstructions remained patent.

Conclusion.—The LPA is an acceptable site for anastomosis of lower extremity bypass grafts.

▶ Femorodistal revascularizations have proceeded in a more distal direction with increasing success. This particular approach is eminently suitable for the diabetic patient with multiple levels of proximal occlusion. The exact technique is illustrated by Andros (1).

Reference

1. Andros G: *Techniques in Arterial Surgery*, Bergan JJ, Yao JST (eds). Philadelphia, WB Saunders Co, 1990, pp 157–168.

Microvascular Pedal Bypass for Salvage of the Severely Ischemic Limb
Gloviczki P, Morris SM, Bower TC, Toomey BJ, Naessens JM, Stanson AW
(Mayo Clinic and Found)
Mayo Clin Proc 66:243–253, 1991   10–13

Background.—Several investigators have reported success with bypass procedures to pedal arteries. Microvascular revascularization to the arteries of the foot was performed in 37 patients with critical, chronic ischemia. The effectiveness of the procedure for salvage of the foot (specifically whether it relieved pain, healed ulcers or gangrenous areas, and restored function of the limb) was assessed.

Methods.—The 37 patients who underwent saphenous vein grafting to the inframalleolar arteries (Fig 10–5) included 21 men and 16 women with a mean age of 69.1 years. Three or more cardiovascular risk factors were present in 57% of patients, and 59% had diabetes. Arteriography showed a suitable pedal artery for use in bypass in all but 1 patient. The greater or lesser saphenous vein was used in all cases. A nonreversed, translocated vein graft was usually done (Fig 10–6). One patient required the use of an arm vein as part of a composite graft. Mean follow-up was 12.3 months.

Results.—There were no perioperative deaths, although there was 1 perioperative myocardial infarction. Graft occlusion occurred within 30 days in 5 cases, 4 of which were revised successfully. In 36 patients, the graft was patent at discharge from the hospital. The primary graft patency rate was 60.8% and the secondary patency rate was 68.8% at 1

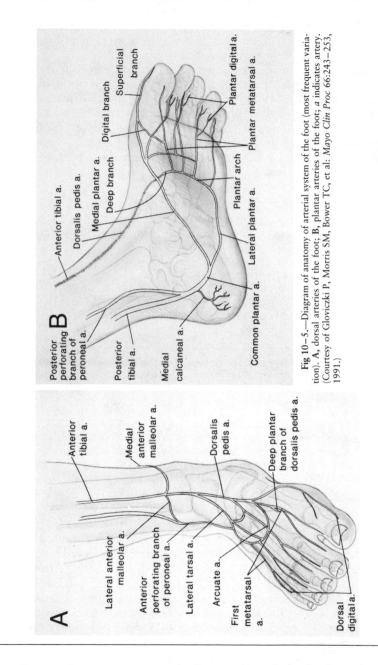

Fig 10–5.—Diagram of anatomy of arterial system of the foot (most frequent variation). **A**, dorsal arteries of the foot; **B**, plantar arteries of the foot; *a* indicates artery. (Courtesy of Gloviczki P, Morris SM, Bower TC, et al: *Mayo Clin Proc* 66:243–253, 1991.)

year. Amputation was necessary in 7 cases (1 early and 6 late) for a cumulative 1-year limb salvage rate of 82.4%. The patency rate was better in grafts that had an intraoperative flow rate of 50 mL/minute or greater. Diabetes had no effect on long-term graft patency. Thirty-four patients

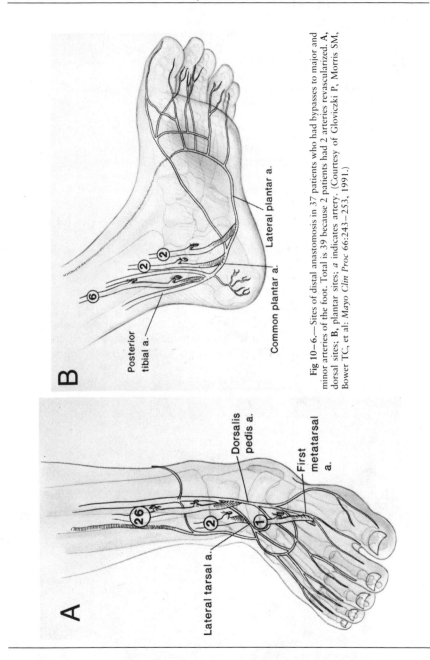

Fig 10–6.—Sites of distal anastomosis in 37 patients who had bypasses to major and minor arteries of the foot. Total is 39 because 2 patients had 2 arteries revascularized. **A**, dorsal sites; **B**, plantar sites; *a* indicates artery. (Courtesy of Gloviczki P, Morris SM, Bower TC, et al: *Mayo Clin Proc* 66:243–253, 1991.)

were alive at follow-up, and 79% of these could walk with the foot, had no pain at rest, and had no substantial loss of tissue.

Conclusions.—For patients with critical, chronic ischemia, pedal bypass should be considered for lower limb salvage. Increased surgical risk and advanced distal atherosclerotic disease should not be considered contraindications. This operation can not only salvage the limb but can also relieve pain and restore function.

▶ With further progression down the arterial tree in femorodistal reconstruction, ancillary measures such as lighting and magnification become extremely important. Although the authors of this study used the dorsalis pedis artery preferentially, they also emphasized the use of the medial and lateral plantar arteries when necessary. Significantly, only 7 anastomoses were distal to the posterior tibial artery in the 37 primary procedures done.

Free Vascularized Tissue Transfer for Limb Salvage in Peripheral Vascular Disease
Greenwald LL, Comerota AJ, Mitra A, Grosh JD, White JV (Temple Univ Hosp, Philadelphia)
Ann Vasc Surg 4:244–254, 1990   10–14

Introduction.—Despite advances in surgical techniques, limb salvage is not possible in many patients with diabetes mellitus and atherosclerotic occlusive disease. Even after adequate arterial reconstruction, the amputation rates may be as high as 40%. A new technique in the management

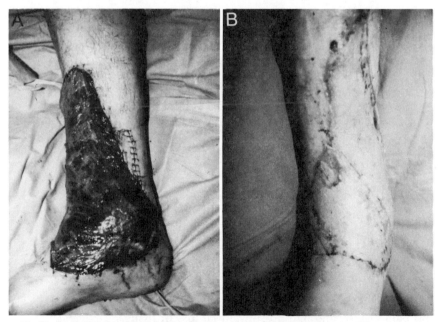

Fig 10–7.—**A**, latissimus dorsi flap in place. **B**, at 1 month postoperatively, complete healing with cosmetic and functional coverage is seen. (Courtesy of Greenwald LL, Comerota AJ, Mitra A, et al: *Ann Vasc Surg* 4:244–254, 1990.)

of tissue defects in such patients, free tissue transfer (FTT), offers higher limb salvage rates.

Patients.—Of 10 patients with a mean age of 62 years, 5 had diabetes and 5 had atherosclerotic occlusive disease. Revascularization was not necessary in 2 patients, both of whom were diabetics with open amputation sites that required coverage. The remaining 8 patients underwent FTT after revascularization for limb salvage.

Surgical Technique.—Before FTT, all of the necrotic soft tissue and exposed or infected bone was débrided radically. The FTTs were performed by vascular and plastic surgery teams. The vascular surgeons selected and exposed the recipient vessels to which the free flap was anastomosed. Recipient vessels were the external iliac artery, saphenous vein bypass grafts, popliteal artery, posterior tibial, and dorsalis pedis vessels. A latissimus dorsi flap was used in 6 patients (Fig 10–7); other donor sites included the gracilis, rectus abdominis, rectus femoris, and scapular muscle flaps.

Outcome.—At a mean follow-up of 20 months, 8 of the 10 flaps were viable. One patient required above-knee amputation 15 months after surgery; another required below-knee amputation 3 years later because of central flap necrosis. The remaining patients were able to resume ambulation.

Conclusion.—Some patients treated previously by amputation alone may be able to keep their limb with FFT in combination with selective revascularization. The FFT offers numerous advantages over other techniques that have been used in patients with diabetes or athersclerotic occlusive disease. An appropriate free flap can be selected from more than 60 potential donor sites on the body.

▶ In addition to the technical points emphasized in earlier abstracts, the final technique described in this abstract requires excellent plastic surgery support. The technique further extends limb salvage to patients whose tissue necrosis has been complicated by profound invasive infection.

Free Tissue Transfers for Limb Salvage Utilizing in Situ Saphenous Vein Bypass Conduit as the Inflow
Chowdary RP, Celani VJ, Goodreau JJ, McCullough JL, McDonald KM, Nicholas GG (Allentown Hosp, LeHigh Valley Hosp, Allentown, Pa)
Plast Reconstr Surg 87:529–535, 1991   10–15

Introduction.—The use of autogenous veins for infrapopliteal bypass to circumvent occluded arterial segments in the lower limb is well established. The in situ bypass is arguably, in the long run, better for grafting to distal segments than the reversed vein technique. In severe ischemia of the lower limb, a good restorative outcome requires that the bones and tendons bared by soft-tissue ulceration receive coverage with well-vascularized grafts; this may be accomplished during bypass surgery. The procedure was used after control of wound sepsis in 8 diabetic patients with either limb-threatening ischemia or tractable soft-tissue defect of the lower limb.

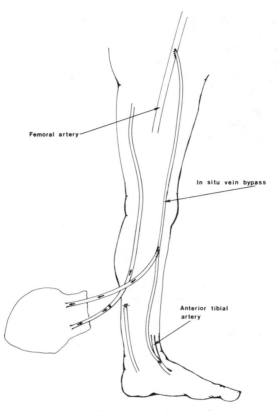

Fig 10–8.—Schematic representation of the in situ vein bypass and microanastomosis to flap vessels. (Courtesy of Chowdary RP, Celani VJ, Goodreau JJ, et al: *Plast Reconstr Surg* 87:529–535, 1991.)

Technique.—After Doppler-mapping, the length of the saphenous vein is exposed, the branches are ligated, valvulotomy is performed, and end-to-side anastomoses is performed with the femoral artery (Fig 10–8). After this stage, arteriography is used to verify free flow through the bypass and to localize potential arteriovenous fistulas, communicating branches that need to be tied off. A radial forearm free flap or latissimus dorsi flap with skin graft is excised simultaneously from the donor site, and vascularized using end-to-side microanastomosis between the inflow vessel of the tissue graft and the in situ saphenous vein. The flap vein and a deep leg vein are anastomosed end-to-end.

Results.—Patients were followed up for an average of 22 months. Of the 8 patients, 6 were healed, and 5 were also ambulatory; 2 later underwent amputation after either clotting of the vein and infection or flap failure leading to osteomyelitis.

Discussion.—Although the operating time is reduced to 6 hours by performing bypass and graft procedures simultaneously; there are some disadvantages. The use of heparin can result in excessive bleeding at the donor site of the flap. Patients should be carefully selected; the healing of postoperative wounds is slow and may be very frustrating for patients with poor circulation. The overall benefit to the patient must be considered because ischemia is often a progressive problem that may necessitate amputation eventually.

▶ The use of free tissue transfers for coverage after successful bypass grafting and debridement is a technique to the applauded. Although use of the bypass as the inflow source insures the vascularization of the transferred tissue, it may compromise the bypass. The transfer of denervated soft tissue to cover an ulcerated area that has its origin in diabetic neuropathy solves the immediate problem; however, long-term observation may reveal recurrence of the same problem for the same reason.

Secondary Femoral-Distal Bypass
Silverman SH, Flynn TC, Seeger JM (Univ of Florida; VA Med Ctr, Gainesville)
J Cardiovasc Surg 32:121–127, 1991   10–16

Introduction.—Because many femoropopliteal and femoral-distal bypasses fail within 5 years of the procedure, new treatment options have been sought for these patients. Most vascular surgeons prefer repeat bypass when possible. The potential risks and benefits of a femoral-distal bypass after the failure of a previous infrainguinal bypass were assessed.

Patients.—The results in 35 patients who underwent 39 secondary femoral-distal bypasses were reviewed and compared with those in 85 patients who underwent 89 primary femoral-distal bypasses. The conduits in the primary procedure included saphenous vein in 7, polytetrafluoroethylene (PTFE)-vein composite in 6, PTFE alone in 18, Dacron in 1, bovine carotid artery in 1, and human umbilical vein in 1; in 5 cases the conduit was unknown. A third of the patients had also undergone previous vascular procedures.

Results.—The graft patency was similar at 2 years for the primary (38%) and secondary (36%) groups. However, early graft failure (within 1 month) was significantly higher in the secondary group (18% vs. 9%). At 6 months, graft patency was 51% for the secondary bypass group and 75% for the primary bypass group. Limb salvage was significantly less for the secondary group, both at 6 months and 2 years. The graft material had a significant effect on outcome. In patients who required a secondary bypass, graft patency was 72% for vein grafts and 24% for composite grafts at 2 years. The 2-year limb salvage rate was 76% with vein grafts and 37% with composite grafts. These differences were not apparent in the patients who underwent primary bypass. Graft patency and limb salvage were lower in both groups for patients who had a previous vascular procedure.

Implications.—In secondary femoral distal bypass, the composite (PTFE/vein) graft is associated with significantly lower graft patency. Patients without an adequate vein for a secondary femoral distal bypass may be candidates for amputation. Secondary procedures using venous conduit do not carry an increased risk of a higher level of amputation if the secondary bypass fails.

▶ If vascular surgery is to succeed in its mission of preventing amputation, a policy of dedication to perform reoperation in patients with a failed distal bypass must be pursued. When an autogenous vein is available, the results will be optimal. Furthermore, the principle of performing a bypass more distally is important to success in the secondary procedures.

Outcomes of Lower Extremity Amputations
Weiss GN, Gorton TA, Read RC, Neal LA (Little Rock Plasma Alliance, Little Rock, Ark; John L. McClellan Mem Veterans Hosp, Little Rock, Ark; Univ of Arkansas, Little Rock)
J Am Geriatr Soc 38:877–883, 1990   10–17

Background.—Complications caused by peripheral vascular disease may result in lower extremity amputation. Despite medical advances, the rates of morbidity, reamputation, and mortality have remained high in elderly patients. To identify the variables that may be used to predict outcomes of amputation, a cohort of 97 veteran amputees with a median age of 64 years was followed.

Methods.—Factors associated with the high incidence and postoperative complications, revision, mortality, and poor quality of life were identified by regression analyses.

Findings.—Both peripheral vascular disease and prolonged preoperative hospitalization were associated with complications. Preoperative gangrene and peripheral vascular disease were associated with the need for revision. Complications, a low body-mass index suggesting malnutrition, and multiple diseases were causes of death. The most important predictor of the quality of life was the ability to perform all of the activities of daily living, not just walking.

Conclusion.—A holistic approach to lower extremity amputation should involve a multidisciplinary team including surgeons, a physiatrist, internist, geriatrician, psychiatrist, social worker, therapist, and hospital administrator, as well as family members. The early identification of patients with potential adverse outcomes and the involvement of the patient or his surrogate in decision making are essential for a favorable outcome.

▶ Amputation is not the last step in the care of the dysvascular patient. It represents only the beginning of rehabilitation.

Persistent Sciatic Artery Aneurysm and Limb Threatening Ischemia
Ranraj M, Southworth M, Goldzer JF (New Rochelle Hosp Med Ctr, New Rochelle, NY)
N Y State J Med 91:111–113, 1991   10–18

Background.—Fewer than 75 cases of persistent sciatic artery (PSA), an embryologic variant of the lower arterial tree, have been described in the literature. This rare vascular anomaly is associated with significant morbidity. In 1 case, the aneurysmal changes in the PSA resulted in limb-threatening ischemia.

Case Report.—Woman, 68, was examined in the emergency room after the sudden onset of severe pain and numbness in the distal left leg. The patient's record included a history of 50 pack-year smoking, chronic alcohol abuse, chronic obstructive pulmonary disease, and deep vein thrombosis of the left leg that was diagnosed 6 weeks before admission. Although the patient's motor function was intact, the left foot was cool and had decreased sensation. Angiography revealed an aneurysm arising from a direct communication of the hypogastric artery and continuing into the thigh. The patient was prepared for embolectomy of the lower extremity arterial tree. An intraoperative angiogram revealed that the superficial femoral artery ended in small collateral circulation above the knee. The popliteal region was explored through a medial incision, confirming the presence of a PSA as the primary blood supply to the extremity. The surgeons successfully created a femoral-popliteal, reversed saphenous vein, above-the-knee bypass. A strongly pulsatile left gluteal mass persisted after surgery, and CT confirmed a PSA aneurysm between 4 cm and 5 cm with laminated thrombus. The region was explored 2 weeks after the original surgery and a 4 cm × 5 cm pulsatile PSA aneurysm was partially dissected. Pulsations in the aneurysm ceased when a large feeding vessel in the sciatic foramen was ligated. The patient underwent a successful transmetatarsal amputation 15 days later.

Conclusion.—In 38% to 45% of the cases reviewed, PSA was associated with aneurysmal dilation. Compression of the sciatic nerve or surrounding tissues often results in pain in the buttock, claudication, and ischemic changes of the distal extremity. Angiography is required for definitive diagnosis. Treatment should be undertaken even in asymptomatic patients because of the high incidence of complications and the possibility of limb loss.

▶ Every busy vascular service will encounter patients with a PSA. This fragile artery enlarges, becomes aneurysmal, contains laminated thrombus, and may present with distal atheromatous embolization as a first symptom. This entity must be a part of the differential diagnosis in patients with distal embolization. Although arteriography will continue to be done in such patients, an equally important and even more informative study will usually involve CT scanning during contrast infusion.

Surgical Treatment of Popliteal Artery Entrapment Syndrome: A Ten-Year Experience
Di Marzo L, Cavallaro A, Sciacca V, Mingoli A, Tamburelli A (Univ of Rome "La Sapienza")
Eur J Vasc Surg 5:59–64, 1991   10–19

Introduction.—Popliteal artery entrapment syndrome is caused by the anomalous interrelationship between the popliteal artery and its surrounding muscular and/or tendinous structures.

Patients.—Between 1979 and 1990, 23 patients with popliteal artery entrapment syndrome were treated surgically. Of the 31 limbs treated, including 8 with bilateral lesions, arteriography showed arterial occlusion in 8, stenosis in 8, and aneurysms in 2, whereas stenosis or occlusion were apparent only after active plantar flexion in 11 limbs. The other 2 limbs did not undergo arteriography because of definitive findings on venography.

Management.—On exploration, 10 anatomical variants were seen, but the medial head of the gastrocnemius was involved in 74.2% of these. Surgical treatment consisted of simple division of the musculotendinous tissue in 16 cases, including 2 in which balloon angioplasty was also used and 12 that had vascular reconstruction; 1 case was explored but not reconstructed.

Results.—During a mean follow-up period of 46 months, patency rate was 94.4% in patients who underwent simple division of the musculotendinous tissue. However, in patients who underwent arterial grafting, the patency rate was only 58.3% during a mean follow-up of 43.5 months.

Summary.—When diagnosed early, popliteal artery entrapment syndrome can be treated effectively by simple division of the offending musculotendinous structure. During late stages, when a stable lesion such occlusion, stenosis and/or aneurysm is present, vascular reconstruction is required in addition to the division of the anomalous musculotendinous tissue.

▶ This entity is more common than was recognized previously. The value of CT scanning has been underemphasized in patients with popliteal artery entrapment syndrome, and this fact is underscored by the absence of CT scanning in the diagnostic protocol detailed in this study.

Value of MRI in the Popliteal Entrapment Syndrome

Lucas C, le Joliff L, Chapuis M, Duvauferrier R, Beschu D, Ramee A (Hôpital Sud, Rennes, France; Centre Hospitalier, Cholet, France)
J Radiol 71:477–480, 1990   10–20

Introduction.—The occurrence of acute or subacute ischemia on effort during recreational athletic activity in young individuals without risk factors for atherosclerotic disease is suggestive of the popliteal artery entrapment syndrome (PAES). Arteriography is the standard diagnostic method for investigating suspected PAES, but young patients are at increased risk of arterial spasm after arteriography. In 1 patient with suspected PAES MRI accurately diagnosed the arterial anomaly of the popliteal artery.

Case Report.—Girl, 12 years, was brought to the emergency department with subacute ischemia of the right leg. Clinical examination revealed a normal left leg

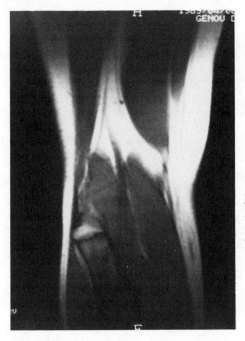
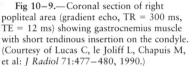

Fig 10–9.—Coronal section of right popliteal area (gradient echo, TR = 300 ms, TE = 12 ms) showing gastrocnemius muscle with short tendinous insertion on the condyle. (Courtesy of Lucas C, le Joliff L, Chapuis M, et al: *J Radiol* 71:477–480, 1990.)

but weak pulses in the popliteal artery. Administration of vasodilators relieved the pain immediately, which strongly suggested a diagnosis of PAES. Doppler ultrasound examination confirmed an interruption of flow in the symptomatic leg, and dynamic phlebography showed extrinsic compression of the popliteal vein. In addition, dynamic arteriography demonstrated compression of the popliteal artery during plantar flexion, and MRI examination showed no sign of an aneurysm or a synovial cyst. However, MRI revealed a partly hypertrophied gastrocnemius muscle with an abnormally short tendinous insertion on the condyle and a vertical course of the popliteal artery (Fig 10–9). The diagnosis was PAES. The patient underwent operation from a posterior approach, and the postoperative course was uneventful.

Conclusion.—Noninvasive examinations such as dynamic echo Doppler and MRI can identify most of the arterial and muscular abnormalities commonly associated with PAES. Magnetic resonance imaging can replace arteriography in young patients, thus eliminating the non-neglible risk of arterial spasm.

▶ Because imaging is key to the accurate diagnosis of this condition, MR must be considered among the imaging modalities. Furthermore, because MR is becoming an imaging method of choice in dealing with joint abnormalities, its use will become increasingly important in uncovering the entrapment syndromes of the popliteal neurovascular bundle.

11 Cerebrovascular Occlusions

Percutaneous Transluminal Angioplasty of the Subclavian Arteries: Long-Term Results in 52 Patients

Hebrang A, Maskovic J, Tomac B (Univ of Zagreb, Yugoslavia; Clinical Hosp "Firule," Split, Yugoslavia; St Johannes Hosp, Hagen, Germany)

AJR 156:1091–1094, 1991   11–1

Background.—Percutaneous transluminal angioplasty (PTA) has been used most often in the subclavian arteries. Only small series of patients have been reported. The technical success, complications, and long-term follow-up of 52 patients who underwent PTA were reported.

Patients.—The patients (mean age, 57 years) all had symptoms of brachial ischemia during exercise or at rest and blood pressure in the arm on the involved side that was at least 30 mm Hg lower than in the opposite arm. The symptoms of vertebrobasilar insufficiency—dizziness, blurred vision, and ataxia—were present in 75% of the patients. Of the 52 patients, 43 were treated for stenosis and 9 were treated for occlusion.

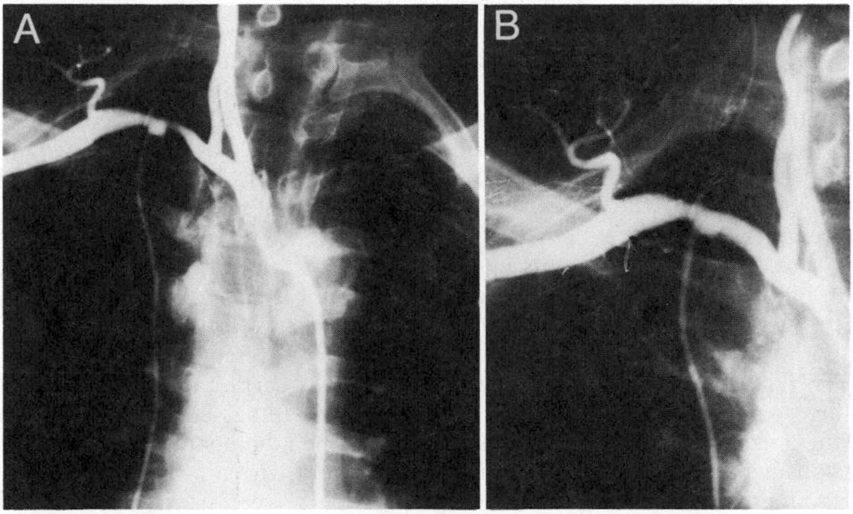

Fig 11–1.—Patient, 52, with 2 stenoses of the right subclavian artery. **A,** initial angiogram shows stenoses distal to the vertebral artery. **B,** angiogram after percutaneous transluminal angioplasty shows a successfully dilated proximal stenosis; distal stenosis was not treated because blood pressure returned to normal after dilatation of proximal stenosis. (Courtesy of Hebrang A, Maskovic J, Tomac B: *AJR* 156:1091–1094, 1991.)

Results.—In 93% of the patients with stenosis and 56% of those with occlusion, PTA was technically successful. Follow-up angiograms in successfully treated patients revealed no narrowing greater than 30% (Fig 11–1). The blood pressure in the 2 arms equalized. After 6 to 48 months of follow-up, the blood pressure in the treated arm remained normal in 91% of the patients and the vertebrobasilar insufficiency symptoms resolved in 72% of the patients.

Conclusions.—Percutaneous transluminal angioplasty appears to be a useful method of treatment for stenosis or occlusion of the subclavian artery. The success rate is lower in patients with occlusion because of the difficulty in passing through the occluded area.The use of heparin during this procedure is not recommended.

▶ Both the original study and the abstract are disturbing because these interventional radiologists are concerned primarily with technical success. Neither in the manuscript nor in the discussion section is there exposition of the neurological complications that occur after this procedure. Nor is there any mention of distal embolization occurring either during or shortly after the procedure. It is hoped that more careful, traditional clinical evaluation of patient status will be used in future studies.

Percutaneous Transluminal Angioplasty of the Innominate, Subclavian, and Axillary Arteries
Insall RL, Lambert D, Chamberlain J, Proud G, Murthy LNS, Loose HWC (Freeman Hosp, Newcastle-upon-Tyne, England)
Eur J Vasc Surg 4:591–595, 1990   11–2

Introduction.—Arterial disease of an upper extremity has traditionally been managed conservatively or surgically. Percutaneous transluminal angioplasty (PTA) of arterial occlusive disease, which has been widely used in the lower extremities and coronary vessels, has yet to be widely accepted for the treatment of brachiocephalic vessels. Data were reviewed on 27 patients who underwent PTA procedures for lesions of upper extremities.

Patients.—These patients underwent 28 procedures for 33 subclavian, 2 innominate, and 2 axillary arterial lesions. Ischemic symptoms were present in 15 patients, neurological symptoms were present in 8, and both ischemic and neurological symptoms were present in 5.

Treatment.—In all of the patients, PTA was carried out via a femoral artery puncture. The guidewire and balloon were passed retrogradely up the aorta under fluoroscopic control. After the administration of intravenous heparin, the balloon was inflated by hand with a 5 mL syringe containing dilute contrast medium. The patients were usually discharged within 2 days, and they were treated with aspirin and dipyridamole for at least 3 months after PTA.

Outcome.—At an average follow-up of 24 months, relief of symptoms was obtained in 25 cases; 19 patients had complete relief and 5 experi

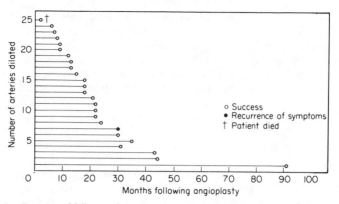

Fig 11–2.—Duration of follow-up for each patient after successful angioplasty represented by *single line commencing at time zero.* (Courtesy of Insall RL, Lambert D, Chamberlain J, et al: *Eur J Vasc Surg* 4:591–595, 1990.)

enced marked improvement (Fig 11–2). In 1 patient who had recurrent ischemia at 30 months, a repeat PTA was successful. The only death in the series resulted from metastatic breast carcinoma. Complications included a femoral artery occlusion, a large groin hematoma, and extension of a contralateral stroke; all complications were managed successfully.

Conclusion.—The incidence of serious complications in brachiocephalic arterial dilatation is as low as that reported for PTA in general. This procedure is readily repeatable if there is failure or recurrence. Percutaneous transluminal angioplasty is recommended as the first line of treatment for arterial disease of an upper extremity.

▶ This study on the clincial status of the patient after PTA emanated from a vascular surgical service and was prepared in cooperation with interventional radiologists. In the discussion section, the authors refer to 400 reported cases of carotid, vertebral, and upper limb PTA in which there were only 2 reported instances of cerebral embolization. The complications that related to the treatment site included only 3 cases of distal embolization into the arm or hand and 3 cases of acute occlusions at the dilation site.

Subclavian Artery Rupture During Transluminal Angioplasty: Treatment by Transcatheter Occlusion and Surgical Bypass
Routh WD, Keller FS, McDowell HA, Vitek JJ (Univ of Alabama)
J Intervent Radiology 5:87–89, 1990   11–3

Introduction.—Vessel wall rupture is a rare complication of percutaneous transluminal angioplasty (PTA). A patient with a left subclavian PTA complicated by acute arterial rupture with pseudoaneurysm formation was assessed.

Case Report.—Woman, 39, had a high-grade stenosis of the proximal left subclavian artery on arch aortography. Other findings included a left vertebral artery with an origin from the aortic arch. A repeat arch aortogram performed after a left subclavian PTA showed resolution of the left subclavian stenosis and extravasation of contrast into a subclavian arterial pseudoaneurysm at the angioplasty site. Because of the imminent risk of free rupture and potentially severe hemorrhage, the subclavian artery was occluded intentionally across the site of the pseudoaneurysm with coil springs, thus obviating the need for a relatively major intrathoracic surgical repair. The finding of a left vertebral artery that rose directly from the aortic arch allowed coil springs to be placed in the proximal subclavian artery without risk of vertebro-basilar thromboembolism. Immediately after the procedure, the patient underwent axilloaxillary bypass grafting and her condition improved.

Summary.—Arterial rupture with subclavian PTA has not been reported previously. Temporary hemostasis of subclavian artery rupture during PTA is similar to angioplasty-related iliac rupture, and can be achieved with either balloon or coil spring occlusion.

▶ It is important to recognize that complications will occur from vascular interventions. It is tragic that what could have been a straightforward surgical repair was rendered so complicated that the patient was left with a clearly inferior reconstruction that, predictably, will fail.

Vertebral Artery Reconstruction: Results in 106 Patients
Habozit B (Clinique Chirurgicale, Chambéry, France)
Ann Vasc Surg 5:61–65, 1991   11–4

Background.—Surgical restoration of the vertebral artery is associated with successful recovery or stable improvement of vertebrobasilar insufficiency in nearly 90% of patients (Table 1). The results of 109 revascularizations of the vertebral artery performed in 106 patients were retrospectively reviewed and compared with those of previous studies (Table 2). There were 98 revascularizations of the proximal vertebral artery and 11 reconstructions of the distal vertebral artery.

Results.—Of the 106 patients, 36 underwent combined carotid and vertebral revascularization procedures. There were 2 deaths and 2 nonfatal cerebral vascular accidents. The rate of complications in isolated ver-

TABLE 1.—Vertebrobasilar Symptoms (104 Patients)

Symptoms	Number of patients	Percent
Acute ataxia	76	73
Acute visual disorders	29	28
Acute vigilance disorders	14	14
Drop attacks	10	10
Acute disorders of speech	8	8
Acute deficits of spinal tracts	2	2
Miscellaneous	13	13

(Courtesy of Habozit B: *Ann Vasc Surg* 5:61–65, 1991.)

TABLE 2.—Surgical Procedures (108 Procedures)

	Total
Proximal surgery	
Reimplantation into common carotid artery	95
direct	92
indirect	3
Reimplantation into subclavian artery	2
Endarterectomy	1
Total	98
Distal surgery	
Carotid-vertebral vein bypass	7
Transposition of external carotid artery	2
Reimplantation into internal carotid artery	2
Total	11

(Courtesy of Habozit B: *Ann Vasc Surg* 5:61–65, 1991.)

tebral artery surgery was less; only 3 nonfatal cerebral vascular accidents occurred in 70 patients. During a mean follow-up of 48 months, 7 patients died. The actuarial 5-year survival was 91%, with patency at 96%.

Conclusion.—A study of the late neurological events showed that 63% of the patients had complete recovery, 30% showed improvement, and 7% had failure or aggravation of symptoms. Associated carotid artery reconstruction is an important factor of early neurological complications in surgery of the vertebral artery. The technical difficulties of distal revascularization result in early patency rates that are lower than those for proximal reconstruction. In selected patients, vertebral artery surgery provides excellent early and late results. Further improvements can be expected with extended indications and better anatomical reconstruction of the distal vertebral artery reconstruction.

▶ The message to be derived from this presentation is clear. No matter how tempting it is to perform simultaneous carotid and vertebral artery reconstruction, and no matter how easy the procedures may be for the surgeon, the morbidity and even the mortality of the combined operation are prohibitively high. Other reports, both from France and from this country, cite morbidity figures similar to the figures found in this abstract (1).

Reference

1. McNamara MF, Berguer R: *J Cardiovasc Surg* 30:161, 1989.

Transesophageal Echocardiography in the Detection of Intracardiac Embolic Sources in Patients With Transient Ischemic Attacks
Pop G, Sutherland GR, Koudstaal PJ, Sit TW, de Jong G, Roelandt JRTC (Univ Hosp Rotterdam-Dijkzigt; Erasmus Univ, Rotterdam, The Netherlands)
Stroke 21:560–565, 1990   11–5

Background.—The heart is a potential source of cerebral emboli in patients with transient ischemic attacks (TIA). The relative efficacy of precordial and transesophageal echocardiography for detecting the potential intracardiac source of cerebral emboli in patients with TIA was compared in a prospective study.

Method.—A group of 72 consecutive patients with a recent unequivocal TIA or nondisabling stroke were studied. Based on clinical cardiological evaluation, the patients were divided into 2 groups: group 1 consisted of 53 patients with clinical cardiac abnormality, and group 2 included 19 patients with abnormal cardiac findings. The mean interval from the onset of neurological symptoms until cardiac evaluation was 8 days.

Findings.—In group 1 patients, precordial echocardiography was normal in all but 1 patient with abnormal thickening of the aortic valve. In 5 patients, transesophageal echocardiography identified abnormalities that were potentially relevant in management. These abnormalities included a left atrial appendage, aortic dissection, mitral valve prolapse, mitral leaflet mass lesion, and aortic valve thickening. In group 2 patients, both precordial and transesophageal echocardiography were normal in 13 patients and abnormal in the other 6. Of the latter patients, 5 had pathological left atrial and/or left ventricular dilatation, but only transesophageal echocardiography identified a left atrial appendage mass lesion in 2. These findings did not affect the therapeutic management of the patients. In 32 of the 72 patients, transesophageal echocardiography identified diffuse thoracic aortic atherosclerotic plaques that were not apparent on precordial echocardiography.

Implications.—In the patients with TIA without clinical cardiac abnormalities, transesophageal echocardiography significantly increases the yield of the cardiac sources of emboli, compared with precordial echocardiography. However, the overall yield of the potential cardiac sources of emboli is relatively small, and the causative relation with TIA cannot be proven. Transesophageal echocardiography also increases the yield of the potential cardiac courses of emboli in patients with clinically cardiac abnormalities; however, these findings are of little clinical relevance in therapeutic management.

▶ This abstract was included to emphasize the utility of transesophageal echocardiography in the detection of aortic atherosclerotic plaques as sources of peripheral embolization.

Cerebrovascular and Neurologic Disease Associated With Antiphospholipid Antibodies: 48 Cases

Levine SR, Deegan MJ, Futrell N, Welch KMA (Henry Ford Hosp, Detroit)
Neurology 40:1181–1189, 1990   11–6

Background.—There is growing evidence of an association between cerebrovascular and neurological disease and antiphospholipid antibodies

Associations With Single, Recurrent, and Transient Ischemic
Cerebrovascular Diseases*

	Single event	Recurrent events	Only transient events	p value
No. patients	13	17	16	
Cigarette use	6	12	4	<0.04†
Hyperlipidemia	4	9	2	<0.05†
Cardiopathy	6	6	4	>0.49
Hypertension	2	5	5	>0.58
Diabetes mellitus	3	1	1	>0.24
SLE	1	5	2	>0.24
+ANA	4	13	6	<0.03†
↓ plt	2	5	6	>0.41
F+ VDRL	0	5	4	>0.10
Other thrombotic events	4	9	7	>0.47

Abbreviations: SLE, systemic lupus erythematosus; *+ANA,* positive antinuclear antibody; *↓ plt,* thrombocytopenia; *F+ VDRL,* false positive VDRL.
*Only patients with cerebral arterial or ocular events or TIA or migrainous events are included in this table (*n* = 46).
†*P* also <.013 on pairwise Fisher's exact tests that were Bonferroni-adjusted for multiple testing, with the level of significance set at *P* <.013.
(Courtesy of Levine SR, Deegan MJ, Futrell N, et al: *Neurology* 40:1181–1189, 1990

(APLAb). These antibodies bind negatively charged or neutral phospholipids and are circulating serum polyclonal immoglobulins. The role of APLAb as markers for increased risk of thrombosis was examined.

Methods.—A group of 48 patients with cerebral or visual disturbances associated with APLAb was studied. Diagnostic, clinical, laboratory, radiological and pathological studies were done to clarify this association. There were 44.4 patient-years of prospective follow-up.

Results.—Diagnostically, most of the patients had transient cerebral ischemia or cerebral infarction, frequently with recurrent and stereotypic events. Amaurosis fugax, retinal or venous occlusion, occipital ischemia, diplopia, and migraine caused presenting visual disturbances. Cigarette smoking, hyperlipidemia, and positive antinuclear antibody value were associated with recurrent eye and brain infarcts (table). The absence of systemic lupus erythematosus was confirmed in 83% of the patients. The angiographic and radiological findings were generally normal in patients with transient dysfunction, but cerebral angiography disclosed some large vessel occlusion and stenosis without vasculitis. The pathological findings disclosed thrombotic occlusive disease without vasculitis.

Conclusions.—Recurrent thrombotic events occurred in most of the patients before detection of the APLAb. One year after the study, almost 50% of the patients had experienced a subsequent stroke. A total of 20% of the patients did not have any other stroke risk factor coexisting with APLAb. Further investigations on the significance and management of

APLAb in ischemic cerebrovascular and neurological disease are being undertaken.

▶ The lupus anticoagulant and anticardiolipin antibodies are closely linked APLAb. These are polyclonal immunoglobulins that are important to vascular surgeons, and they should be a part of the coagulopathy screen when we look at young individuals with either venous or arterial thrombotic events.

Pictural Creations of a Painter With Left-Sided Neglect
Vigouroux RA, Bonnefoi B, Khalil R (Clinique de Neurologie, Marseilles, France)
Rev Neurol (Paris) 146:665–670, 1990   11–7

Introduction.—A study documented the changes in the paintings and drawings of a painter from the time he had a complete left-sided stroke at age 66 until his death 12 years later. The painer continued to draw and paint throughout his illness. The work produced during his illness was analyzed.

Case Report.—Man, 66, an artist, was taken to the hospital on the day a stroke occurred, and he remained there for 3 months. He had a history of poorly

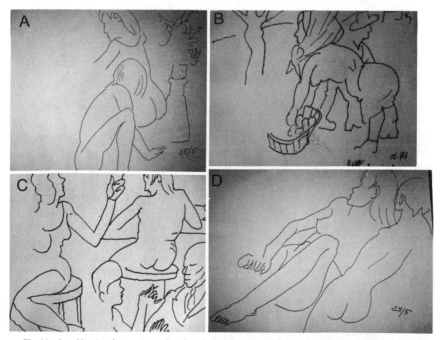

Fig 11–3.—Hemineglect may involve the whole left part of the drawing (**A**) or some of its elements, such as the basket (**B**) or the left side of the figures (**C**). The hand is poorly structured on the left side (**D**). It is also found in the left portions of some objects or figures: the flower bouquet (**A**), the peasant's shoulder (**B**), or the female customer seated in a bar (**C**). (Courtesy of Vigouroux RA, Bonnefoi B, Khalil R: *Rev Neurol (Paris)* 146:665–670, 1990.)

controlled arterial hypertension and diabetes, weighed 110 kg, and abused alcohol and tobacco. During his hospital stay, the painter lost more than 40 kg and his glycemia was normalized. After discharge, he became severely depressed. This was reflected in his work. He tried to commit suicide by taking an overdose of clonazepam but was discovered in time by his family. He was then taken to a neurological clinic where he received trimipramine for his depression. His neurological status and mood both improved, and his work reflected this improvement. During this period, he still showed excellent spatial organization in his drawings, and his style remained well recognizable. The shapes and volumes of his favorite topics were unchanged, but the left side of the paper on which he drew was empty and the left side of his drawings lacked detail, documenting unilateral neglect as a consequence of the left-sided lesion (Fig 11–3). Aware that he could not finish the left side of his drawings, he would sometimes turn the paper around and fill in the empty spaces. The painter deteriorated slowly and made a second suicide attempt. Extrapyramidal side effects caused his hand to tremble. His drawings became less and less structured and his spatial organization also deteriorated. Even his signature eventually became almost illegible. However, in rare moments of clarity, he would create drawings showing that his esthetic capabilities and artistic talent had remained intact. His very last drawings were totally unstructured. The artist died in 1985 in a long-term nursing care facility in the setting of arteriopathical dementia.

▶ This is a sad but very instructive documentation.

Screening of the Internal Carotid Arteries in Patients With Peripheral Vascular Disease by Colour-Flow Duplex Scanning
Klop RBJ, Eikelboom BC, Taks ACJM (Stichting Doetinchemse Ziekenhuizen, Doetinchem; St Antonius Ziekenhuis Nieuwegein, The Netherlands)
Eur J Vasc Surg 5:41–45, 1991   11–8

Objective.—Little is known about the prevalence of carotid artery disease in patients with peripheral arterial disease (PAD). A total of 416 consecutive patients (aged 32–91 years) with PAD were screened for carotid artery disease using color-flow duplex scanning.

Findings.—Major internal carotid artery disease (MICAD), defined as 75% stenosis and/or occlusion, occurred in 62 (14.9%) patients (Fig 11–4), and most of these patients (84%) had unilateral disease. Of these, 32 (7.7%) had a stenosis of 76% to 99%. Of the 30 (7.2%) patients with occlusions, 20% had a contralateral stenosis of 76% to 99%, indicating that 1.5% of all patients had high-grade stenosis and contralateral occlusion. There was no correlation between the severity of PAD and the prevalence of MICAD. The prevalence of MICAD was significantly higher in patients with obstructive atherosclerosis (16%) than in patients with aneurysms (4.7%) (Fig 11–5). There was no correlation between MICAD and known risk factors for atherosclerosis (such as hypertension, gender,

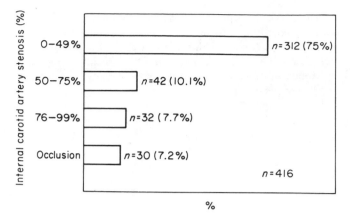

Fig 11–4.—Prevalence of various degrees of carotid artery disease in 416 patients with peripheral arterial disease. (Courtesy of Klop RBJ, Eikelboom BC, Taks ACJM: *Eur J Vasc Surg* 5:41–45, 1991.)

age, diabetes mellitus, hypercholesterolemia, smoking, and ischemic heart disease).

Summary.—A high prevalence of MICAD in patients with PAD was demonstrated. If surgery should be found beneficial in patients with high-grade stenosis, it would be useful to start a screening program using non-invasive methods to reduce the morbidity and mortality associated with strokes.

▶ This paper is important in defining the incidence of high-grade carotid stenosis in patients with peripheral arterial disease. The high-grade stenosis has an increased risk of stroke that does not end with occlusion of the artery. The surgical prevention of carotid occlusion is a worthwhile effort.

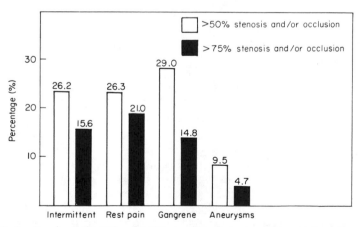

Fig 11–5.—Prevalence of >50% and >75% stenosis/occlusion in patients with intermittent claudication (282), rest pain (38), gangrene (54), and aneurysms (42). (Courtesy of Klop RBJ, Eikelboom BC, Taks ACJM: *Eur J Vasc Surg* 5:41–45, 1991.)

Prevalence of Hemodynamically Significant Stenosis of the Carotid Artery in an Asymptomatic Veteran Population
Fowl RJ, Marsch JG, Love M, Patterson RB, Shukla R, Kempczinski RF (Cincinnati VA Med Ctr; Univ of Cincinnati Med Ctr)
Surg Gynecol Obstet 172:13–16, 1991   11–9

Introduction.—A recent study reported a low prevalence of hemodynamically significant carotid artery stenosis among an asymptomatic volunteer population from a local church. However, this group had a low incidence of atherosclerotic risk factors and was not representative of the patients seen by most vascular surgeons. Therefore, a similar study was performed in an asymptomatic population of veterans with a much more representative distribution of atherosclerotic risk factors.

Methods.—A group of 269 patients underwent Duplex scanning of 538 carotid arteries. There were 255 men and 14 women (mean age, 64.4 years). Of these patients, 153 were treated for nonvascular problems and 16 had significant arterial occlusive disease of the lower extremities. All of the patients were questioned about a history of transient ischemic attacks, cardiac disease, hypertension, diabetes mellitus, tobacco use, peripheral vascular disease, and previous vascular operations.

Findings.—Asymptomatic, hemodynamically significant carotid artery lesions were found in 25 of the 269 patients. A total of 20 patients had a unilateral lesion, and 5 had bilateral lesions. The prevalence of carotid lesions was 6.5% among the patients treated for nonvascular problems and 12.9% among those treated for lower extremity occlusive disease. The presence of hypertension, diabetes, or previous vascular operation were not significant risk factors for high-grade carotid artery lesions. However, cardiac disease was significantly associated with carotid artery stenosis. The correlation between smoking and carotid artery disease approached statistical significance. Significant carotid artery lesions were present in 7 of the 40 patients in whom cardiac disease, peripheral vascular disease, and smoking were present. In contrast, none of the 32 patients in whom all 3 risk factors were absent had a significant carotid artery lesion.

Conclusion.—Asymptomatic patients with a history of cardiac disease, smoking, and peripheral vascular disease (either alone or in combination) have an increased risk for asymptomatic, hemodynamically significant stenosis of the carotid arteries. These patients should be monitored closely for disease progression and for the occurrence of neurological symptoms.

▶ In this study, significant stenosis was defined as greater than 50% diameter stenosis. Even at this less dangerous degree of stenosis, the incidence of carotid disease in this elderly population would not justify routine screening.

Extracranial Carotid Artery Stenosis: Prevalence and Associated Risk Factors in Elderly Stroke Patients
Admani AK, Mangion DM, Naik DR (Northern Gen Hosp, Sheffield, England; Barnsley District Gen Hosp, Barnsley, England)
Atherosclerosis 86:31–37, 1991   11–10

Background.—The risk of stroke increases with the increasing severity of extracranial carotid artery stenosis (ECAS). Because age is an important risk factor for ECAS, the prevalence of ECAS and associated risk factors in elderly stroke victims was analyzed.

Methods.—A duplex pulsed wave ultrasound system was used to assess the degree of arterial stenosis in the right and left extracranial carotid arteries of 118 stroke patients aged 65 years and older. Of the 118 patients 66 were men. Overall, 28% of the patients had severe stenosis; 14%, moderate stenosis; and 58%, little or no stenosis. A total of 34% of the strokes occurred in the presence of moderate or severe stenosis in the ipsilateral extracranial carotid artery.

Results.—According to multivariate logistic regression, there was a significant positive correlation between ECAS in either artery and ischemic heart disease, systolic blood pressure, and the male sex. When the analysis was repeated for ECAS in the clinically significant arteries only (those with maximal stenosis ipsilateral to the stroke) similar results were obtained. However, the relationships were weak.

Conclusions.—Carotid and coronary atherosclerosis share common risk factors, and systolic blood pressure and male sex are independent risk factors for ECAS. However, the relationships demonstrated in this study are weak, suggesting that other factors that have not yet been identified may be important.

▶ The data that emerge from screening studies reveal that patients with peripheral arterial occlusive disease are at risk for carotid stenosis, but patients who are aged or those with stroke may not be at risk.

Evaluation of the Associations Between Carotid Artery Atherosclerosis and Coronary Artery Stenosis: A Case-Control Study
Craven TE, Ryu JE, Espeland MA, Kahl FR, McKinney WM, Toole JF, McMahan MR, Thompson CJ, Heiss G, Crouse JR III (Wake Forest Univ Med Ctr, Winston-Salem, NC; Univ of North Carolina, Chapel Hill)
Circulation 82:1230–1242, 1990   11–11

Background.—Population-based studies have shown that people with signs and symptoms of coronary artery disease (CAD) have a higher risk of cerebrovascular disease than unaffected people. A group of 343 patients with CAD and 167 unaffected patients were evaluated for extent of carotid atherosclerosis by computation of a B-mode score using a Biosound compact real-time imager. All of the patients had undergone coronary angiography and were evaluated for CAD risk factors. Statistical analyses tested for an association between asymptomatic carotid artery atherosclerosis and CAD and evaluated whether the extent of carotid atherosclerosis would be useful in classifying CAD status.

Results.—Among male and female patients both older and younger than 50 years of age, the B-mode scores were significantly higher in those with CAD than in the unaffected control patients. After correction for age, logistic regression analysis showed that the association remained significant for all groups except men younger than 50 years. In a univariable analysis, the extent of carotid atherosclerosis was correlated significantly with many other CAD risk factors. A step-wise logistic regression analysis showed that the B-mode score was significantly and independently associated with coronary status in men and women older than 50 years. In an analysis of men and women older than 50 years, the B-mode score resulted in increased sensitivity and specificity of a logistic model for classification of CAD status. Recursive partitioning implied that the B-mode score was the most important individual parameter for classification of coronary status.

Conclusions.—This case-controlled study provides evidence that, among men and women older than 50 years, the B-mode score is the most important classifier of CAD status. It is possible that the association between carotid and coronary atherosclerosis is caused by shared risk factors not evaluated here.

▶ It is apparent that age, high-density lipoprotein, and pack-years of smoking correlate with the severity of both CAD and carotid artery occlusive disease.

Thickness of Carotid Artery Atherosclerotic Plaque and Ischemic Risk
Dempsey RJ, Diana AL, Moore RW (Univ of Kentucky; VA Hosp, Lexington, Ky)
Neurosurg 27:343–348, 1990   11–12

Background.—Recent studies of the predictors of stroke emphasize the importance of evaluating plaque likely to produce emboli, as well as the flow dynamics of arteries. In some cases, the hemorrhage of a plaque and the extrusion of emboli through the ulcerated endothelial surface may be more important than the vessel diameter in determining ischemic symptoms. The contribution of atherosclerotic plaques at the bifurcation of the common carotid artery to a history of cerebrovascular, systemic vascular, or cardiac disease was assessed. The relationship of the thickness of the plaques to known atherosclerotic risk factors was also assessed.

Methods.—Noninvasive standard duplex ultrasound exams with 7.5 MHz and 10 MHz probes were done in multiple planes in 286 successive symptomatic and asymptomatic patients who were referred to a central diagnostic laboratory for suspicion of atherosclerotic pathology. Extensive medical histories were correlated with plaque thickness and degree of vessel stenosis in the common (CCA), external, and internal carotid arteries (ICA), and the CCA-ICA bulb complex. The predictors of ipsilateral ischemic events were studied independently for the 547 arteries examined. The carotid cerebrovascular events included ipsilateral stroke and transient ischemic attacks (TIAs) when carotid artery plaque was present.

Results.—A total of 66.5% of this population were smokers, many with more than 50 pack-years of use. The cholesterol levels were greater than 230 in nearly half of the 51.2% of patients for whom the data were available. More than 65% of the patients had manifestations of systemic atherosclerotic disease. The range of plaque thickness was from 0–8 mm, with 40.4% of the arteries having moderately thick plaque of 2 mm–3 mm. Atherosclerotic plaque thickness correlated with vessel stenosis, and both of these parameters were independent predictors of cerebrovascular events. Patient age and pack-years were independent predictors of plaque thickness (heavy smokers younger than 55 years had the thickest plaques), and pack-years and plaque thickness were independent predictors of systemic atherosclerotic disease. The best predictor of prior TIAs was plaque thickness, but vessel stenosis predicted prior stroke more reliably.

Discussion.—Patients with a moderate level of plaque and a 38% stenosis insufficient to compromise cerebral tissue evidenced systemic atherosclerotic disease and distribution strokes of the carotid artery. Emboli and resultant ischemia may derive from a plaque that is yet too small to impede flow. Thus, embolic risk is not determined by the severity of carotid artery stenosis. A noninvasive duplex study capable of detecting small lesions is of value in predicting patients who are at risk for systemic atherosclerosis and in determining those patients in whom risk factors must be energetically modified.

▶ This study emphasizes that although neurologists and internists are interested in the degree of carotid stenosis, they overlook the important fact that strokes result from carotid artery plaques that narrow the carotid artery less than 50%.

Pulsatile Two-Dimensional Flow and Plaque Formation in a Carotid Artery Bifurcation
Nazemi M, Kleinstreuer C, Archie JP Jr (North Carolina State Univ, Raleigh, NC)
J Biomech 23:1031–1037, 1990   11–13

Background.—Physical and biochemical factors such as the influence of hemodynamics and particle transport play an important role in atherogenesis and thrombosis.

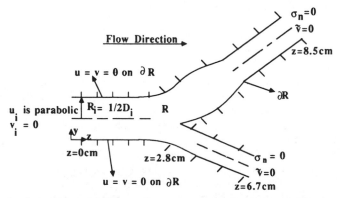

Fig 11–6.—System schematics with coordinate system (graph is not to scale). (Courtesy of Nazemi M, Kleinstreuer C, Archie JP Jr: *J Biomech* 23:1031–1037, 1990.)

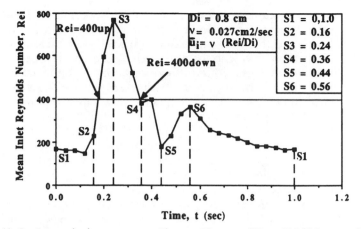

Fig 11–7.—Input pulse for common carotid artery. (Courtesy of Nazemi M, Kleinstreuer C, Archie JP Jr: *J Biomech* 23:1031–1037, 1990.)

Study Design.—Realistic input pulse, velocity and pressure fields, streamlines, and wall shear stress distributions were numerically obtained for 2-dimensional, steady and pulsatile flow in a carotid artery segment (Figs 11–6 and 11–7). An advanced plaque formation model was used.

Findings.—On the basis of results with the validated plaque formation model, transient 2-dimensional rigid conduit flow modeling is an important initial step in the simulation of hemodynamic factors that are relevant in atherogenesis. The plaque formation model predicts plaque sites in branching arteries under pulsatile flow conditions, making it a useful predictive tool for improved surgical reconstructions.

▶ The carotid artery bulb does not seem to have been designed particularly well.

Variability of Flow Patterns in the Normal Carotid Bifurcation

Steinke W, Kloetzsch C, Hennerici M (Heinrich-Heine-Univ, Düsseldorf, Germany; Ruprecht-Karls-Univ, Heidelberg, Germany; Klinikum Mannheim, Mannheim, Germany)
Atherosclerosis 84:121–127, 1990   11–14

Introduction.—Because atherosclerotic plaques tend to occur at the carotid bifurcation, numerous studies have investigated the hemodynamic flow velocity patterns in the carotid bifurcation; however, the findings remain inconclusive. A systemic study was initiated to document the shift from normal to abnormal flow patterns in the carotid bifurcation at the onset of atherosclerosis.

Methods.—Doppler color flow imaging (DCFI) provides real-time, color-coded, plain images of both intravascular blood flow and vessel wall structures at the carotid bifurcation. The spatial and temporal distribution of blood flow, its direction and velocity, and the flow separation phenomena at the carotid bifurcation can be superimposed simultaneously on the display of tissue and vascular structures and can then be stored on videotape. Fifty-six individuals (aged 17–81, years) without clinical or sonographic evidence of atherosclerotic carotid disease underwent DCFI studies of 109 carotid bifurcations. Only 3 bifurcations were excluded from analysis because of poor display quality. The videotapes were examined to detect and characterize the flow separation patterns.

Findings.—Flow separation was seen in 102 (93.6%) carotid bifurcations, but it could not be detected in 6 right (5.5%) and 1 left (.9%) bifurcations. Although the spatial and temporal distribution and the extent of secondary flow within the carotid bulb were highly variable, different patterns could be distinguished. Separated flow was found in the proximal external carotid artery (ECA), the internal carotid artery (ICA), or both. In some of the arteries, the zones of secondary flow extended from the ICA into the ECA around the flow divider, and in others the distribution was diffuse. Only 3 patients had symmetric separation zones in both

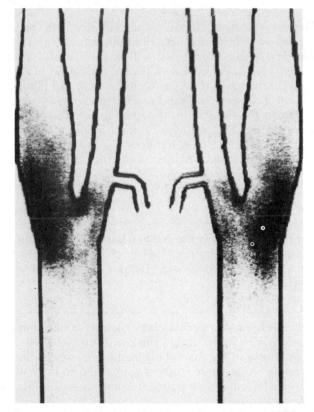

Fig 11–8.—Computer-assisted superimposition of separation zones in carotid bifurcations averaged from 48 right *(R)* and 54 left *(L)* bifurcations. *Darkness* correlates with the frequency of blue coded flow signals. On the left side the separation zone in the internal carotid artery is larger, extending more distally, and secondary flow is more pronounced at the flow divider. (Courtesy of Steinke W, Kloetzsch C, Hennerici M: *Atherosclerosis* 84:121–127, 1990.)

carotid sinuses. The largest zone of secondary flow was located at the outer wall of the carotid sinus and extended into the ICA; however, smaller centers were found at the flow divider and the origin of the ECA (Fig 11–8).

Conclusion.—The unexpectedly variable spatial and temporal patterns of secondary flow phenomena contrast with the concepts established in earlier in vitro flow studies. Doppler color-flow imaging is presently the most promising technique available for the further study of blood flow patterns in the human carotid bifurcation.

▶ In vitro studies such as those mentioned reported in Abstract 11–13 are important in defining concepts. However, this study reinforces our knowledge that the best study subject for human diseases is man.

Morphological Characterization of Carotid Artery Stenoses by Ultrasound Duplex Scanning
Widder B, Paulat K, Hackspacher J, Hamann H, Hutschenreiter S, Kreutzer C, Ott F, Vollmar J (Univ of Ulm, Germany)
Ultrasound Med Biol 16:349–354, 1990   11–15

Background.—Several studies suggest that plaque ulceration and/or intraplaque hemorrhage increase the risk of an ischemic event in patients with carotid artery stenoses. The efficacy of duplex scanning in predicting plaque morphology was studied.

Method.—Plaque border, plaque density, and plaque structure on duplex scanning were compared with intraoperative morphological findings in 169 consecutive carotid endarterectomies.

Results.—A total of 2% of the sonograms were inadequate, and 20% showed poor image quality—particularly with increasing degree of stenoses. Regular plaque borders on sonography had smooth or, at most, minimally ulcerated surface in 92%, whereas irregular plaque borders revealed grossly ulcerated stenoses in only 27%. In detecting ulcerations, sonography had a sensitivity of 29%, specificity of 50%, and diagnostic accuracy of 43%. Plaque borders were not visible in 35% of the cases. Simple fibro-atheromatous plaques were echogenic in 72% of the cases. Echolucency occurred in 80% of stenoses with intraplaque hemorrhage, but the positive predictive value for echolucent plaques was only 43%. On the other hand, sensitivity and specificity were high, being 72% for the detection of intraplaque hemorrhages and 80% for the assessment of simple fibro-atheromatous plaques.

Summary.—Duplex scanning can reliably detect smooth, fibro-atheromatous stenoses, but it cannot reliably detect the existence of ulcerations. Furthermore, duplex scanning cannot reliably differentiate intraplaque hemorrhage from atheromatous debris.

▶ It is disappointing to repeatedly find a lack of correlation between the diagnosis of carotid ulceration and the findings of surgery.

Clinical Significance of Carotid Plaque Hemorrhage

Bornstein NM, Krajewski A, Lewis AJ, Norris JW (Univ of Toronto)
Arch Neurol 47:958–959, 1990   11–16

Introduction.—Although extracranial carotid atheromatous plaque was first identified as a cause of stroke nearly 40 years ago, the precise mechanism underlying the process is poorly understood. In addition, the importance of intraplaque hemorrhage in the genesis of ischemic hemispheric events remains unresolved. The clinical role of intraplaque hemorrhage in the pathogenesis of transient ischemic attacks (TIAs) and stroke was investigated.

Methods.—During a 30-month period, 51 men and 20 women with a mean age of 67 years underwent a total of 77 carotid endarterectomies for angiographically confirmed internal carotid artery stenosis. Symptoms included TIAs and transient monocular blindness. All of the carotid plaques specimens removed at endarterectomy were examined for appearance, including ulceration and the presence and estimated age of any hemorrhages or luminal thrombus. The time delay between symptoms and operation was also recorded.

Findings.—Intraplaque hemorrhage was seen in 66 (86%) of the 77 plaques. There were 83 hemorrhages in the 66 hemorrhagic plaques, of which 52 were deeply located and 31 were subintimal plaques. Only 11 subintimal hemorrhages were connected with the lumen (Fig 11–9). Intraplaque hemorrhages were seen predominantly in plaques with greater than 90% stenosis, but the finding of intraplaque hemorrhages had no relationship to the timing of symptoms. Luminal thrombus was seen infrequently and was always microscopic.

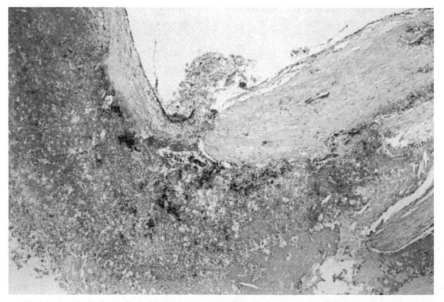

Fig 11–9.—Intraplaque hemorrhage communicating with the lumen through a fissure in the fibrous cap. (Courtesy of Bornstein NM, Krajewski A, Lewis AJ, et al: *Arch Neurol* 47:958–959, 1990.)

Conclusion.—Hemorrhage into the carotid plaque appears to be an index of stenosis severity and plaque instability, and it does not seem to have a direct role in the pathogenesis of TIAs or stroke.

▶ Intraplaque hemorrhage may reduce residual lumen rapidly, thereby converting a seemingly trivial degree of stenosis into a dangerous degree of stenosis.

Rupture of Atheromatous Plaque as a Cause of Thrombotic Occlusion of Stenotic Internal Carotid Artery
Ogata J, Masuda J, Yutani C, Yamaguchi T (Natl Cardiovascular Ctr, Osaka, Japan)
Stroke 21:1740–1745, 1990   11–17

Background.—Clinical imaging techniques and histological analysis have been used to characterize the structure of atherosclerotic plaques of the internal carotid artery (ICA), but reports that address the mechanism of fatal thrombotic occlusion of the ICA are scarce. The plaque complications that can lead to blockage and stroke mechanisms were analyzed in a retrospective analysis.

Patients.—During an 11-year period at this facility, 5 of 48 patients had autopsy-verified ICA occlusion and died within 60 days after evidencing blockage by a clot of the ICA. The cause of death was tentorial herniation caused by cerebral infarct in 3 cases, congestive heart failure in 1, and bleeding gastric ulcer in 1. At autopsy the brains and extracranial arteries of these 5 hypertensive patients were fixed and prepared for serial histological analysis at 3-mm intervals.

Results.—Although the probable mechanisms of stroke were varied (Fig 11–10), 2 features were evident in the histological analysis of the

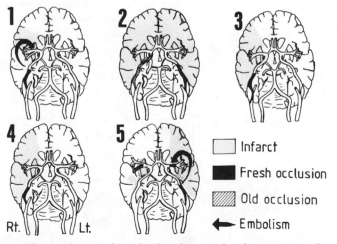

Fig 11–10—Schematic drawing of postulated mechanisms of strokes in 5 autopsied patients with thrombotic occlusion of the internal carotid artery. (Courtesy of Ogata J, Masuda J, Yutani C, et al: *Stroke* 21:1740–1745, 1990.)

blocked ICAs in all 5 cases: tight constriction of the artery caused by atheromatous plaques and breakage of the fibrous lining that covered a gruel of atheroma at or proximal to the region of greatest constriction. The arterial lumen was filled with this gruel, and blocked by a fibrin clot in 4 cases. Recent hemorrhage was evident inside the ruptured lining in 3 cases. At the location of the plaque rupture, the shortest average diameter of the ICA lumen was 1.5 mm.

Discussion.—The rupture of the fibrous lining of atheroma is known to cause thrombotic occlusion of the cerebral and coronary arteries; these results demonstrate that despite the normally greater diameter of the carotid artery, a thrombus formed by the same mechanism can block the artery when it is constricted. Prospective trials that include anticoagulant or antiplatelet therapy to treat carotid stenosis should reduce the incidence of constricted ICA blockage by clots. They should also reduce the incidence of stroke resulting from decreased cerebral perfusion or artery-to-artery embolism.

▶ Plaque rupture and plaque hemorrhage may narrow the carotid artery rapidly and cause it to become totally obstructed. Neither event is predictable, but both are associated with hypertension.

Duplex Imaging and Incidence of Carotid Radiation Injury After High-Dose Radiotherapy for Tumors of the Head and Neck
Moritz MW, Higgins RF, Jacobs JR (Wayne State Univ; Harper Hosp, Detroit)
Arch Surg 125:1181–1183, 1990   11–18

Introduction.—High-dose radiation therapy (RT) has induced disease of the arterial system in patients who have received treatment for advanced carcinomas of the head and neck. Sequential duplex ultrasound examination is suggested for follow-up in these patients.

Methods.—A total of 91 patients were studied; 53 had received RT and 38 had not. High-resolution, real-time B-mode ultrasonic imaging was used for examination of the extracranial carotid arteries, and Doppler spectrum analysis assessed the velocities.

Results.—Moderate or severe carotid artery lesions were found in 30% of the irradiated group and in 5.6% of the nonirradiated group. Of the 53 patients who received RT, 5 were symptomatic. The findings relating carotid artery disease to prior chemotherapy and radical or modified radical neck dissection were not significant.

Discussion.—High-dose RT for head and neck tumors increases the risk for carotid artery disease. These patients should be followed closely with frequent duplex scanning to detect any early irregularities that may still be asymptomatic.

▶ Because we are used to seeing advanced atherosclerotic occlusive disease in arteries that have been subjected to radiation, it is surprising that only 30% of the arteries in this study had such lesions.

Aspirin in Stroke Prevention: An Overview
Barnett HJM
Stroke 21(Suppl IV):40–43, 1990   11–19

Background.—Early pilot observations found aspirin beneficial in patients with cerebral ischemic events. Later randomized prevention trials
studied patients with transient ischemic attacks (TIAs) and minor stroke.
Various studies that have had an impact on the clarification of aspirin's
role in patients at risk for stroke were reviewed.

Review.—Ten randomized trials with a total of 7,684 patients have
evaluated and compared aspirin with placebo in the prevention of stroke.
In 1,311 patients (4 trials) no benefit from aspirin was detected. However, in 1 trial a maximum dose of 75 mg of aspirin was used; in another
study, patients who had already experienced major stroke were included.
No regimen of very-low-dose aspirin (40 mg–75 mg) has positive results
in secondary stroke-prevention studies. Two trials have compared the
benefit of aspirin and warfarin with that of placebo in patients with atrial
fibrillation without rheumatic valvular disease. One study yielded benefit
for warfarin but not for aspirin; however, more than half of the subjects
were older than age 74 years. The other study found benefit for both aspirin and warfarin, compared with placebo. In this trial the older patients
benefited least, if at all. In 3 studies that evaluated the benefit of platelet
inhibitors after myocardial infarction, the principal goal was to reduce
the risk of subsequent myocardial infarction. The subgroups analyzed for
stroke showed not-quite-significant reductions in stroke in 2 studies and
significant stroke reduction in a third. Three trials that included both
men and women tested aspirin against placebo in patients with unstable
angina; 1 of these also tested sulfinpyrazone against placebo. These studies showed risk reduction ranging from 51% to 72% with aspirin. Equal
benefit was found with doses of 325 mg/day and 1,300 mg/day. Two
large studies of 22,071 and 5,139 normal individuals found no stroke reduction with doses of 325 mg of aspirin taken every other day. Both trials raised the possibility of an increased risk for hemorrhagic stroke with
aspirin, but the numbers were very small, and neither study defined cerebral hemorrhage. It seems unlikely that aspirin poses a risk of any consequence in causing hemorrhagic stroke.

Conclusions.—Aspirin appears to be effective in secondary stroke prevention. Early evidence that women respond less well than men may result from the fact that women already have better prognoses after TIA or
stroke. Although the optimum dose of aspirin has not been established,
evidence has not shown that a larger dose (1,000 mg–1,300 mg) is less
beneficial. The benefit of aspirin has been established in patients at risk
for stroke from arteriosclerosis of the major cerebral arteries, those with
previous myocardial infarction, and those with atrial fibrillation. The
benefits relative to warfarin and ticlopidine have not been established,
and the concern about hemorrhagic infarction merits further study.

▶ This abstract states that the benefits of warfarin anticoagulation and ticlopidine as an antiplatelet agent have not been established in prevention of stroke.

A careful look at the studies cited indicates that the benefits were for the combined stroke and death morbidity rather than for the prevention of stroke alone in patients treated with aspirin. This calls into question the actual benefit of antiplatelet agents in the prevention of stroke.

Free-Floating Thrombus of the Extracranial Internal Carotid Artery
Combe J, Poinsard P, Besancenot J, Camelot G, Cattin F, Bonneville J-F, Moulin T, Henlin J-L, Chopard J-L, Cotte L (Jean Minjoz Univ Hosp Ctr, Besançon, France)
Ann Vasc Surg 4:558–562, 1990   11–20

Background.—Free-floating blood clots in the internal carotid artery (ICA) are often handled by emergency surgery or, more recently, by thrombolysis. The success of a noninvasive acute treatment with heparin followed by elective secondary surgery was appraised.

Patients.—In 6 patients, a regular, pedicled, nonocclusive filling defect at least 10 mm long was observed in the proximal ICA during biplanar

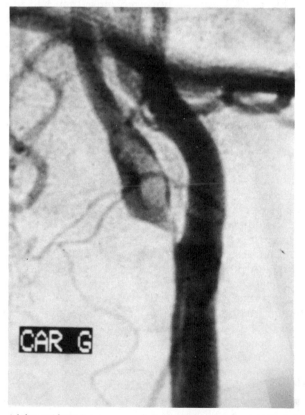

Fig 11–11.—A left carotid arteriogram upon admission showing free-floating clot and tight stenosis of the carotid artery. (Courtesy of Combe J, Poinsard P, Besancenot J, et al: *Ann Vasc Surg* 4:558–562, 1990.)

arteriography. The patients had been admitted at a mean of 15 hours after the onset of ipsilateral neurological symptoms of fixed (3 patients) or evolving (3 patients) stroke. Thrombus was suspected in only 1 patient after ultrasound studies. Focal hypodensities were found in 3 patients by CT at admission. Arteriograms obtained by retrograde catheterization of the affected ICA detected all 6 clots (Fig 11–11). The procedure aggravated neurological symptoms in 1 patient. Intravenous heparin therapy of all patients lased from 2 to 5 weeks and consisted of 3 mg/kg to 4 mg/kg of heparin daily via electric infusion pump.

Outcome.—In all of the heparin-treated patients, the initial neurological symptoms improved, and no further neurological accidents occurred. Clot dissolution, assessed by successive arteriograms and by surgery, was complete in 4 patients 25–38 days after heparin therapy was begun. Partial lysis was seen in 1 patient, and the remaining patient had moderate extension of the thrombus. Five patients later elected secondary endarterectomy. Results were good, and there were no postoperative neurological events.

Discussion.—Heparin is effective for the treatment of free-floating extracranial ICA clots in the acute phase. Because arteriography may pose an additional hazard during this phase, when sonographic studies suggest the presence of a clot, the arteriograms should be delayed until heparin therapy has been in progress for 3 weeks. Emergency surgery may not only be unnecessary but may also increase the risk of iatrogenic embolism when the clots are very friable, as in the acute phase. Heparin therapy poses little risk during the acute phase, and it offers time for a more considered approach to subsequent surgery.

▶ In this abstract it is unclear which of the patients with CT evidence of cerebral infarction had preocclusive carotid stenoses and which had ulcerated plaque. If a patient has no clinical symptoms of stroke and no CT or MRI evidence of infarction, then urgent carotid thromboendarterectomy is certainly more appropriate than 4–6 weeks of continuous intravenous heparin because of the inherent risks of cerebral hemorrhage and/or embolization.

However, when a CT or MRI scan demonstrates infarction, the age, location and extent of the infarct must be correlated with the patient's clinical neurological status. If the patient's neurological status is stable, then urgent digital subtraction arteriography with selective vessel catheterization, nonionic contrast agents, and reduced dye loads can be performed safely. Meticulous carotid dissection to prevent embolization is essential when operation is indicated, the common and external carotid arteries should be cross-clamped and an arteriotomy should be made, with the internal carotid artery allowed to back-bleed freely in the hope of removing any thromboembolic material. If no back-bleeding occurs, gentle thromboembolectomy with a Fogerty catheter is mandatory. once back-bleeding has been established, a temporary shunt should be inserted to ensure the restoration of cerebral blood flow.

If the patient has a fixed deficit, evidence of infarction by CT or MRI scan, and a "free-floating" thrombus in a patent internal carotid artery, the surgeon may be forced to operate, recognizing the increased risk for a postoperative neurological deficit. If no prograde internal carotid artery flow is demonstrated, then the intravenous heparin regimen recommended by the authors may be beneficial in retarding thrombus organization and/or proliferation of the thrombus until the infarct and the patient's neurological status stabilize before possible thrombectomy. Further evaluation of this management schema is warranted, and a multicenter-national study from France may answer the question of how best to manage these infrequent, but difficult patients.— David Rosenthal, M.D., Atlanta, Ga

---

Implications of the Angiographic String Sign in Carotid Atherosclerosis
Fredericks RK, Thomas TD, Lefkowitz DS, Troost BT (Wake Forest Univ)
Stroke 21:476–479, 1990   11–21

Objective.—Slim sign, string sign (SS), and atherosclerotic pseudo-occlusion are synonyms for a narrowing, post-stenotic region of conspicuously reduced diameter (Fig 11–12) that is associated with a high-grade lesion of the internal carotid artery (ICA) in angiograms. Patency of the lumen may be difficult to demonstrate. Nonatherosclerotic conditions may also produce SS. The clinical appearance, angiographic results, atherosclerotic risk factors, response to surgical intervention, and survival were compared in patients with ICA lesions with and without SS.

Methods.—The records of 60 patients (average age, 62.6 years) with at least 95% carotid stenosis as measured by angiography, were reviewed retrospectively. Of these patients, 28 had SS. The patients had been studied by cranial CT, delayed and subtraction angiography, continuous-wave Doppler studies, and real-time ultrasonography. The average follow-up was 8 months in the 26 SS patients and 7.3 months in the 21 non-SS patients who underwent endarterectomy.

Results.—Patients with and without SS did not differ significantly in demographics, presentation, prevalence of atherosclerotic risk factors, diameter of endarterectomy samples, or rate of perioperative complications. In patients with SS, bimodal continuous-wave Doppler frequencies were either less than 6 KHz or more than 16 KHz; in those without SS, the range was 9 KHz– 16 KHz. The Doppler studies tended to incorrectly indicate occlusion in SS patients.

Discussion.—The presence or absence of angiographic SS had no significance for the clinical appearance or outcome of patients with high-grade carotid lesions. Although real-time ultrasonography was 83% effective in showing a patent lumen, angiography may still be required to avoid unnecessary surgery.

▶ This is a curious report in which the findings contradict those of the prospective, randomized trials that have proven the dangerous nature of severe carotid artery stenosis.

Normal Angiograms and Carotid Pathology
Senkowsky J, Bell WH III, Kerstein MD (Tulane Univ, New Orleans)
Am Surg 56:726–729, 1990   11–22

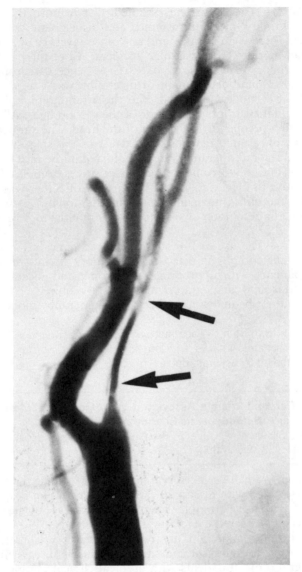

Fig 11–12.—Carotid arteriogram demonstrating long segment of poststenotic narrowing *(arrows)* consistent with string sign. (Courtesy of Fredericks RK, Thomas TD, Lefkowitz DS, et al: *Stroke* 21:476–479, 1990.)

Introduction.—Transient ischemic attacks, amaurosis fugax, and stroke may result from nonstenotic ulcerated atherosclerotic plaques of the carotid arteries. These symptoms have traditionally been investigated by ultrasound and arch aortography angiograms of the carotid bifurcation. Ultrasound is the better procedure to detect and delineate these lesions. The ultrasound findings in patients whose arteriograms were negative were analyzed.

Observations.—The 21 patients studied all had normal angiograms, abnormal real-time B-mode ultrasound, and hemispheric transient ischemic attacks. There were 15 men and 6 women, average age 66 years, 1 of whom had a prior cerebrovascular accident. All of the patients had a history of coronary artery disease or ECG evidence of coronary artery disease.The ultrasound determinant of ulceration was irregularity of the carotid wall on B-mode ultrasound, and the arteriographic determinant was wall irregularity or loss of contour of the carotid bulb. All of the patients also had a preoperative CT scan of the head. The surgical findings confirmed the ultrasound diagnosis of 20% to 50% stenosis and ulcerative plaques. The arteriograms were reevaluated in the face of these surgical findings, but only 3 could be read as positive. Computed tomography was positive in the 4 patients with a history of cerebrovascular accident and showed old lacunar infarcts in an additional 3 patients. All of the patients had a resolution of symptoms at 6 months to 3 years postoperatively.

Conclusions.—The use of B-mode ultrasound appears to be superior to the use of angiography in detecting nonstenotic lesions of the carotid artery. In patients with appropriate symptoms and ulcerative plaque shown by ultrasound, angiography may not be required before surgery. Surgery should not be done on the basis of angiography alone.

▶ The message from both the abstract and the original article is that patients with transient ischemic attacks who are found to have normal arteriograms should be re-studied by accurate duplex imaging.

Small Deep Cerebral Infarcts Associated With Occlusive Internal Carotid Artery Disease: A Hemodynamic Phenomenon?

Waterston JA, Brown MM, Butler P, Swash M (The London Hosp, London)
Arch Neurol 47:953–957, 1990   11–23

Introduction.—Small deep cerebral infarcts, or lacunae, have been traditionally associated with disease of the small perforating vessels, particularly with hypertensive arteriolar sclerosis. Any disease of the carotid arteries has been considered coincidental. However, up to 40% of the patients with lacunar infarction are not hypertensive. Therefore, other mechanisms such as embolism and carotid occlusive disease may be important. A group of 10 patients with atypical clinical findings in whom small deep cerebral infarcts were associated with ipsilateral internal carotid artery (ICA) occlusive vessel disease were evaluated.

Patients.—During a 2-year period, 7 men and 3 women (aged 42–62 years) received a diagnosis of small deep cerebral infarcts associated with severe ipsilateral ICA occlusive disease. Severe occlusive disease of the contralateral ICA was also diagnosed in 7 patients. Severe carotid stenosis was defined as a more than 75% reduction in luminal diameter. Nine patients were cigarette smokers, 6 patients had hypercholesterolemia, 4 patients had hypertension, and 4 patients had ischemic heart disease.

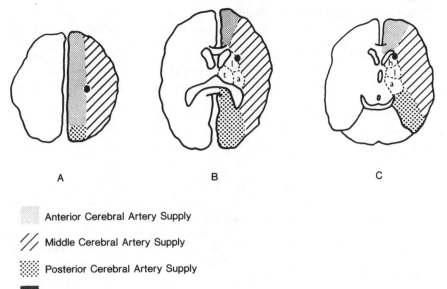

A   B   C

Anterior Cerebral Artery Supply

Middle Cerebral Artery Supply

Posterior Cerebral Artery Supply

Area of Infarction

Fig 11–13.—*Abbreviations: l* indicates lenticulostriate branches (middle cerebral artery); *t,* thalamo-perforating, thalamogeniculate, and posterior choroidal branches (posterior cerebral artery); *a,* anterior choroidal and additional branches of internal carotid artery; and *h,* Heubner's artery (anterior cerebral artery). Topography of the small deep cerebral infarcts in 10 patients, related to the arterial supply of deep border zone areas **A,** centrum semiovale and corona radiata infarction. **B,** capsular infarction. **C,** infarction in the caudate head and anterior limb of the internal capsule. (From Damasio H: *Arch Neurol* 40:138–142, 1983. Courtesy of Waterston JA, Brown MM, Butler P, et al: *Arch Neurol* 47:953–957, 1990.)

Findings.—Radiological areas of infarction on CT corresponded to the deep irrigation zones of the ICA. Most of the infarcts were located in the region of the centrum semiovale and the corona radiata. This territory is supplied by the long penetrating vessels that arise from the pial vessels. It is a border zone located between the deep cortical branches of the anterior and the middle cerebral arteries (Fig 11–13). In 3 of the patients, the infarcts were located in the region of the anterior limb of the internal capsule and the caudate head. A total of 5 patients had clinical symptoms that were highly suggestive of hemodynamic compromise. Three patients had transient limb shaking and 1 patient had syncope. Both symptoms are suggestive of an acute hemodynamic disturbance of cerebral perfusion.

Conclusion.—The clinical and radiological features in these 10 patients were consistent with hemodynamically mediated cerebral ischemia. Occlusive ICA disease in patients with hemodynamic cerebral ischemia may be more common than was recognized previously. Small cerebral infarcts in the deep arterial border zone areas appear to be an important manifestation of this process.

▶ This is an interesting study in which extracranial arteriosclerosis is found to be an important cause of lacunar infarction.

Prognosis of Asymptomatic Carotid Occlusion

Rautenberg W, Mess W, Hennerici M (Klinikum Mannheim, Univ of Heidelberg, Mannheim, Germany)
J Neurol Sci 98:213–220, 1990   11–24

Introduction.—The management of asymptomatic carotid occlusion remains controversial.

Patients/Study Design.—As part of a prospective study of neurologically asymptomatic patients with extracranial arterial disease, 94 patients with occlusion of the internal carotid artery (ICA) were followed for a mean 44 months. An additional 27 patients in whom stenosis progressed to occlusion were followed up for a mean 47.5 months.

Outcome.—Of the 94 asymptomatic patients with ICA occlusion, 16% had a stroke and 11.7% had transient ischemic attacks (TIAs). About half of these events occurred ipsilateral to the occluded ICA. The annual stroke rate was 4.4% and the annual TIA rate was 3.2%, with an annual mortality rate of 11.3%. In contrast, of the 27 asymptomatic patients whose extracranial arterial disease progressed to occlusion during follow-up, 7.4% had a stroke and 18.5% had TIAs. This represented an annual stroke rate of 1.9% and an annual TIA rate of 4.7%. Thus, although the annual stroke rate was lower, the TIA rate was higher compared with the post-occlusive rates.

Conclusions.—These data suggest an increased risk of stroke in patients with progressive high-degree carotid stenosis that continues after occlusion. Carotid endarterectomy is recommended for selected asymptomatic patients with progressing carotid stenoses.

▶ The dangerous nature of ICA occlusion is now recognized and, as the authors say, "This may favor carotid endarterectomy for selected patients in the preocclusive state because medical treatment has not been shown to prevent progression of stenosis to occlusion."

The Diminishing Role of Diagnostic Arteriography in Carotid Artery Disease: Duplex Scanning as Definitive Preoperative Study

Wagner WH, Treiman RL, Cossman DV, Foran RF, Levin PM, Cohen JL (Cedars-Sinai Med Ctr, Los Angeles)
Ann Vasc Surg 5:105–110, 1991   11–25

Background.—Most surgeons still require a carotid arteriogram before performing a carotid endarterectomy (CEA), but this requirement is debated. Some researchers have reported doing CEA without arteriography in specially selected patients. The results of 260 CEAs performed without prior arteriograms were assessed.

Methods.—Between January 1984 and December 1989, 612 patients underwent 753 CEAs, 98% of which were elective. The mean age for the 294 men and 318 women was 71 years. A total of 10 patients had a combined CEA and coronary artery bypass. Stenosis in the common, external, and internal carotid arteries was assessed by Fast Fourier Transform spectral analysis. The endarterectomy results were divided into these procedures performed after duplex scans alone and those performed after arteriography.

Findings.—The percentage of CEAs performed without angiography has continued to increase since 1984. During 1988 and 1989, 32% of CEAs were done after arteriography, and most of these were ordered by the referring physician and not the surgeon. Eleven of the patients had arteriograms without any prior noninvasive procedures. At endarterectomy, the presurgical scan results were confirmed in each patient in the duplex scan group, all 225 of whom had significant bifurcation pathology. The indications for surgery for the duplex scan group and for the arteriography group were similar. Patients who left the hospital with a new central neurological deficit were considered to have had a stroke. No statistically significant differences in stroke incidence or mortality were observed between the diagnostic groups.

Conclusions.—When duplex scans are used by appropriately trained technicians they can accurately evaluate a patient's cervical carotid bifurcation. With selective use of cerebral arteriography, one can minimize neurological local, and systemic morbidity and contain cost without compromising the patient's surgical outcome.

▶ At this point in the progression of our knowledge of preoperative carotid imaging, we can conclude that excellent duplex scans can effectively obviate the need for arteriography. The next step, of course, is for excellent MR angiography to replace standard contrast, invasive arteriography. Because MR tends to overread atherosclerotic occlusive disease, the duplex scan will undoubtedly remain a part of the diagnostic armamentarium.

Carotid Surgery Without Arteriography: Noninvasive Selection of Patients
Gertler JP, Cambria RP, Kistler JP, Geller SC, MacDonald NR, Brewster DC, Abbott WM (Massachusetts Gen Hosp, Boston)
Ann Vasc Surg 5:253–256, 1991   11–26

Background.—Arteriographic complications are well recognized in using this technique to diagnose carotid disease. Noninvasive criteria were established to identify situations in which arteriography was not required before carotid endarterectomy (CEA). These criteria were based on the correlation between carotid stenosis in CEA specimens and spectral frequency results.

Methods.—A group of 40 symptomatic and 104 asymptomatic internal carotid arteries were studied by arteriography and noninvasive techniques between 1985 and 1987. The noninvasive studies included duplex scanning, spectral frequency analysis, and ocular-pneumoplethysmography-Gee or supraorbital Doppler assessments. The studies were re-reviewed prospectively and in blinded fashion.

Results.—Using peak frequency, 39 of 40 symptomatic internal carotid arteries were identified noninvasively to be appropriate for CEA. All had arteriographically confirmed internal carotid artery stenosis of greater than 50%, and 22 met the noninvasive surgical criteria of a peak systolic frequency-internal carotid artery greater than 14 mHz, a carotid index greater than 7, and an abnormal ocular-pneumoplethysmography-Gee or supraorbital Doppler. Stenosis greater than 80% on arteriographic examination had been confirmed in all of these.

Conclusions.—More than 1 noninvasive modality should be used in evaluation of the carotid disease, and stringent criteria must be met before arteriography is rendered unnecessary. Each patient must be judged on an individual basis.

▶ Abstracts 11–25 and 11–26 stress the need for routine CEA in every preoperative case; however, is this true?

Significance of Transcranial Doppler CO₂ Reactivity Measurements for the Diagnosis of Hemodynamically Relevant Carotid Obstructions
Reith W, Pfadenhauer K, Loeprecht H (Zentralklinikum Augsburg, Augsburg, Germany)
Ann Vasc Surg 4:359–364, 1990   11–27

Introduction.—Transcranial Doppler ultrasonography allows noninvasive and simple measurement of CO_2 reactivity in the large basal cerebral arteries.

Study Design.—Using transcranial Doppler ultrasonography, the mean blood flow velocities in the middle cerebral arteries were determined during normocapnia, hypercapnia after inhalation of a mixture of 5% CO_2 and 95% oxygen, hypocapnia under hyperventilation, and normocapnia again. The CO_2 reactivity was expressed as the percentage increase in mean flow velocity between 40 mm Hg and 46.5 mm Hg of PCO_2. This was called the normalized autoregulatory reserve (NAR). Studies were performed in 49 normal individuals (mean age, 43.2) and 218 patients with documented stenoses or occlusions of the internal carotid artery.

Findings.—The mean NAR value in the normal population was 31.3; the lowest value measured was 16. When an NAR value of 15 was used as the lower limit of normal, patients with internal carotid artery obstructions were well separated from the normal controls. Stenoses of the internal carotid artery that were ≥70% resulted in a significant decrease of NAR in the ipsilateral middle cerebral artery, which could be normalized by the removal of the upstream flow obstacle by carotid thromboendarterectomy. In severe internal carotid obstructions, the scatter of NAR values indicated the variability of collateral circulation. In patients with ischemic deficits, the clinical symptoms correlated significantly with reduced NAR values in the ipsilateral supply area of the internal carotid artery.

Conclusion.—Transcranial Doppler ultrasonography can be used to determine CO_2 reactivity in the large basal cerebral arteries. The CO_2 reactivity of the middle cerebral artery correlates with the degree of stenosis of the ipsilateral carotid artery and with ipsilateral ischemic symptoms.

▶ This article by Reith et al. is a well-designed and authoritative study on the increasing awareness of the necessity to perform physiological studies examining the effects that extracranial arterial occlusive disease might have on intracranial blood flow. These possible effects have been overestimated in the past because the predominant mechanism of stroke is not low flow effect but thromboembolic. However, despite this, there is a small subgroup of patients who experience cerebral insufficiency, strokes, and ischemic eye disease that are caused by critically reduced cerebral blood flow. As the study points out, the variability of the cerebral collateral system via the circle of WIllis prevents us from making physiological determinants based on the degree of extracranial stenosis alone. Critical decisions, including those of surgery, must be based on hemodynamic information.

A number of reports that are now in the literature (including this recent publication) demonstrate this important point. All of these studies identify true cases of cerebrovascular insufficiency in which cerebral blood flow is insufficient to maintain adequate compensation. These patients may benefit from surgical measures to improve flow, such as extracranial intracranial bypass surgery, carotid endarterectomy, or even other recanalization techniques. The identification of this subgroup of stroke prone individuals must be based on the detection of exhausted cerebrovascular reserve, not on the extent of extracranial vascular disease.

Cerebrovascular physiologists have long been aware of the ability to identify this group of patients and they have done so by a number of techniques, including regional cerebral blood flow and positron emission tomography. Despite this available information, these studies have not been commonly used, possibly because of their invasiveness, expensiveness, or availability. Perhaps transcranial Doppler ultrasonography will fill this gap.

Although transcranial Doppler ultrasonography has some inherent problems that are appropriately pointed out in this study, it lends itself nicely to these examinations. Using measures of CO_2 reactivity avoids the inherent problems of flow versus velocity and measures what we really need to know, such as the patient's vascular reserve. Until a method like this can be utilized regularly, we will not be able to make authoritative decisions regarding the efficacy and risk of vascular recanalization techniques. This study demonstrates the ease and accuracy of transcranial Doppler ultrasonography vasomotor testing, and it should be read by all surgeons who are involved in this type of vascular work. See also Reference 1.—S.M. Otis, M.D., Head, Division of Neurology, Scripps Clinic and Research Foundation, La Jolla, California

Reference

1. Ringelstein EB, et al: *Stroke* 19:963, 1988.

Pre- and Intraoperative Transcranial Doppler: Prediction and Surveillance of Tolerance to Carotid Clamping

Benichou H, Bergeron P, Ferdani M, Jausseran J-M, Reggi M, Courbier R (Fondation Hôpital Saint-Joseph, Marseilles, France)
Ann Vasc Surg 5:21–25, 1991   11–28

Background.—Transcranial Doppler (TCD) scanning can directly measure blood flow velocity in the main cerebral arteries, particularly the middle cerebral artery (MCA). The ability of TCD to predict hemodynamic tolerance to carotid cross-clamping, to correlate velocity with mean stump pressure (SP), and to monitor shunt function was evaluated in 100 carotid revascularizations in 91 patients, aged 49–85 years. The revascularizations were performed during a 1-year period.

Methods.—The TCD was performed preoperatively, intraoperatively, and postoperatively in 85 patients. Based on the results of the preoperative examination, patients were classified into 2 groups. Group A comprised 72 procedures in 65 patients who did not require an intraoperative indwelling shunt. Group B comprised 20 procedures in 20 patients who required a shunt. When the mean SP after cross-clamping was less than 50 mm Hg, a shunt was inserted. In group A, all of the patients had satisfactory collateral circulation with 1 functional anterior and 1 or 2 posterior communicating arteries. No communicating arteries were seen on TCD in the group B patients, 17 of whom had a shunt because of SP less than 50 mm Hg.

Results.—Scanning with TCD was able to predict whether a shunt was required in 88 (95.6%) of 92 cases, the mean MCA velocity was 37 cm/second in group A and 13 cm/second in group B. Shunt insertion increased the mean MCA velocity from 13 cm/second to 36 cm/second. In addition, TCD discovered 4 cavernous and 2 MCA stenoses that were hemodynamically significant. When correlated with arteriographic findings, the sensitivity of TCD was 70% and the specificity was 90%.

Conclusion.—When used preoperatively, TCD can measure the velocities of the main cerebral arteries and the collateral capacity of the circle of Willis. It is also useful in predicting the patient's tolerance to carotid cross-clamping. When used intraoperatively, TCD can correlate the flow velocity in the MCA with SP, thus allowing shunt surveillance. Scanning with TCD may provide useful data for the pathophysiological study of neurological events.

▶ Time will tell whether or not TCD information is important.

Carotid Endarterectomy for Asymptomatic Carotid Stenosis: An Update

Thompson JE (Baylor Univ Med Ctr)
J Vasc Surg 13:669–676, 1991   11–29

Background.—The advisability of performing arteriography and carotid endarterectomy on patients with asymptomatic carotid stenosis is controversial. The factors that currently seem to predict an increased incidence of stroke in patients with symptomatic carotid stenoses were reviewed in an attempt to better define the indications for carotid endarterectomy.

Discussion.—The literature suggests that, after noninvasive screening and arteriography, several specific indications for carotid endarterectomy can be identified. These indications are the presence of severe unilateral stenosis of greater than 70%; bilateral stenoses greater than 50%; unilateral stenosis and contralateral occlusion; stenosis progressing to more than 50%; positive noninvasive tests, such as duplex scan, spectral analysis, ocular pneumoplethysmography (OPG), and possibly CT and MRI; and a markedly ulcerated plaque. Carotid endarterectomy should be performed before other major surgery if the noninvasive tests and arteriography are strongly positive.

Conclusions.—When patients are selected properly, the angiography is done by skillful clinicians, and the appropriate surgery is performed by experienced operators, operative mortality and morbidity rates associated with carotid endarterectomy are low and the immediate results are excellent. When these conditions are met, asymptomatic patients seem to have better outcomes than their nonoperated counterparts in terms of subsequent cerebral ischemic episodes.

▶ Now that we have received the prospective, randomized trial results, the prophetic words of Jesse Thompson are interesting to reread.

Carotid Endarterectomy for Asymptomatic Carotid Stenosis: A Ten-Year Experience With 120 Procedures in a Fellowship Training Program
Anderson RJ, Hobson RW II, Padberg FT Jr, Pecoraro JP, DeGroote RD, Jamil Z, Lee BC, Breitbart GB, Franco CD (University of Medicine and Dentistry of New Jersey-New Jersey Med School)
Ann Vasc Surg 5:111–115, 1991   11–30

Introduction.—The use of the carotid endarterectomy procedure to treat asymptomatic carotid stenosis is controversial, possibly because of the lack of data from prospective and randomized clinical trials testing this technique. The immediate and long-term results of the carotid endarterectomy for the asymptomatic condition were assessed in 120 patients during the past decade to test the theory that the success of this treatment depends on the technical skill of the surgeon and the perioperative care of the patient.

Methods.—Between January 1979 and January 1989, 512 carotid endarterectomies were performed; 120 of these were in asymptomatic patients. The pre-operative and postoperative noninvasive techniques used to assess the patients included ocular pneumoplethysmography (OPG-Gee) only before 1980 and, after 1980, OPG-Gee and real-time B-mode ultrasonography and Doppler spectrum analysis. All of the patients underwent biplanar arteriography before the carotid endarterectomy.

Technique.—Important details of the surgery included the use of arterial lines in all patients to measure arterial pressure and to control hypotensive or hypertensive variations during anesthesia induction, the operative procedure, and the postoperative period. The dissection of the artery was aided with visualization and protection of the cranial nerves. A routine shunt was installed, the placement of which was rehearsed before the surgery. Then the total endarterectomy surface was cleared of smooth muscle fibers to avoid embolization of debris.

Results.—Of the 120 patients who underwent this procedure, 22 (18%) were women and 98 (82%) were men (average patient age, 65.6 years). Restenosis during the postoperative period did not produce any overt symptoms. Although no perioperative strokes or deaths occurred, 2 patients experienced transient neurological events (1 case of amaurosis fugax and 1 of right hemiparesis). The overall survival 6 years after surgery in this series of 120 patients was 79%.

Implications.—These findings support the conclusion that carotid endarterectomy performed on asymptomatic carotid stenosis patients is an effective and safe procedure. Low morbidity resulted from close attention to technical proficiency during the operative procedure.

▶ The wisdom derived from focused retrospective studies is valuable and much less costly than that derived from prospective, randomized, multi-institutional trials.

New Triple Coaxial Catheter System for Carotid Angioplasty With Cerebral Protection
Theron J, Courtheoux P, Alachkar F, Bouvard G, Maiza D (Ctr Hospitalier Universitaire de Caen, Caen, France)
Am J Neuroradiol 11:869–874, 1990   11–31

Introduction.—The fear of dislodging an embolus from an ulcerative plaque in patients undergoing percutaneous transluminal angioplasty (PTA) of a stenotic carotid artery has led to the development of a catheter system designed to protect the cerebral circulation during PTA. With this technique, the flow within the internal carotid artery is arrested temporarily during the manipulation of the ulcerated plaques. A new triple coaxial catheter system was developed to simplify the technique.

Patients.—A total of 13 patients, aged 55–77 years, with stenosis of a carotid artery ranging from 70% to more than 95% underwent PTA with the complete triple coaxial system. The angiograms of 5 patients showed obviously ulcerated plaques. All of the patients underwent Doppler studies before and after treatment. The mean follow-up period was 8.5 months.

Results.—In 10 of the 13 patients, a normal or subnormal diameter of the dilated carotid artery was obtained. The aspirated blood was analyzed for 6 patients. Large cholesterol crystals of 600 μm–1,200 μm was seen in 4 samples. Of the 3 patients in whom a normal or subnormal diameter was not obtained, 1 had a 30% residual stenosis on the immediate postangioplasty angiogram. However, the arterial wall had a smooth appearance and there was no residual hemodynamic modification at Doppler examination. The second patient had a persistent 50% stenosis of the internal carotid artery that was hemodynamically significant at Doppler. The third patient had a 20% residual stenosis that was not significant at Doppler. None of the patients experienced local or neurological complications during or after angioplasty, and none had further symptoms since undergoing the procedure.

Conclusion.— The new triple coaxial catheter system for carotid angioplasty that incorporates cerebral protection appears to prevent iatrogenic emboli from reaching the cerebral circulation.

▶ One can't help but be troubled by the statement that this method prevents *most* emboli from reaching the cerebral circulation.

Carotid Endarterectomy for Chronic Retinal Ischemia
Rubin JR, McIntyre KM, Lukens MC, Plecha EJ, Bernhard VM (Case Western Reserve Univ School of Medicine; Univ of Arizona Medical Center)
Surg Gynecol Obstet 171:497–501, 1990   11–32

Background.— Carotid arterial disease can cause a number of ischemic ocular problems that could lead to permanent blindness. Investigators have reported variable results with carotid endarterectomy (CEA) performed for ischemic oculopathy. A total of 18 patients who underwent carotid arterial reconstruction for chronic retinal ischemias studied to determine the effectiveness of restoring normal ophthalmic arterial flow.

Methods.— Of the 18 patients, 13 were men, 14 were hypertensive, 6 had diabetes mellitus, 12 were cigarette smokers, 5 had coronary arterial disease, and 1 had renal failure. Whereas 11 patients had either visual loss or decreased visual acuity, 5 had pain. The patients underwent macular photostress testing, ophthalmodynamometry, axial CT, and duplex scanning. Whereas 12 patients underwent standard CEA, 3 underwent bilateral staged CEA, 2 underwent external CEA and Barnett's stump ligation, and 1 underwent staged ipsilateral internal and contralateral external CEA.

Results.— None of the patients had preoperative stroke or died within 30 days of surgery. Fourteen of 16 eyes had subjective improvement in periorbital and eye pain, as well as visual improvement. One patient had recurrent episodes of amaurosis fugax that resolved after 14 days. Another had continued visual deterioration and eye pain. After a mean 21-month follow-up, visual acuity had improved in 6 patients and was unchanged in 11 patients; 1 patient had deterioration in acuity alone. Macular photostress testing showed attenuation in the visual evoked response in 14 of 16 eyes that had previously had prolonged recovery times. Despite medical treatment, intraocular pressures continued to increase in 1 patient, and panretinal laser photocoagulation was required. Intraocular pressures decreased subsequently, and visual impairment stabilized—but only after substantial loss.

Conclusions.—Carotid arterial reconstruction is an effective treatment for ischemic oculopathy. It is most effective when performed early, before irreversible neurovascular glaucoma occurs.

▶ When retinal ischemia is the indication for carotid endarterectomy, it must be remembered that worsening of neovascular glaucoma can occur, presumably secondary to the increased blood flow to the ciliary body. This causes an increased aqueous humor production and an obstructed filtering and absorption angle.

Carotid Endarterectomy for Elderly Patients: Predicting Complications
Brook RH, Park RE, Chassin MR, Kosecoff J, Keesey J, Solomon DH (Rand Corp, Santa Monica, Calif; Univ of California, Los Angeles Ctr for the Health Sciences; Value Health Sciences, Los Angeles)
Ann Intern Med 113:747–753, 1990   11–33

Objective.—The efficacy of carotid endarterectomy remains controversial. Whether the complication or death rate from carotid endarterectomy for elderly patients can be predicted from hospital and physician structural variables was investigated.

Method.—The records of 1,032 patients, 65 years and older, who underwent carotid endarterectomy in 3 geographic areas in the United States during 1981 were reviewed. After controlling for the severity of patients' illness and comorbid conditions, regression analyses were used to predict the postoperative stroke, heart attack, and 30-day mortality rate as a function of patient, physician, and hospital characteristics.

Findings.—A total of 11% of the patients had a postoperative stroke, heart attack, or died within 30 days of operation. The risk for adverse outcomes after carotid endarterectomy was not significantly related to patient age, race, income, and gender; physician volume, board certification status, and age; and hospital size, profit status, ownership, and teaching status. The probability of complication was higher when the endarterectomy was performed by a surgeon who was a graduate of a foreign, but not a Western European or Canadian, medical school.

Summary.—It appears that complications after carotid endarterectomy, in general, cannot be predicted from the structural variables defining physician or hospital characteristics. Physicians should consider the surgeon's and hospital's actual postoperative complication and death rate when referring patients for carotid endarterectomy.

▶ To put it another way, the complications of carotid surgery are in the hands of the surgeon.

Community Hospital Carotid Endarterectomy in Patients Over Age 75
Maxwell JG, Rutherford EJ, Covington DL, Churchill P, Patrick RD, Scott C, Clancy TV (Univ of North Carolina School of Medicine; New Hanover Memorial

Hosp, Wilmington, NC; Area Health Education Ctr, Wilmington, NC)
Am J Surg 160:598–603, 1990   11–34

Background.—The number of carotid endarterectomies performed yearly in the United States has increased 500% in the past decade. This increase has been accompanied by mounting concern over whether the benefits outweigh the risks and complications, especially in elderly patients who have anticipated higher risks of surgery. The outcome of carotid endarterectomy performed by general surgeons in a community hospital was examined.

Methods.—The prevalence of stroke and death in patients older than 75 years was compared with that in patients younger than 75 years. A total of 133 patients older than 75 years underwent 170 endarterectomies, whereas 501 patients younger than 75 years underwent 640 procedures.

Results.—Of the older patients, 3 (2%) had strokes, whereas 9 (1%) of the younger patients had strokes; 8 (5%) of the older patients and 14 (2%) of the younger patients died. A logistic regression model, controlled for the possible effects of prior stroke, diabetes, history of angina, prior carotid artery disease, history of myocardial infarction, previous vascular surgery, preoperative hypertension requiring medication, and female gender revealed that patients aged 75 or older were no more likely to have stroke or death than younger patients.

Conclusions.—Age alone is not a contraindication for the safe performance of endarterectomy. However, elderly patients may have risk factors not found in a younger population. In this study, risk factors were a history of myocardial infarction and hypertension requiring medication. There was no evidence that surgeons who perform occasional carotid endarterectomy have worse outcomes than surgeons who perform the procedure frequently.

▶ Data show that there is no patient age at which this operation cannot be done safely.

Cerebral Vasoreactivity and Blood Flow Before and 3 Months After Carotid Endarterectomy

Russell D, Dybevold S, Kjartansson O, Nyberg-Hansen R, Rootwelt K, Wiberg J (Rikshospitalet, The National Hosp, Univ of Oslo)
Stroke 21:1029–1032, 1990   11–35

Background.—The effects of carotid endarterectomy on cerebral blood flow (CBF) and intracranial hemodynamics have not been established. Therefore, 14 selected patients who experienced cerebral transient ischemic attacks (TIA) caused by ipsilateral internal carotid artery (CA) stenosis were studied.

Methods.—Regional CBF (rCBF) was assessed using xenon-133 inhalation with single photon emission computed tomography, and cerebral vasoreactivity was assessed using the acetazolamide test both before and 3 months after carotid endarterectomy. The median interval from the last TIA to carotid endarterectomy was 15 days (range, 10–33 days). None of the patients had clinical or cerebral CT evidence of infarction. A group of 25 healthy subjects served as controls.

Findings.—Before endarterectomy, the baseline rCBF was symmetrical and did not differ significantly from that of controls. Cerebral vasoreactivity in the middle cerebral artery (CA) and/or anterior CA territories was significantly reduced on the symptomatic side, compared with the contralateral side and controls. Three months after surgery, the rCBF remained unchanged, but cerebral vasoreactivity in the middle CA and/or anterior CA were symmetrical and within normal limits.

Conclusion.—These data strongly suggest that ICA stenosis causes a reduction in cerebral perfusion reserve that improves with carotid endarterectomy. Although the clinical implications of these findings are not clear, they may prove important in the assessment of prognosis and selection of patients for carotid endarterectomy.

▶ It is reassuring to note that clinical improvement is now corroborated by objective measurements of CBF.

Vein Patch Rupture After Carotid Endarterectomy: A Survey of the Western Vascular Society Members
Tawes RL, Treiman RL (San Mateo, Calif)
Ann Vasc Surg 5:71–73, 1991   11–36

Background.—Vein patch angioplasty has been used for closure of the carotid artery after endarterectomy. The rupture or blowout of the patch is uncommon, and most surgeons have had little experience with this complication. The members of the Western Vascular Society were surveyed to determine the prevalence, demographics, and morbidity of vein patch ruptures.

Methods.—Of the 90 vascular surgeons surveyed, 48 reported experience in 23,873 carotid operations, including use of a vein patch in 1,760 operations. Rupture occurred from a split in the saphenous vein patch in 13 patients. There were 2 ruptures on postoperative day 1, 6 on day 2, 3 on day 3, 1 on day 8, and 1 on day 21.

Findings.—Death was caused by airway obstruction in 1 patient, hemorrhagic cerebral infarction in 1, and myocardial infarction in 2; 3 patients survived a stroke, 1 had a retinal embolus, and 5 underwent uneventful reoperation.

Conclusion.—The incidence of vein patch rupture is low, but when it occurs, there is significant mortality and morbidity. To facilitate immediate re-operation, patients with a vein patch should be observed in the hospital for 3 days after endarterectomy.

▶ The vein was harvested from the ankle in 12 of the 13 vein patch ruptures.

Distal Internal Carotid Exposure: A Simplified Technique for Temporary Mandibular Subluxation
Dossa C, Shepard AD, Wolford DG, Reddy DJ, Ernst CB (Henry Ford Hosp, Detroit; St Clair Shores, Mich)
J Vasc Surg 12:319–325, 1990   11–37

Introduction.—Distal internal carotid artery (ICA) exposure remains a technically demanding procedure even for experienced vascular surgeons. Temporary mandibular subluxation (TMS) is the simplest and least debilitating approach among the several procedures suggested to facilitate distal ICA exposure. However, current techniques for maintaining TMS for distal ICA exposure are time consuming and associated with complications. A new simplified technique of TMS for distal ICA exposure was used in 14 patients.

Surgical Technique.—Unilateral TMS is maintained by interdental wiring from the ipsilateral mandibular bicuspids to the contralateral maxillary bicuspids in patients with healthy teeth, and with diagonal wiring between maxillary and mandibular Steinmann pins in edentulous patients or in those with periodontal disease. The mandibular condyle should be positioned onto or just beyond the articular eminence of the zygoma because further displacement forward will result in dislocation of the condyle into the infratemporal fossa. Both techniques require less than 10 minutes to complete.

Results.—Distal ICA exposure was necessary for extended carotid endarterectomy in 8 patients, carotid body tumor excision in 2, repair of distal ICA trauma in 2, and repair of post-endarterectomy pseudoaneurysm in 2. Exposure of the distal ICA was adequate for all vascular procedures, and none of the patients experienced malocclusion, dental injury, or infection. Three patients had transient postoperative cranial nerve dysfunction, and another 3 had transient ipsilateral temporomandibular joint pain. Two patients had permanent cranial nerve dysfunction that was not related to TMS.
Summary.—Unilateral TMS by diagonal wiring technique is safe, expeditious, and effective for facilitating distal ICA exposure.

▶ Although temporary mandibular subluxation may be useful, it may also be dangerous. This danger occurs when extreme condylar dislocation results in a compression of the contralateral carotid sheath between the mandible and the transverse vertebral processes when the head is turned for performance of the operation.

Does Carotid Restenosis Predict an Increased Risk of Late Symptoms, Stroke, or Death?
Bernstein EF, Torem S, Dilley RB (Scripps Clinic and Research Found, La Jolla, Calif)
Ann Surg 212:629–636, 1990   11–38

Background.—The identification of carotid restenosis as an unexpected late complication of carotid endarterectomy may be important as a source of new cerebral symptoms, stroke, or death. A 9% rate of carotid restenosis has previously been verified postoperatively by angiography. The ramifications for later stroke and death were examined in restenoses verified by duplex scanning.

Methods.—Vascular and clinical data from 430 patients who underwent 484 carotid endarterectomies were collected at 1, 3, 6, and 12 months, then annually for an average of 41.9 months. Of these patients, 64% were male, 76.4% were smokers, and 12.4% were diabetic. The degree of stenosis at the carotid bifurcation was determined by spectral analysis of duplex scans. This noninvasive method has an overall accuracy rate of 86%, and a sensitivity of 90% for discerning lesions of 50%

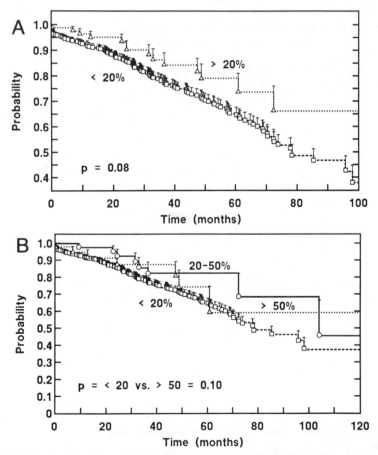

Fig 11–14.—A, effect of any degree (more than 20%) of carotid restenosis on the probability of remaining free of any subsequent cerebrovascular event (amaurosis fugax, anterior or posterior transient ischemic attack, stroke, or death). **B,** probability of remaining free of subsequent cerebrovascular events is plotted against degrees of carotid restenosis. (Courtesy of Bernstein EF, Torem S, Dilley RB: *Ann Surg* 212:629–636, 1990.)

to 99% compared with formal contrast angiography. The absence of an internal carotid flow signal indicated occlusion.

Results.—In 63.2% of the arteries, carotid bifurcations were normal in duplex scans throughout the follow-up period. However in a restenosis group (10.1% of arteries), at least a 50% restenosis was verified some time after the normal postoperative evaluation. Restenosis or occlusion occurred significantly more often in females (14.5%), than in males (8%). Among the 49 patients in the restenosis group, life expectancy improved significantly with increasing restenosis; those patients with 50% or greater or 20% or greater restenosis lived longer than those with no stenosis or mild stenosis. The effects of restenosis on subsequent fatal plus nonfatal cerebrovascular events are illustrated in Figure 11–14. Most of the restenoses were identified at an early stage of development during the first postoperative year.

Discussion.—These data suggest that asymptomatic carotid restenosis is a benign event, and that affected patients may gain some degree of protection against subsequent cerebrovascular events. Recurrent stenosis, as distinct from residual stenosis, should be treated conservatively. Surgery is not recommended unless the threat of occlusion is imminent or symptoms appear.

▶ Restenosis after carotid endarterectomy is a fact of life. Therefore, it is helpful to know that the process may be quite benign and that it is therefore considerably different from atherosclerotic stenosis.

Redo Endarterectomy for Recurrent Carotid Artery Stenosis
Gagne PJ, Riles TS, Imparato AM, Lamparello PJ, Giangola G, Landis RM (New York Univ Med Ctr)
Eur J Vasc Surg 5:135–140, 1991   11–39

Introduction.—Many variables are used to calculate the incidence of recurrent stenosis after carotid endarterectomy; this is reflected in the broad range (1.5% to 49%) of reported prevalence. The effect of operative technique on restenosis was examined and the long-term outcome of secondary endarterectomy was assessed.

Methods.—Between 1970 and 1988, 2,406 carotid bifurcation reconstructions were performed on 1,818 patients with an average age of 65 years. Of these patients, 29 (1.6% of the total group) underwent both primary operations and re-operation for recurrent stenosis during this period; data from these 29 patients were evaluated. The technique of the original surgery was endarterectomy with vein-patch angioplasty in 26 patients and endarterectomy with primary closure in the remainder. There was no evidence of residual stenosis in the 16 patients who were tested shortly after primary surgery. Re-operation was performed for the reappearance of neurological symptoms in 23 patients, and for asymptomatic restenosis of at least 80% in 6 patients. Repeat endarterectomy and patch angioplasty were done in 27 patients, and patch angioplasty alone was done in 2.

Results.—Patients who had restenosis were significantly younger (average age, 59 years) at the time of their primary surgery, and they were the same age as the larger group at re-operation an average of 5.5 years later. No differences in the interval to re-operation were attributable to the original surgical techniques. In contrast, the pathology of the restenosis appeared to influence this interval to reoperation; in the 27% with myo-intimal hyperplasia, the average interval was 29 months, compared with 84 months in the 53% with atherosclerosis and 65 months among the 17% with thrombus and vessel dilation. Patients required a third operation at 55, 79, and 129 months after the second operation. The incidence of tertiary restenosis was 21%. Short-term mortality was 0; 6 patients died of causes other than cerebrovascular disease during the average 50-month follow-up period after the second surgery, and 1 died of stroke.

Discussion.—The relatively low incidence of restenosis in this study may be caused by the customary use of the vein patch technique at this institution; this would be consistent with the results of several studies that have found this approach to be superior to others. The relative youth of patients who have restenosis suggests that they may have a more malignant form of the disease. The high incidence of tertiary restenosis, implies that the risk is 10 times greater after secondary surgery than after primary endarterectomy. It is not yet known whether this is attributable to host factors or to failure of the second operation.

▶ In this study, a recurrence of neurological symptoms was the chief reason for re-operation. In 5 of these 23 patients, the symptoms were monocular, and in 10, motor and speech symptoms were present. A total of 8 patients had cerebrovascular accidents, suggesting that Abstract 11–38 may have been looking

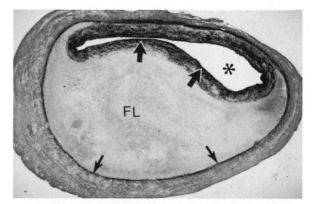

Fig 11–15.—Cross-section of a segment of an elongated dissecting aneurysm (posttraumatic in this case) demonstrates section through the internal carotid artery (ICA) and the related dissecting aneurysm. Note that the aneurysm is formed within the media. The external elastic lamina *(thin arrows)* surrounds both the true lumen of the ICA *(asterisk)* and the thrombus-filled false lumen of the aneurysm *(FL)*. The false lumen has compressed the true lumen *(thick arrows)*. (Courtesy of Mokri B: *J Neurol* 237:356–361, 1990.)

at a different patient category. Carotid restenosis may not be a benign pathological process.

Traumatic and Spontaneous Extracranial Internal Carotid Artery Dissections

Mokri B (Mayo Clinic and Found)
J Neurol 237:356–361, 1990

11–40

Background.—Although both traumatic and spontaneous extracranial internal carotid artery (ICA) dissections usually have a good prognosis, the 2 types were compared for clinical and angiographic features and outcome to determine which was more favorable.

Methods.—A group of 21 patients with traumatic and 70 patients with spontaneous extracranial ICA dissections were evaluated clinically

Frequency of Symptoms and Signs in 70 Patients With Spontaneous and 21 Patients With Traumatic Dissections of Extracranial Internal Carotid Arteries

Symptom or sign	Patient group			
	Spontaneous		Traumatic	
	No.	%	No.	%
Headache	59	84	8	38
Focal cerebral ischemic symptoms	43	61	15*	71
TIAs	24		2	
Stroke	13		11	
TIAS and stroke	6		2	
Oculosympathetic paresis	37	53	7	33
Bruits (subjective, objective, or both)	32	46	8	38
Neck pain	16	23	1†	
Light-headedness	15	21		
Syncope	8		2	
Amaurosis fugax	8		1	
Scalp tenderness	5			
Neck swelling	3			
Dysgeusia	2			
Lower cranial nerve palsies	2			
Asymptomatic ‡	1			
Sensation of pulsation in neck	1		1	

Abbreviation: TIA, transient ischemic attack.
*Often delayed after the accident: within 30 minutes to 12 hours in 6 patients; within 4–20 days in 3; in 2 months in 1; and after 6–10 years in 5.
†Excluding any neck pain in connection with the original trauma.
‡Symptoms related to a concomitant vertebral artery dissection.
(Courtesy of Mokri B: *J Neurol* 237:356–361, 1990.)

and angiographically. Angiographic follow-ups were done in 60% of the spontaneous group and in 71% of the traumatic group.

Results.—Compared with the spontaneous dissection group, the traumatic dissection group was more likely have significant neurological deficits. Angiography demonstrated that the traumatic group also had more aneurysms (Fig 11–15) and more stenoses progressing to occlusion. Finally, a significantly higher percentage of patients who underwent spontaneous dissections were asymptomatic at follow-up compared with those who underwent traumatic dissections. The frequency of symptoms in both patient groups is outlined in the table.

Conclusions.—The prognosis for traumatic dissection patients appears to be somewhat less favorable than the prognosis for spontaneous dissection patients.

▶ Magnetic resonance angiography is revealing an increasing incidence of carotid dissections. Blunt injury to the carotid artery may be a particularly disfavored cause.

Carotid Artery Reconstruction Following Extracorporeal Membrane Oxygenation
Crombleholme TM, Adzick NS, deLorimier AA, Longaker MT, Harrison MR, Charlton VE (Univ of California, San Francisco)
Am J Dis Child 144:872–874, 1990   11–41

Introduction.—Several centers have reported a significant incidence of right hemispheric brain injury in surviving neonates treated with veno-arterial extracorporeal membrane oxygenation (ECMO). The injury is probably secondary to right carotid artery ligation. Right carotid artery reconstruction was performed after ECMO decannulation in 5 infants.

Technique.—The edges of the arteriotomy are débrided and inspected for the presence of an intimal flap. Under ×3.5 surgical loop magnification, the arteriotomy site is re-anastomosed with interrupted 7-0 absorbable sutures applied transversely to maximize the transluminal diameter.

Patients.—The right carotid artery was reconstructed at the time of decannulation after successful ECMO in 4 of 5 infants. Both duplex and transcranial Doppler ultrasound scanning showed excellent antegrade blood flow in all 4 infants. None of the infants had signs of unilateral brain injury at discharge or at 3–7 months' follow-up. The neonate in whom ECMO was successful underwent carotid artery ligation because of extensive arterial intimal disruption.

Conclusion.—Carotid artery reconstruction after ECMO is a technically simple procedure that may reduce the incidence of right hemispheric brain injury and avoid the long-term consequences of compromised right hemispheric perfusion.

▶ Although several small series have suggested an increased incidence of right-sided brain lesions in neonatal ECMO patients, larger studies have failed to show convincing evidence linking carotid artery ligation to adverse developmental outcome. Nevertheless, there is growing concern over the potential short-term and long-term risks of asymmetric cerebrovascular development. These risks include abnormal right cerebral hemispheric development (1) above the ligated right common carotid artery, and the potential adverse consequences of atherosclerosis or trauma on the left carotid artery in later life (1).

The results of this study indicate that right common carotid artery reconstruction is technically feasible after neonatal ECMO. However, there are several important issues that must be addressed before widespread acceptance of this potentially injurious and therapeutically unproven procedure occurs. These issues include: identification of the absolute and relative contraindications to arterial repair (intimal disruption during arterial cannulation, a suspected wound infection, or preexistent right- or left-sided cerebral hemorrhage); proof of the optimal means for vascular repair (primary closure, excision of the arteriotomy site with end-to-end anastomosis, or vein patch); recognition of those most qualified to undertake and follow-up such repairs; proper management of early and late complications (early asymptomatic stenosis or late symptomatic occlusion); the overall risks of adverse neurological outcome caused by technical misadventure; and objective proof that the benefits of the procedure outweigh the risks. Until more information becomes available, permanent ligation of the right common carotid artery remains an accepted form of practice at the time of veno-arterial cannulation for extracorporeal life support.—Steven L. Moulton, M.D., Surgical Resident, Department of Surgery, University of California, San Diego.

Reference

1. Lott IT, et al: *J Pediatr* 116:343, 1990.

Carotid Body Tumors
Kraus DH, Sterman BM, Hakaim AG, Beven EG, Levine HL, Wood BG, Tucker HM (Cleveland Clinic Found)
Arch Otolaryngol Head Neck Surg 116:1384–1387, 1990   11–42

Purpose.—The diagnosis and management of carotid body tumors were studied in a retrospective review of 15 patients seen between June 1979 and June 1987.

Data Analysis.—The mean age of the patients was 45 years (range, 24 to 72 years). A total of 7 patients had multiple paraganglionomas. Bilateral carotid angiography was very reliable in the diagnosis. Fifteen carotid body tumors were resected in 14 patients. One of these patients underwent staged bilateral surgery; the remaining patient received radiation therapy. Vascular or neural structures were sacrificed in 10 of 15 procedures to achieve complete tumor resection. All of the patients with primary repair had patent carotid arteries, but 2 of the 3 saphenous vein interposition grafts became occluded. None of the patients had symptoms of cerebral ischemia, and none showed evidence of tumor recurrence during a mean follow-up of 36 months. Two patients underwent true vocal cord Teflon injection for vagus nerve paralysis.

Conclusions.—Surgery remains the preferred treatment for carotid body tumors. Surgical management involves the identification and preservation of vascular and neural structures adjacent to the tumor. Bilateral carotid angiography is the benchmark of preoperative evaluation. Small or moderately sized tumors can be resected with little morbidity. Resection of large tumors places neurovascular structures at greater, but acceptable, risk. Tumor resection is facilitated by dissection in the subadventitial plane. Primary repair of arteriotomies or shunting with saphenous vein grafts is preferred when carotid arteriotomy is unavoidable. Postoperative intravenous digital subtraction angiography allows evaluation of the arterial repair.

▶ Carotid arteriography is not essential to evaluation of carotid body tumors. Good quality duplex scans are definitively diagnostic, and they sometimes show the blood supply from the external carotid artery.

Carotid Body Tumours: Report of Six Cases and a Review of Management
Keating JF, Miller GA, Keaveny TV (St Vincent's Hosp, Dublin)
J R Coll Surg Edinb 35:172–174, 1990   11–43

Background.—Carotid body tumors are rare, accounting for less than .5% of all tumors. A total of 6 patients were treated for carotid body tumors between 1972 and 1988.

Patients.—All 6 patients (2 men and 4 women mean age, 46 years) were initially seen with a neck mass. In addition, 1 patient had Horner's syndrome and another had tinnitus. One woman who had previous surgery for a contralateral carotid body tumor had a sibling with the same tumor. The diagnosis was confirmed by ultrasound and angiography in all patients.

Management.—A group of 5 patients underwent surgical resection; 1 elderly patients at risk for surgery was managed nonsurgically. At follow-up ranging from 6 months to 12 years, none of the patients who underwent surgery had any recurrence, and the patient managed conservatively had only a slight increase in tumor size.

Discussion.—Surgery remains the preferred treatment for these tumors. Preoperative embolization may be a useful adjunct in difficult cases because it has low complication rates. Angiography is the definitive preoperative investigation. Although the risk of perioperative stroke has decreased considerably, injury to the cranial nerves remains a major hazard of surgery. A conservative approach may be justified in elderly patients when the risks of surgery are high.

▶ Wisdom may be found in this study, which suggests that the tumor may be treated expectantly in older patients.

Familial Occurrence of Carotid Body Tumors
Shedd DP, Arias JD, Glunk RP (Roswell Park Mem Inst, Buffalo, NY)
Head Neck 12:496–499, 1990   11–44

Introduction.—Carotid body tumors are rare. Four of these tumors were encountered in 1 family.

Patients.—Carotid body tumors were diagnosed in 4 related patients aged 27–50 years, including 2 siblings and 2 children. Two of the patients had bilateral tumors; none had metastasis. The tumors were excised; the ansa hypoglossi was encased by the tumor in 1 patient and had to be resected along with the external carotid artery. The postoperative courses were uneventful.

Discussion.—The carotid body is located in the adventitia of the posterior medial surface of the common carotid artery bifurcation. The tumor may present either in the more common sporadic form or in the familial form that is transmitted via an autosomal-dominant pattern. There is a 32% incidence of bilateral tumors. As the tumor enlarges, it displaces the internal and carotid arteries laterally, which is a pathognomonic sign of carotid body tumors on bilateral cerebral angiography. The vagus nerves, the hypoglossal nerves, and occasionally the sympathetic chain may be displaced or encased by the tumor. Metastasis occurs in about 5% of the cases and involves the regional lymph nodes, lungs, and bones. These tumors recur locally, and they may grow relentlessly if not resected. The associated morbidity includes progressive cranial nerve palsies, dysphagia, airway obstruction, and extension to the base of the skull with infiltrations of the central nervous system. The mortality rate is 8% in untreated patients. It is recommended that all carotid body tumors should be excised unless there are contraindicating medical or technical reasons.

▶ Tumors of the carotid body are spontaneous, familial, or secondary to living at high altitude.

12 Visceral Circulation

Current Status of Duplex Doppler Ultrasound in the Examination of the Abdominal Vasculature
Eidt JF, Harward T, Cook JM, Kahn MB, Troillett R (Univ of Arkansas; Univ of Texas Health Science Ctr, Houston)
Am J Surg 160:604–609, 1990   12–1

Background.—Although duplex scanning has been widely used to diagnose a number of vascular disorders, the role of duplex Doppler ultrasound in the evaluation of intra-abdominal vascular disease remains unclear. Therefore, the current status of duplex scanning in the investigation of renal arteries, mesenteric arteries, and the portal venous system was investigated.

Review.—In some centers, duplex scanning has been successful as a screening test for renovascular hypertension; however, there are technical problems that currently limit its widespread use. These problems include a requirement for considerable expertise and time. Also, as many as 22% of patients with renovascular hypertension may have multiple renal arteries or branch stenosis, neither of which is usually detectable by duplex scanning. In a series of 35 patients who underwent duplex scanning for chronic mesenteric insufficiency, all of the stenoses greater than 50% were identified correctly. Mesenteric arterial duplex scanning also provides important physiological information that cannot be derived from arteriography alone in patients with weight loss, postprandial abdominal pain, and episodic diarrhea associated with an epigastric bruit. Duplex examination has been used to evaluate portal hypertension, liver transplantation, transplant anatomy, and both the function and patency of hepatic and portal anastomoses. As with other forms of deep abdominal duplex scanning, examination of the portal vein requires patience and persistence. The pitfalls include mirror-image or "flip" artifacts, an inability to obtain Doppler signals from small vessels identified on ultrasound, and an inability to analyze important vascular channels because of ascites or bowel gas.

Conclusions.—Duplex scanning can be an accurate method for imaging the portal system in hospitals with high volumes of patients. In the average vascular laboratory, the technique presently has only a limited role for the detection of occult portal hypertension or the evaluation of an occasional patient requiring porto-systemic shunt. Duplex scanning appears to be useful for determining the patency of the portal vein and its major branches, and it may also be helpful in the postoperative evaluation of portal decompression surgical procedures.

▶ Although this abstract suggests that the role of duplex ultrasound in the evaluation of intra-abdominal vascular disease is unclear, the reverse is actually true. Ultrasound is an important screening test for mesenteric vascular insufficiency. However, it is true that technical problems limit the technique in the evaluation of the renal arteries.

Chronic Intestinal Ischaemia

Marston A (Middlesex Hosp; Univ College, London; Middlesex School of Medicine, London)

Acta Chir Scand Suppl 555:237–243, 1990   12–2

Background.—Although stenoses and blockages of the visceral arteries are quite common, intestinal angina is rare. Furthermore, the clinical diagnosis of chronic intestinal ischemia remains difficult.

Discussion.—In chronic intestinal ischemia, circulatory impairment progresses gradually to total occlusion. At the same time, a collateral circulation builds up, ensuring that bowel infarction does not occur under normal circumstances. However, this process is unable to produce the hyperemia demanded by digestion. The patient often has generalized, crampy abdominal pain after meals, and loss of weight occurs as a consequence of low food intake. Aortography confirms the diagnosis. The "meandering mesenteric artery" of Moskowitz and hypertrophy of the pancreatic arcades are the most important radiological features. Surgical reconstruction is considered when food-related abdominal pain persists and the presence of an arterial block has been established.

Management.—In the Bloomsbury Vascular Unit, approximately 100 patients were examined for suspected intestinal angina during a 25-year period. Of these, 41 underwent surgical reconstructions and were followed up from 3 to 160 months (Fig 12–1). A total of 32 patients sur-

Intestinal Angina : Bloomsbury Vascular Unit 1962-1990

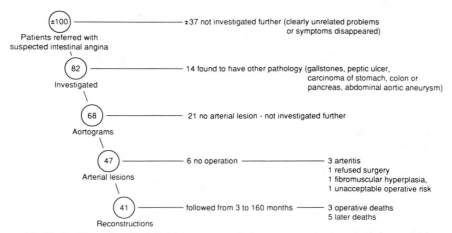

Fig 12–1.—Bloomsbury Vascular Unit patients with chronic intestinal ischemia. (Courtesy of Marston A: *Acta Chir Scand Suppl* 555:237–243, 1990.)

Bloomsbury Vascular Unit: Intestinal Angina 1962-1990

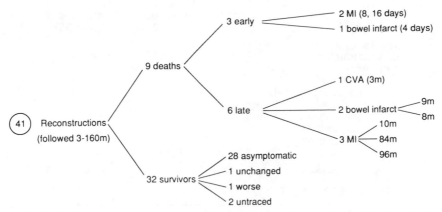

Fig 12–2—Outcome of reconstructive procedures. (Courtesy of Marston A: *Acta Chir Scand Suppl* 555:237–243, 1990.)

vived, and 28 became asymptomatic (Fig 12–2). There were 3 operative deaths and 6 late deaths, including 3 from bowel infarction.

Conclusion.—Chronic intestinal ischemia is a syndrome with widely differing modes of presentation. In addition, narrowing of the visceral arteries has not been definitely associated with the alimentary dysfunctions. Although surgical reconstruction of the involved arteries has relieved symptoms in a number of patients, distinguishing between the life-threatening and the insignificant vascular blocks remains difficult.

▶ Both the original article and the abstract fail to emphasize 2 important facts. First, this syndrome occurs in young women, often younger than age 45, in whom the double effects of smoking and the contraceptive pill act to produce visceral artery narrowings. In addition, the syndromes of chronic visceral ischemia lead to bowel infarction. Timely diagnosis can prevent catastrophic calamities.

Superior Mesenteric Artery Embolism: Eighty-Two Cases
Batellier J, Kieny R (Hôpital Central, Strasbourg, France)
Ann Vasc Surg 4:112–116, 1990   12–3

Background.—Embolization to the superior mesenteric artery (SMA) can cause acute mesenteric ischemia syndrome (AMIS), which will lead to mesenteric infarction if not promptly treated. Because the symptoms of AMIS are highly variable, the policy at 1 hospital was to perform mesenteric arteriography whenever a high-risk patient complained of abdominal pain, even if the pain was atypical.

Patients.—During a 22-year period, 1,650 patients had peripheral arterial embolization. Of these patients, 82 (5%) had embolization to the

Cause of Death After Surgical Treatment

	AMIS (n = 34)	Mesenteric infarction (n = 31)	Overall results (n = 65)
Irreversible lesions*		9	9
SMA rethrombosis†	4	6	10
Recurrence			
SMA embolus	1		1
embolus in another site	2	3	5
Cardiac	2	1	3
Pulmonary embolism	1		1
Multiple organ failure	2		2
Intestinal hemorrhage		1	1
Intestinal fistula		1	1

*Exploratory laparotomy.
†Mesenteric infarction.
(Courtesy of Batellier J, Kieny R: Ann Vasc Surg 4:112–116, 1990.)

SMA; the patients were 43 men and 39 women, aged 29–90 years. In 2 of the patients, the diagnosis was made when intestinal discoloration and absence of SMA pulses were observed suddenly during infrarenal aortic surgery. Another 61 patients (74.5%) experienced abdominal pain. The remaining 19 patients (23%) had either no or atypical abdominal pain. Seventy-nine patients had embologenic pathological findings. In 74 patients, the embolism originated in the left heart chambers, and 65 of these patients had total arrhythmia caused by atrial fibrillation. A group of 29 patients had had 1 or more arterial embolic episodes. All of the embolic episodes, except the 2 that occurred during operation, were diagnosed by selective mesenteric arteriography.

Outcome.—A total of 65 patients were operated on—31 for mesenteric infarction and 34 for AMIS without intestinal necrosis. Of the patients operated on for mesenteric infarction, 21 (68%) died; 12 patients (35%) operated on for mesenteric ischemia also died (table). The mean duration of ischemia before operation was 21 hours for patients with mesenteric infarction and 13 hours for those with AMIS. Of the 17 medically treated patients, 2 (12%) also died. The overall mortality was 43%.

Conclusion.—Survival after SMA embolization is related directly to early diagnosis and treatment. The routine practice of urgent mesenteric arteriography in all patients with a clinical suspicion of embolization to the SMA increased the overall survival rate to 57%. The survival rate in patients operated on during the first 13 hours of ischemia was 65%.

▶ Because mesenteric artery embolization presents a dramatic clinical syndrome and appears as a major cause of acute bowel infarction, a thorough knowledge of its pathogenesis and treatment must be a part of the intellectual resource of every vascular surgeon.

Aortic Reimplantation of the Superior Mesenteric Artery for Atherosclerotic Lesions of the Visceral Arteries: Sixty Cases
Kieny R, Batellier J, Kretz J-G (Hôpital Central, Strasbourg, France)
Ann Vasc Surg 4:122–125, 1990   12–4

Background.—Complete 3-artery vascularization of the visceral arteries is recommended whenever possible to prevent symptomatic relapse. When vascularization is not technically possible, there is no agreement as to which artery is the most important to revascularize. A total of 87 patients underwent revascularization of the superior mesenteric artery (SMA).

Patients.—A group of 60 reconstructions that were direct or indirect reimplantations of the SMA into the aorta were reviewed. The patient group included 51 men and 9 women with a mean age of 54.9 years. Of the patients, 7 underwent emergency surgery for acute intestinal ischemia, 31 were operated on for chronic mesenteric ischemia, and 22 underwent prophylactic mesenteric reconstruction during other procedures. Most of the patients (97%) had 2- or 3-artery disease.

Outcome.—Twenty-two reimplantations of the SMA were direct and 38 were indirect; all reimplantations involved the use of a short prosthetic segment. Revascularization of the SMA was isolated in 51 patients, associated with that of the celiac artery in 6 cases, and associated with the inferior mesenteric artery in 2 cases. Only 2 patients died after revascularization. At a mean follow-up of 8.5 years, 29 more patients had died. The 5-year survival rate was 69.6% (Fig 12–3), and 21 of the patients who were available for follow-up had good functional results.

Conclusions.—The results of isolated reimplantation of the SMA on the anterior aspect of the infrarenal artery are satisfactory in terms of

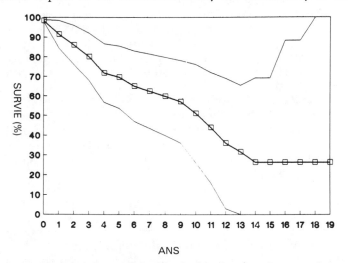

Fig 12–3.—Actuarial survival curve after aortic reimplantation of superior mesenteric artery for atherosclerotic lesions of visceral arteries in 60 patients. (Courtesy of Kieny R, Batellier J, Kretz J-G: *Ann Vasc Surg* 4:122–125, 1990.)

survival, patency, and symptomatic relief. The technique is useful in weakened patients for whom the low risk of minimal revascularization is preferable to the high operative risk of complete 3-artery revascularization.

▶ Reimplantation of the mesenteric arteries is a technique that has fallen largely into disuse in this country. Now that French vascular surgeons are reporting their results in the English language, it is refreshing to see large experiences such as those described in this abstract and in Abstract 12–3.

Clinical Characteristics Useful in Screening for Renovascular Disease
Svetkey LP, Helms MJ, Dunnick NR, Klotman PE (Duke Univ)
South Med J 83:743–747, 1990   12–5

Introduction.—Renovascular hypertension is identified diagnostically by its relief after surgical correction of a renal artery stenosis (RAS). Therefore, the first step in diagnosis is the identification of hypertensive patients with a significant narrowing of the lumen of a main renal artery. Abdominal bruit and malignant hypertension are both associated with renovascular disease. The predictive values of additional clinical signs were tested.

Procedure.—A total of 100 ambulatory adult hypertensives who were assessed by physical examination, medical history, and laboratory tests met 1 or more of the study entry criteria. The criteria included the presence of abdominal or flank bruit, hypertension refractory to antihypertensive therapy, severe hypertension, a recent onset of hypertension or recently worsened hypertension, and late or early onset of hypertension. All of the patients were assessed for the presence of RAS by arteriography.

Data Analysis.—The predictive values of the different clinical signs are listed in the table. The selected population had an 18% rate of angiographically verified RAS. Of the 18 patients with RAS, the hypertension of 13 was significantly relieved by surgery; thus, these patients did have renovascular disease. Bruit predicted 10 of the 18 patients with RAS, but it also occurred in 8 patients without RAS. Of the 32 patients with refractory hypertension, 6 also had RAS.

Conclusions.—The frequency with which abdominal bruit and refractory hypertension reflect the presence of RAS is unclear. All of the other clinical features examined failed as predictors. Better laboratory and clinical screening criteria are needed to identify patients with RAS and select patients for angiography.

▶ Refractory hypertension should lead to renal arteriography.

Renal Duplex Sonography: Evaluation of Clinical Utility
Hansen KJ, Tribble RW, Reavis SW, Canzanello VO, Craven TE, Plonk GW Jr, Dean RH (Bowman Gray School of Medicine, Winston-Salem, NC)
J Vasc Surg 12:227–236, 1990   12–6

Introduction.—The diagnosis of critical stenosis of the main renal artery (RVD) often requires angiography. Recent studies suggest that renal duplex sonography (RDS) can be a useful substitute for the screening for RVD.

Patients.—To further investigate its clinical utility, renovascular disease defined by RDS criteria was compared prospectively with angiogra-

Associations Between Clinical Features and the Presence of RAS in 100 Patients with Hypertension (HTN)

Clinical Feature	Feature Present		Feature Absent		P Value (Fisher's Exact Test)	Odds Ratio *
	RAS Present (a)	RAS Absent (c)	RAS Present (b)	RAS Absent (d)		
Bruit	10	8	8	74	<.0005	11.6
Refractory HTN	6	26	2	48	.051	5.5
Progressively severe HTN	5	27	3	47	.25	2.9
Severe HTN	3	45	5	29	.27	.39
Recent onset of HTN	2	13	6	61	.63	1.6
Early onset of HTN	1	19	7	55	.67	.41
Late onset of HTN	1	13	7	61	1.0	.67

*Odds ratio = $a(d)/b(c)$.
(Courtesy of Svetkey LP, Helms MJ, Dunnick NR, et al: *South Med J* 83:743–747, 1990.)

phy during a 10-month period. A total of 74 consecutive patients with 77 comparative RDS and standard angiographic studies of the arterial anatomy to 148 kidneys were studied. Of these patients, 26 had severe renal deficiency and 67 had hypertension; 14 patients had 20 kidneys with multiple renal arteries. Bilateral disease occurred in 22 of the 44 patients with significant RVD.

Findings.—In 6 of the kidneys, RDS was considered inadequate for interpretation. Of the remaining 142 kidneys, 122 had single renal arteries. Renal duplex sonography correctly identified 67 of 68 kidneys with <60% renal artery stenosis, 35 of 39 kidneys with ≥60% to 99% renal artery stenosis, and 15 of 15 renal artery occlusions. In the presence of single renal arteries, RDS was 83% sensitive, 98% specific, had a positive predictive value of 98%, a negative predictive value of 94%, and an overall accuracy of 96%. These results were affected adversely when kidneys with multiple (polar) renal arteries were examined. A group of 35 patients underwent surgical renal revascularization. Although the end-diastolic ratio was related inversely to the serum creatinine level, the low end-diastolic ratio did not preclude beneficial blood pressure or renal function response after renal revascularization.

Conclusions.—Renal duplex sonography can be a valuable screening test for the detection of significant RVD, particularly in patients with single renal arteries that cause global renal ischemia and secondary renal insufficiency (ischemic nephropathy). However, RDS does not identify polar renal arteries or predict clinical response after the correction of RVD.

▶ Unfortunately, renal artery ultrasonography is a difficult art that is best performed by very experienced technicians who have access to many patients. Therefore, the value of renal artery ultrasonography in screening is limited in the community hospital. Renal arteriography is the most common technique in such hospitals (see Abstract 12–5). Renovascular hypertension is often associated with polar renal artery stenosis, in which case arteriography becomes doubly mandatory.

Extrinsic Compression of the Renal Artery by Diaphragmatic Crus
Clément C, Ruiz R, Costa-Foru B, Nicaise H (Hôpital Robert Debrè, Reims, France)
Ann Vasc Surg 4:305–308, 1990   12–7

Introduction.—Few cases of extrinsic compression of the renal artery have been reported in the literature. The most frequent extrinsic compression of the renal artery, a fibromuscular band originating in the diaphragm, was discovered in a patient with both systemic hypertension associated with stenosis and kinking of the renal arteries.

Case Report.—Woman, 26, had intermittent systemic hypertension; she had taken an estrogen-progestin contraceptive for a brief period of time. Stenosis and kinking of 1 renal artery were documented with intravenous digital sutration ar-

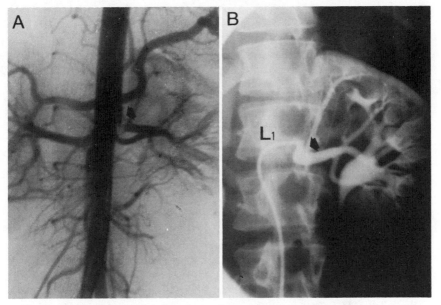

Fig 12–4.—**A**, preoperative digital arteriogram (anteroposterior view) showing stenosis of left superior renal artery (*arrow*). **B**, selective renal arteriograms: stenosis with kink and poststenotic dilatation. (Courtesy of Clément C, Ruiz R, Costa-Foru B, et al: *Ann Vasc Surg* 4:305–308, 1990.)

teriograms (Fig 12–4). Because the lesion suggested fibromuscular dysplasia, percutaneous transluminal angioplasty was used. However, the catheter was unable to penetrate the stenotic area. Selective renal arteriograms defined the characteristics of the stenosis. An extrinsic compression of the left superior renal artery was identified and approached using Kocher's maneuver. The renal artery originated posteriorly and was compressed by an internal fibromuscular band. Resection of the band caused the kink to disappear, the expansion of the artery to return to normal, and the patient's hypertension to disappear.

Discussion.—Data on only 6 such patients have been found in the literature. Because transluminal angioplasty is not effective in the treatment of stenosis, surgery is always required. The possible signs of extrinsic compression of the renal artery by diaphragmatic crus include young age, hypertension, bruit variable with position and increasing with inspiration after exercise, and arterial stenosis a few millimeters lateral to the border of the spine with a kink or post-stenotic dilatation just distal to the ostium.

▶ This very rare condition may have been overlooked in the past.

Surgical Treatment of Renovascular Hypertension and Respective Late Results: A Twenty Years Experience
Poulias GE, Skoutas B, Doundoulakis N, Prombonas E, Haddad H, Papaioannou K, Sendekeya S (Red Cross Gen Hosp; Athens Med Ctr, Athens, Greece)
J Cardiovasc Surg 32:69–75, 1991   12–8

Introduction.—Careful patient selection is necessary to gain the maximal benefit from surgery for renovascular hypertension. The wider availability of effective antihypertensive drugs and the advent of angioplasty have prompted a more selective use of surgery.

Study Design.—Renovascular reconstruction was performed in 115 hypertensive patients from March 1968 to October 1988. A total of 54 patients had a segmental renal artery lesion; 23 of these patients had fibromuscular disease and 31 had atherosclerosis. A group of 37 patients had more diffuse atherosclerotic disease, and 38 had an abdominal aortic lesion treated at the same time.

Results.—Two of the patients died after aortorenal reconstruction. The overall survival rate was 78% at 5 years and 61% at 10 years. Better results were achieved in the patients with fibromuscular dysplasia. Persistent hypertension adversely influenced late survival. Patency rates of 73% to 82% were achieved with dacron, polytetrafluoroethylene, and saphenous vein grafts. Four patients required late nephrectomy.

Conclusions.—These findings affirm the beneficial effect of reconstructive surgery in patients with renovascular hypertension. Renal function is preserved and dialysis is avoided. Despite some degree of irreversible ischemic renal damage, it is usually possible to control the blood pressure postoperatively.

▶ The long-term follow-up of patients with renovascular hypertension reveals a striking survival rate, a very slight appearance of uremia as a cause of late death, and remarkable success with prosthetic graft reconstruction of the renal arteries.

Occlusive Disease of the Renal Arteries and Chronic Renal Failure: The Limits of Reconstructive Surgery
Mercier C, Piquet P, Alimi Y, Tournigand P, Albrand J-J (Hôpital de la Conception, Marseille, France)
Ann Vasc Surg 4:166–170, 1990   12–9

Background.—Renal arterial restoration for chronic renal failure of ischemic origin has not been advocated routinely because of the high rate of associated mortality and the lack of pre-operative functional or pathological criteria to identify suitable patients. The long-term results of 48 renal revascularizations in 43 patients with chronic renal failure and associated occlusive lesions of the renal arteries were reported.

Method.—Diagnosis of kidney failure was based on 2 consecutive determinations of serum creatinine levels greater than 120 μmol/L. The patients were divided into 4 groups according to increasing levels of creatinine; group IV contained 2 patients with chronic renal failure who required hemodialysis.

Findings.—A total of 37 patients had hypertension. Restoration of the renal artery was unilateral in 38 patients and bilateral in 5. Of the 24 patients who had renal artery surgery associated with reconstruction of the infrarenal aorta, 3 died. In groups I and II, 69.5% of the patients had stabilized or improved kidney function. The preoperative serum levels of creatinine in these groups were between 120 μmol/L and 350 μmol/L.

Conclusion.—A preoperative serum level of creatinine that is less than 350 μmol/L and a kidney size greater than 8 cm are the best predictors of improved renal function after restoration. Because mortality is closely associated with the magnitude of the surgical procedure, the associated aortic restoration should be performed only when absolutely necessary.

▶ Good practice of nephrology includes the use of renal arteriography in patients who are being considered for permanent renal dialysis. Although vascular surgery can prevent strokes in some patients, extend comfortable life expectancy in individuals with aneurysm disease, and prevent amputation in individuals with limb-threatening ischemia, it can also improve the quality of life of patients whose renal failure is caused by total renal artery occlusions. This abstract helps to clarify the various conditions that will respond to renal revascularization.

Hepatorenal and Splenorenal Artery Bypass for Salvage of Renal Function
Rigdon EE, Durham JR, Massop DW, Wright JG, Smead WL (Ohio State Univ)
Ann Vasc Surg 5:133–137, 1991   12–10

Introduction.—Aortic surgery can pose high risks to patients who have had previous cardiac dysfunction, aortic grafts, or severe atherosclerosis in the aorta. Although aortorenal bypass is the most commonly used operation, both renal bypass by anastomosis of the splenic artery to the left renal artery and hepatic-to-right renal artery bypass are also being used in these patients. The results of these methods of renal bypass were assessed in 8 high-risk patients with axotemia.

Methods.—Between July 1988 and January 1990, 25 patients underwent renal revascularization, 14 of whom did not have accompanying aortic reconstruction. Of these patients, 8 (3 women and 5 men; mean age, 62 years) had hepatorenal and splenorenal bypasses. The mean preoperative serum creatinine level was 2.7 mg/dL. Five of the patients had unilateral revascularization and 3 patients underwent bilateral revascularization.

Results.—The serum creatinine levels improved significantly in all of the patients immediately after surgery. Renal function improved in the 2 patients who had a unilateral revascularization procedure with a normal contralateral renal artery. Of the 5 patients with severe hypertension, 4 had improvement in their medical management because the number of medications they received to maintain normal blood pressure before surgery was significantly reduced after the operation. One patient was judged as completely cured, and 1 patient failed to improve and needed hemodialysis. Renal bypass patency was confirmed by arteriography or by an isotope perfusion scan in 6 patients. In half of the patients, the gastroduodenal artery served as the inflow vessel and was attached by end-to-end anastomoses to the right renal artery (Fig 12–5). No postoperative liver or pancreatic dysfunction or complications related to the hepatorenal bypass were observed. One patient had a splenectomy for an injured spleen; another had a splenic infarction that required a splenectomy. In addition, 3 patients had a myocardial infarction; 1 patient died as a result.

Implications.—These findings indicate that hepatorenal and splenorenal artery bypass surgery can salvage renal function and improve renovascular hypertension. Modifications of reported methods have simplified the techniques, thereby reducing the risk of injury to the spleen during the procedure. The use of hepatorenal and splenorenal bypass by experienced vascular surgeons is recommended in patients with previous aortic reconstruction, cardiac disease, or a seriously diseased aorta.

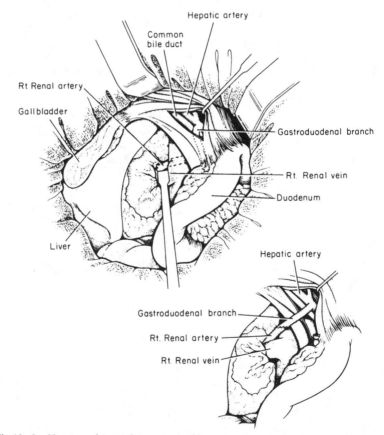

Fig 12–5.—Hepatorenal artery bypass is possible in many cases with primary anastomosis of the gastroduodenal branch of the hepatic artery to the renal artery, which should be divided as near as possible to its origin from behind or left of the vena cava to provide the maximum length of usable artery. (Courtesy of Rigdon EE, Durham JR, Massop DW, et al: *Ann Vasc Surg* 5:133–137, 1991.)

▶ Nonaortic sources of inflow are being used increasingly in renal artery reconstruction. This limits the magnitude of the operative procedure and decreases mortality in patients who are frequently a poor operative risk.

Renal Artery Revascularization With Polytetrafluoroethylene Bypass Graft
Cormier J-M, Fichelle J-M, Laurian C, Gigou F, Artru B, Ricco J-B (Hôpital St Joseph, Paris)
Ann Vasc Surg 4:471–478, 1990   12–11

Methods.—Polytetrafluoroethylene (PTFE) that is used as a prosthetic material in femoropopliteal bypass revascularization is reliable in most instances. A total of 68 patients with 74 PTFE grafts were studied. Emergency surgery for a ruptured suprarenal aneurysm or acute thrombosis was done in 8 patients (9 revascularizations). Elective surgery was performed in 60 patients (19 renal revascularizations and 46 combined aortic and renal revascularizations). The reinforced expanded PTFE prosthetic graft was used in all of the procedures.

Outcome.—Only 1 patient survived emergency surgery, and at 6-year follow-up both revascularizations were patent on arteriography. Patients who had elective surgery were followed from 12 to 76 months. Early follow-up demonstrated occlusion in 6 reconstructions. Later follow-up arteriograms showed 2 more late occlusions and 2 distal anastomotic stenoses. At 72 months, the actuarial patency was 85% ± 10% (Fig 12–6).

Discussion.—This success with PTFE in renal bypass grafts is promising. Its use is recommended in anastomoses with large-caliber renal arteries in normal-sized kidneys.

▶ As shown in an earlier abstract, prosthetic renal artery reconstruction is eminently satisfactory. This very experienced group from Paris confirms that the most modern of prostheses yields quite acceptable results.

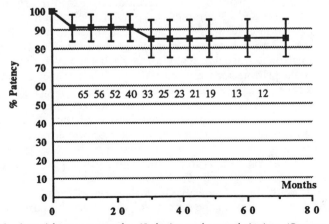

Fig 12–6.—Actuarial patency curve for 65 elective renal revascularizations. (Courtesy of Cormier J-M, Fichelle J-M, Laurian C, et al: *Ann Vasc Surg* 4:471–478, 1990.)

Improved Results of Vascular Reconstruction in Pediatric and Young Adult Patients With Renovascular Hypertension

Martinez A, Novick AC, Cunningham R, Goormastic M (Cleveland Clinic Found)
J Urol 144:717–720, 1990   12–12

Background.—Although renal revascularization has been used effectively for more than 25 years to treat adult renovascular hypertension, the initial outcome of this surgery in children was less successful. The improvement in the outcome for young patients who were operated on during the past decade was evaluated, and the basis for the improvement was investigated.

Patients.—Two chronological groups were analyzed. The first group consisted of 28 patients who underwent surgery between 1955 and 1977, whereas the second group included 28 patients who were treated between 1978 and 1988. Patient age ranged from 10 months to 21 years, and 53 of the 56 patients had severe hypertension that was associated with renal artery disease caused by fibrous dysplasia. Patients were considered cured when medication was no longer administered and blood pressure was normal for age. Those patients with normal blood pressure on medication or with a diastolic decrease of 15 mm Hg or more were classified as improved.

Results.—There were 2 significant preoperative differences between patients in the 2 groups; the first group had more severe hypertension for a shorter period than did the second group. Surgical revascularization was the most common procedure in both groups. Although a variety of techniques were used in the early group, 45% were done by aortorenal bypass and 55% were done by renal autotransplantation in the later group. There was a technical failure of the primary revascularization in 39% of the patients in the first group, but in only 3% of those in the second group. The rates of failure or partial or complete cure of hypertension did not differ significantly between the 2 groups. However, significantly more improvements or cures were achieved through revascularization (96%) as opposed to complete or partial nephrectomy (4%) in the second group, compared with 48% and 52% in the first group.

Discussion.—Those surgical advances of the past decade that permit extracorporeal microvascular repair of branch renal artery lesions have made revascularization accessible to patients who, in earlier eras, would have had total or partial nephrectomies, or been considered inoperable. Despite recent improvements in antihypertensive therapy, a life-long commitment to drug treatment with risk of loss of renal function caused by disease progression is not an appropriate option for young patients. Percutaneous transluminal angioplasty may not be technically feasible. Aortorenal bypass using a graft of autologous hypogastric artery is the technique of choice, although saphenous vein may be used in postpubertal children. With the current advances in surgical revascularization, renovascular hypertension in the young individual can be cured while protecting renal function.

▶ The fact that cure or improvement of hypertension was achieved in 96% of these youngsters treated since 1978, with only 1 patient requiring nephrectomy, is a remarkable accomplishment. Advances in microvascular techniques and improvements in surgical approaches are exemplified by a decrease in the technical failure rate after primary renal revascularization from 39% in patients treated prior to 1978 to 3% in the more contemporary patient group. Interestingly, these advances parallel technical improvements in other areas of vascular surgery, notably distal bypass grafting. These data provide additional convincing evidence that most young patients with renovascular hypertension are best treated surgically.—Charles S. O'Mara, M.D., Jackson, Mississippi

---

Renal Autotransplantation in Children: A Successful Treatment for Renovascular Hypertension
Merguerian PA, McLorie GA, Balfe JW, Khoury AE, Churchill BM (Hosp for Sick Children, Toronto)
J Urol 144:1443–1445, 1990   12–13

Introduction.—Pediatric renovascular hypertension caused by renal artery occlusive disease is rare; until recently it was corrected by nephrectomy. Vascular surgical techniques refined in renal transplant surgery have made reconstructive vascular procedures feasible as a new option. Preservation of function, rather than ablation, is especially important in children because the disease is frequently bilateral. The results of renal autotransplantation performed during a 10-year period in 10 kidneys in 7 renally hypertensive children were reviewed.

Technique.—A central venous line monitored central venous pressure; it was also used for hydration and postoperative parenteral nutrition. Core cooling was maintained at 4° C through the use of a cooling jacket and perfusion of the kidney with cold Collin's or Belzer's solution. Autotransplantation consisted of end-to-side anastomosis of each renal artery to the common iliac artery, and end-to-side anastomosis of each renal vein to the common iliac veins. In 1 child with a stenotic lesion in the posterior branch of the left renal artery, a saphenous vein patch was used in a bench procedure; in all of the other patients, the ureter was untouched.

Results.—The average follow-up was 4.2 years. All 3 patients with bilateral disease were cured and were able to maintain normal blood pressure in the absence of medication. Of 4 children with unilateral disease, 3 were cured; the remaining child, whose preoperative hypertension had persisted with 6 different antihypertensive medications, maintained normal pressure on a low-dose antihypertensive therapy after renal autotransplantation. These results represent an 86% cure rate for hypertension and a 100% improvement rate.

Discussion.—Many renovascular reconstructive techniques that are successful in adults, including splenorenal bypass, saphenous vein grafts, synthetic grafts, and arterial grafts, are not reliably positive in the outcome in children. This renal autotransplantation procedure had better results than those reported for other reconstructive methods in children, and it is clearly preferable to life-long drug therapy with the risk of progressive disease.

▶ This technique of treating renovascular hypertension in children has been with us for 20 years, and it has proven itself time and time again. The technique was introduced by a fine urologist, Dr. Joseph Kaufman of Los Angeles.

Long-Term Results After Percutaneous Transluminal Angioplasty of Atherosclerotic Renal Artery Stenosis—The Importance of Intensive Follow-Up
Weibull H, Bergqvist D, Jonsson K, Hulthén L, Mannhem P, Bergentz S-E (Lund Univ; Malmö Gen Hosp, Sweden)
Eur J Vasc Surg 5:291–301, 1991   12–14

Background.—Many reports have suggested that percutaneous transluminal renal angioplasty (PTRA) should not be done for atherosclerotic renal artery stenosis. However, good results have been reported with the procedure. The long-term results of PTRA on isthmus and juxta-aortic atherosclerotic renal artery stenoses were studied.

Methods.—A total of 71 atherosclerotic renal artery stenoses were treated in 65 patients. All of the patients (38 men and 27 women; mean age, 65 years) had renovascular hypertension, and 37 also had impending renal insufficiency. The diagnostic studies included angiography and measurements of pressure gradient and renal venous renin. The patients were seen at least 4 times yearly. The indication for reevaluation and possible reintervention was a deterioration in either blood pressure or renal function. The median follow-up was 56 months.

Results.—The PTRA treatment was successful in 59 stenoses and 2 occlusions; 10 procedures failed. The primary patency rate at follow-up was 55%. There were 27 restenoses and 4 occlusions, all but 2 occurring within 1 year. Further PTRA was done in 17 stenoses and surgical reconstruction was done in 8. After all interventions, the secondary patency was 90%. A total of 33% of patients died; 80% of these patients died of cardiovascular disease. Survival was reduced significantly in patients with multilocular atherosclerosis, renal insufficiency, contralateral renal artery stenosis, and ischemic heart disease. Blood pressure problems were cured or improved in 90% of the patients. Renal function was improved in 50% of the patients with impending renal insufficiency, but remained unchanged in 39%. Only 1 PTRA was needed in 55% of the patients, whereas a repeat procedure was needed in 25%, and operation was done in 20%.

Conclusions.—It appears that PTRA may be used as the initial treatment for atherosclerotic renal artery stenosis. Follow-up must be intensive, including angiography if symptoms or signs of recurrence are seen.

A repeat procedure or reconstructive surgery should be done if the PTRA is a technical failure or if the condition recurs.

▶ The high mortality during early follow-up in this group of patients suggests a population different from that reported in Abstract 12–8. Prevalence of atherosclerotic occlusive disease as a cause of death further suggests that more elderly patients with serious comorbid conditions are being subjected to balloon dilation of renal artery lesions. The reported rate of secondary patency is commendable, but the primary patency rate is quite low—even at 12 months.

Renal Artery Stent Placement with Use of the Wallstent Endoprosthesis
Wilms GE, Peene PT, Baert AL, Nevelsteen AA, Suy RM, Verhaeghe RH, Vermylen JG, Fagard RH (Univ Hosps, Leuven, Belgium)
Radiology 179:457–462, 1991   12–15

Introduction.—The placement of an intravascular endoprosthesis is sometimes used to treat the restenosis of lesions resistant to angioplasty or its complications. The results of placing the Wallstent endoprosthesis in 12 renal arteries in 11 patients were evaluated.

Methods.—A total of 11 patients (2 women and 9 men), aged 42–82 years, received a Wallstent endoprosthesis for the treatment of restenosis after dilation and for insufficient result after dilation from previous angioplasty. The 11 patients had 15 stents placed in 12 renal arteries. The mean follow-up was 6.7 months. The Wallstent endoprosthesis that was used in these procedures had been coded with a so-called less thrombogenic Biogold coating. Bifemoral arterial puncture was performed, with the stent introduced over the guide wire in the renal artery and the doubled-over rolling membrane retracted during insertion.

Results.—Dilation of the renal artery stenosis succeeded in 6 of the 12 insertions. The introduction of the delivery catheter was successful in all cases. After stent release, residual stenosis of less than 20% occurred in 10 of the 12 renal arteries treated (Fig 12–7). Two patients had complications from stent insertion: 1 patient with 1 kidney had deterioration of renal function and required temporary hemodialysis related to massive cholesterol embolization in the kidney; another patient had unexplained microscopic hematuria and proteinuria for 1 week, but renal function later returned to normal. In 1 patient with a relapse of hypertension after 2 months, the stent shortened. This resulted in restenosis, and the patient received a second stent. Of the 10 patients with hypertension, 4 were cured, 4 improved, and 2 remained unchanged after the placement of the stent. In addition, 10 of the 11 patients continued to have unchanged serum creatinine levels.

Implications.—The feasibility of placing a renal artery stent using the Wallstent endoprosthesis is supported, although some difficulties exist for positioning the stent with respect to the aortic wall. A fourth marker for the delivery of the catheter helped to solve this problem. The clinical out-

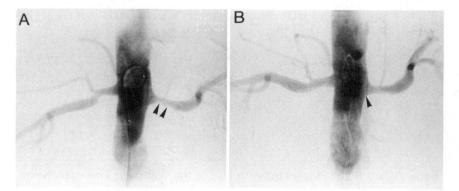

Fig 12–7.—Renal artery stent placement. **A**, angiogram obtained before renal artery stent placement shows moderate postostial stenosis of the right renal artery and severe postostial stenosis of the left renal artery (*arrowheads*). **B**, angiogram obtained after left renal artery stent placement and right renal artery angioplasty shows that the stent (*arrowheads*) is perfectly aligned with the aortic wall. Notice excellent result of angioplasty on the right. (Courtesy of Wilms GE, Peene PT, Baert AL, et al: *Radiology* 179:457–462, 1991.)

come of these patients requires further observation before any conclusions about this technique can be made.

▶ This is not a very encouraging report.

Surgical Treatment of Renal Artery Stenosis After Failed Percutaneous Transluminal Angioplasty
Martinez AG, Novick AC, Hayes JM (Cleveland Clinic Found)
J Urol 144:1094–1096, 1990   12–16

Introduction.—There are concerns that percutaneous transluminal angioplasty may compromise the performance or outcome of subsequent surgical renovascular reconstruction. To address those concerns, 53 patients with renovascular hypertension who underwent surgical treatment after failed initial percutaneous transluminal angioplasty were studied.

Data Analysis.—Renal artery stenosis was caused by fibrous dysplasia in 17 patients and by atherosclerosis in 36. Surgical revascularization was performed because of an inability to dilate the stenotic lesion in 32 patients, acute renal artery occlusion or dissection from attempted percutaneous transluminal angioplasty in 10, and recurrent renal artery stenosis after initially successful percutaneous transluminal angioplasty in 11. Follow-up ranged from 5 to 91 months.

Results.—Successful surgical revascularization was achieved in 50 patients. The remaining 3 patients underwent nephrectomy because of a noviable kidney after complete renal artery occlusion in 2 patients and a subtotal occlusion with intramural dissection in 1 after attempted percutaneous transluminal angioplasty. There was no significant fibrosis or inflammation around the previously dilated renal artery in any patient, and only 1 patient required a more complicated revascularization.

Conclusion.—Patients treated with percutaneous transluminal angioplasty may have persistent or recurrent renal artery obstruction that necessitates surgical revascularization. If the kidney is viable at operation, renovascular reconstruction is not more technically difficult than when done primarily. In addition, the same excellent results can be achieved.

▶ This very experienced group did not find that renal artery reconstruction was more difficult after balloon dilation of the renal artery. Other experienced surgeons have found the opposite to be true. Nevertheless, difficult or not, surgical repair is mandatory if hypertension is to be relieved or renal function is to be improved when balloon angioplasty has failed.

13 Upper Extremity Ischemia

Translumbar Arch Aortography: A Retrospective Controlled Study of Usefulness, Technique, and Safety
Bakal CW, Friedland RJ, Sprayregen S, Calligaro KD, Cynamon J, Veith FJ (Albert Einstein College of Med, New York)
Radiology 178:225–228, 1991   13–1

Introduction.—Axillofemoral bypass grafting is a safe alternative to aortofemoral bypass in the poor-risk patient. However, axillary artery stenosis has recently been recognized as a more important cause of axillofemoral graft failure in patients with advanced atherosclerosis than was previously believed. Classification of the degree of stenosis is problematic because noninvasive techniques such as duplex Doppler ultrasonography are not diagnostic. The safety and efficacy of a simple technique for visualizing the innominate, subclavian, and axillary arteries during conventional translumbar aortography were assessed in 31 patients with advanced lower extremity ischemia and 70 controls.

Methods.—The patients underwent preoperative aortofemoral runoff and arch studies through the translumbar route (TLR-arch), whereas the controls underwent conventional translumbar runoff (TLR) arteriography without arch studies. The arch arteries were assessed by exchanging the initial 16-gauge sheath for a 5-F pigtail catheter. The arterial lesions were defined as significant if there was at least 50% luminal narrowing.

Findings.—Of 33 attempts in 30 patients, 32 diagnostic TLR-arch aortograms were obtained. Exchange of the catheter failed in 1 patient. Of the 71 attempts in 70 controls, 69 diagnostic TLR aortograms were obtained. There were 8 significant innominate, subclavian, or axillary artery stenoses identified on the TLR-arch aortograms of 7 patients (23%); 1 patient had bilateral stenoses. In 5 of the 7 patients, the stenosis was found on the side of the ischemic leg and the choice of the inflow site was altered subsequently. There were 2 major complications in 1 patient who underwent TLR-arch and 11 major complications in 10 patients who had conventional TLR.

Conclusion.—In patients undergoing axillofemoral bypass procedures, arch aortography yields important preoperative information about the status of the innominate, subclavian, and axillary artery inflow. The procedure can be performed safely as an adjunct to conventional translumbar examination of the aorta and peripheral vessels.

▶ Although translumbar arch aortography sounds like a formidable procedure, it can be done effectively and safely by experienced radiologists. However, clinical examination supplemented by bilateral arm blood pressure estimations may obviate the need for such aortography.

White Fingers After Excessive Motorcycle Driving: A Case Report
Stark G, Pilger E, Klein GE, Melzer G, Decrinis M, Bertuch H, Krejs GJ (Karl Franzens Univ, Graz, Austria)
VASA 19:257–259, 1990   13–2

Background.—Vibration-induced white finger disease, also known as vibration-induced Raynaud's phenomenon, is common in workers who handle power vibration tools. A motorcyclist was found to have comparable vibration-induced white finger syndrome.

Case Report.—Man, 18, had pain and impaired circulation in the fingers of his right hand. He first noticed this while driving a motorcycle during motorcross training. Except for coolness of the fingers and delayed capillary filling, clinical and laboratory findings were normal. His only hobby was off-street motorcycling for an average of 4 hours a day for the past 4 years. Angiography showed occlusion of the proper palmar digital arteries of the second, third, fourth, and fifth fingers, a small aneurysm of the distal ulnar artery of the right hand (Fig 13–1), and stenosis of the deep palmar arch of the left hand. These angiographic findings were consistent with vibration-induced raynaud's phenomenon. The symptoms of ischemia resolved after treatment with intra-arterial prostaglandins, but they recurred promptly when the patient resumed motorcycle driving.

Conclusion.—Vibration-induced white finger disease can occur after excessive motorcycle driving.

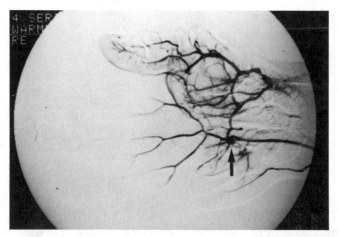

Fig 13–1.—Digital subtraction angiogram of the right hand showing an aneurysm of the distal ulnar artery (*arrow*) and occlusions of the proper digital arteries. (Courtesy of Stark G, Pilger E, Klein GE, et al: *VASA* 19:257–259, 1990.)

▶ Previous studies have suggested that vibration-induced white finger disease is associated with motorcycle riding. The association is very much unrecognized. This study stresses that the primary cause of Raynaud's phenomenon appears to be motorcycle handlebar vibration.

Buerger's Colour
Kimura T, Yoshizaki S, Tsushima N, Sano M, Hanai G (Fujita Health Univ, Nagoya City; Natl Cardiovascular Ctr Hosp, Suita City, Osaka, Japan)
Br J Surg 77:1299–1301, 1990   13–3

Background.—Patients with Buerger's disease have cyanotic hands and feet. This cyanosis is called "Buerger's color." The pinkish appearance results from a network of small thin-walled vessels located about 1 mm below the surface of the skin. The reactions of the subpapillary venous plexus in 14 patients with Buerger's disease and in 13 healthy controls were studied.

Methods.—The fractional blood volume of tissue was analyzed using a visible light reflective spectrophotometer. An intravital video-microscopic system was used to examine capillary morphology.

Findings.—Compared with the normal controls, the nailbeds of the patients with Bureger's disease had an increase in the number of loops, a change in cyanotic color, and dilation. Incompetence of venular tonus and regurgitation at venular valves were both observed in the patients.

Conclusions.—Chronic ulceration of the hands and feet in patients with Buerger's disease is not produced by a reduction in arterial blood flow alone. Chronic congestion in the subpapillary venous plexus is also involved.

A Cellist With Arm Pain: Thermal Asymmetry in Scalenus Anticus Syndrome
Palmer JB, Uematsu S, Jankel WR, Arnold WP (Johns Hopkins Univ; Good Samaritan Hosp, Baltimore)
Arch Phys Med Rehabil 72:237–242, 1991   13–4

Background.—A variety of musculoskeletal and neurological problems in musicians may result from playing their instruments. A cellist had arm pain and significant cooling of the bowing arm while playing. Abnormal thermographic studies revealed intermittent compression of the subclavian artery. To extablish the effect of arm exercise on thermal asymmetry of the hands, healthy volunteers and the cellist with arm pain were studied.

Methods.—The subjects were 57 healthy noncellist controls, a cellist with arm pain, and a cellist with no apparent difficulty. Thermography was performed at rest and during elbow flexion and cello-playing exercises in all subjects. The temperature difference (ΔT) between 1 hand and the other was used to define temperature asymmetry.

Results.—At rest, the mean ΔT in controls was .309° C. Neither elbow flexion exercises nor mimicking of cello playing significantly affected ΔT in these individuals. Findings in the cellist without arm pain were similar. In the cellist with arm pain, ΔT was 3.6° C, which was 10 times the values in controls. Angiography revealed extrinsic compression of the subclavian artery, which occurred only after cello playing. The pain was relieved by sympathetic ganglion block. Abnormal skin temperature may have reflected sympathetic vasomotor hyperactivity.

Conclusions.—In scalenus anticus syndrome, intermittent neurovascular compression and sympathetic hyperactivity appear to be important factors. Because radiological confirmation is usually lacking, this condition may be treated as a nonspecific musculoskeletal pain syndrome until irreversible dystrophic changes have occurred. Angiographic and thermographic stress testing may aid diagnosis.

▶ Manifestations of the thoracic outlet syndrome can occur in a variety of musicians, especially those who play the violin. The provocative position for thoracic outlet symptomatology is the position commonly used in violin playing. In this careful study of peripheral skin temperature after stress testing, decreased cutaneous blood flow is emphasized as causing aggravation of the syndrome. Further studies in other patients are necessary to corroborate these findings.

Recurrent Thoracic Outlet Syndrome After First Rib Resection
Lindgren K-A, Leino E, Lepäntalo M, Paukku P (Kuopio Univ Central Hosp, Kuopio, Finland; Helsinki Univ Central Hosp)
Arch Phys Med Rehabil 72:208–210, 1991   13–5

Work History and Clinical Findings in a Follow-up Examination
After First Rib Resection for TOS

	Asymptomatic (n = 31)	Recurrent TOS (n = 11)		Residual symptoms (n = 42)
Female/male	18/13	9/2		22/20
Desk work	10 (32%)	8 (73%)	*	14 (33%)
Heavy labor	11 (35%)	2 (18%)		13 (31%)
Roos test +	8 (26%)‡	10 (91%)		27 (64%)
		NS		
Tinel test +	9 (29%)*	8 (73%)	NS	22 (52%)
Neurologic deficiencies	5 (16%)‡	10 (91%)	NS	23 (55%)

Abbreviations: NS, nonsignificant (*t*-test); *n*, number of first ribs resected.
*P < .05.
†P < .01.
‡P < .001.
(Courtesy of Lindgren K-A, Leino E, Lepäntalo M, et al: *Arch Phys Med Rehabil* 72:208–210, 1991.)

Introduction.—Thoracic outlet syndrome (TOS) is often relieved by resection of the first rib, regardless of the site of compression. Primary results have been excellent, ranging from 80% to 99%. Data on 77 patients (aged 19–61 years) who underwent transaxillary first rib resection for long-term brachialgia in 84 limbs were reviewed retrospectively.

Methods.—The patients had previously undergone bilateral resection of the first rib for TOS. The duration of follow-up was 2.5–13.5 years (average, 6 years) after operation. Examination of the mobility of the spine, upper extremities, and the neurological functions was done.

Results.—For up to 6 months postoperatively, 42 limbs (50%) were asymptomatic. At long-term follow-up, 31 limbs were still asymptomatic (table) and 11 had preoperative symptoms. Of these 11 patients with recurrent TOS, 9 had monotonous desk jobs that could have caused kinesiological abnormalities in the thoracic aperture. Cervical rotation-lateral-flexion tests disclosed that 7 of 11 first rib stumps were subluxated in patients with recurrent TOS.

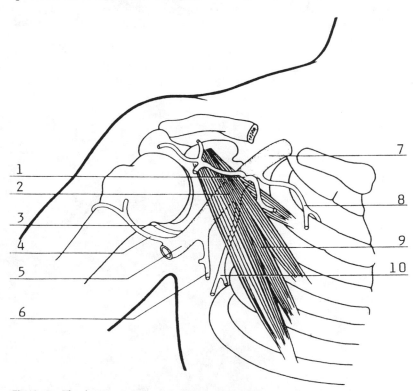

Fig 13–2.—The close anatomical relationship from the axillary artery and its branches to the proximal humerus, the muscle framework, and the brachial plexus is demonstrated. *1*, thoracoacromial artery; *2*, middle axillary artery segment; *3*, posterior humeral circumflex artery; *4*, anterior humeral circumflex artery; *5*, distal axillary artery segment; *6*, subscapular artery; *7*, proximal axillary artery segment; *8*, proximal thoracic artery; *9*, minor pectoral muscle; *10*, lateral thoracic artery. (Courtesy of Nijhuis HHAM, Müller-Wiefel H: *J Vasc Surg* 13:408–411, 1991.)

Discussion.—These findings demonstrate that a subluxated stump may be an indication of persistant problems for patients undergoing first rib resection. Additionally, desk-type jobs may contribute to TOS symptoms, even after the surgical resection of the first rib. Individuals with these types of jobs are urged to perform shoulder exercises.

▶ There are many causes of recurrent symptomatology after first rib resection for the neurological symptoms of thoracic outlet syndrome.

Occlusion of the Brachial Artery by Thrombus Dislodged From A Traumatic Aneurysm of the Anterior Humeral Circumflex Artery
Nijhuis HHAM, Müller-Wiefel H (St Johannes-Hosp, Duisburg, Germany)
J Vasc Surg 13:408–411, 1991   13–6

Purpose.—Isolated injury of the axillary artery is unusual because of the proximity of the artery to the brachial plexus (Fig 13–2). A traumatic aneurysm of the anterior humeral circumflex artery was treated successfully.

Case Report.—Man, 22, had a history of coolness, paleness, and pain in his right hand and forearm, especially after playing fistball. On examination, there was no numbness of the right arm; however, the radial, ulnar, and brachial arter-

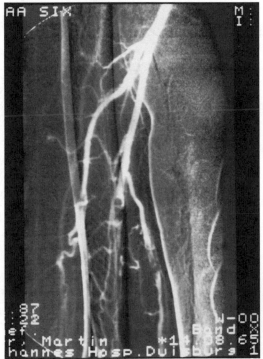

Fig 13–3.—Occlusion of the brachial artery in the right upper arm with collateral vessels progressing after occlusion. (Courtesy of Nijhuis HHAM, Müller-Wiefel H: *J Vasc Surg* 13:408–411, 1991.)

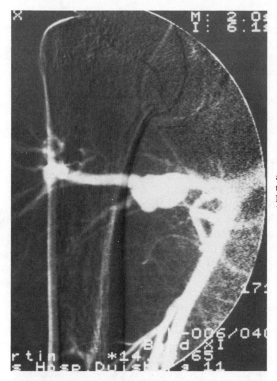

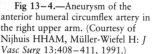

Fig 13–4.—Aneurysm of the anterior humeral circumflex artery in the right upper arm. (Courtesy of Nijhuis HHAM, Müller-Wiefel H: *J Vasc Surg* 13:408–411, 1991.)

ies were not palpable. Angiography revealed an occlusion of the brachial artery (Fig 13–3) and an aneurysm of the anterior humeral circumflex artery (Fig 13–4). The aneurysm was resected and a thromboembolectomy was performed. After operation, both arteries in the right forearm were palpable, and angiography showed no irregularities of the brachial artery and no aneurysm.

Conclusions.—Successful therapy for this patient consisted of ligation of the anterior humeral circumflex artery proximal and distal to the aneurysm, resection of the aneurysm, and transcubital thromboembolectomy. The unusual retrograde embolization of the content of the aneurysm appeared to be caused by a forceful compression of the aneurysm during fistball.

▶ The syndrome described in this abstract is very likely overlooked in most patients. Only carefully performed arteriography will reveal a lesion and dictate appropriate treatment.

Surgical Management of Ulnar Artery Aneurysms
Rothkopf DM, Bryan DJ, Cuadros CL, May JW Jr (Massachusetts Gen Hosp; Harvard Univ)
J Hand Surg 15-A:891–897, 1990   13–7

Background.—Ulnar artery aneurysms are rare vascular lesions, and the best approach to surgical treatment remains controversial. Whereas hand surgeons without microsurgical training favor conservative therapy or simple aneurysm excision, surgeons trained in microsurgery advocate excision and microsurgical reconstruction. The results of selective microsurgical reconstruction of these lesions were reviewed.

Patients.—During a 10-year period, 9 male patients (aged 6–51 years) were treated for 10 ulnar artery aneurysms. Blunt trauma was responsible for 7 aneurysms, puncture wounds for 2, and no apparent traumatic cause could be found for 1 aneurysm. There were 6 true aneurysms, 2 pseudo-aneurysms, and 2 thrombotic ulnar artery aneurysms. All of the patients underwent diagnostic arteriography. Three of the aneurysms were seen initially as asymptomatic masses of 4 weeks or less duration, and they showed no evidence of emboli. The other 7 aneurysms were associated with vascular symptoms of 6 weeks or more; they showed definite clinical and radiographical evidence of digital emboli (Fig 13–5).

Treatment.—Intraoperative digital plethysmography was used to assist in the surgical decision making. Five of the aneurysms were treated with resection and end-to-end microvascular repair after mobilization of the proximal and distal arterial segments, 4 lesions were resected without microvascular repair, and 1 aneurysm was treated medically with an anticoagulant because the patient refused operation.

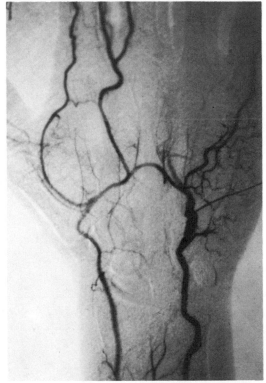

Fig 13–5.—Arteriogram of the left hand shows fusiform aneurysm of ulnar artery with embolic occlusion of ring finger digital arteries. (Courtesy of Rothkopf DM, Bryan DJ, Cuadros CL, et al: *J Hand Surg* 15-A:891–897, 1990.)

Results.—After an average follow-up of 40 months, all of the patients showed uniform improvement of their vascular symptoms without loss of jeopardized tissues. Five hands were asymptomatic, and the other 5 hands had mild digital cold intolerance.

Conclusion.—With careful preoperative and intraoperative radiographical study, ulnar artery aneurysms can be treated successfully with selective microvascular reconstruction.

▶ Traumatic ulnar artery aneurysms are particularly suitable for aneurysmectomy and direct arterial repair without interposition grafting.

Ulnar Artery Thrombosis and the Role of Interposition Vein Grafting: Patency With Microsurgical Technique
Mehlhoff TL, Wood MB (Mayo Clinic and Found, Rochester, Minn)
J Hand Surg 16-A:274–278, 1991   13–8

Background.—Pharmacological or mechanical sympathectomy has been used to treat ulnar artery thrombosis in the past, but there is little concordance on the optimal treatment. Recent data indicate that the reestablishment of pulsatile flow to painful digits may produce the best clinical outcome. The outcome of microsurgical reversed autogenous interpositional vein grafts used to treat symptomatic chronic ulnar artery thrombosis was reviewed retrospectively.

Patients.—The series consisted of 8 men (average age, 40 years) with a history of trauma and painful Raynaud's symptoms in the digits of the dominant hand (in 5 men) or the nondominant hand (in 3 men) caused by ulnar artery thrombosis that was verified by arteriograms or intraoperatively. Of the 8 patients, 5 were smokers. Preoperative and postoperative Doppler studies and Allen's test results were compared. The preoperative 2-point discrimination and the ulnar and median nerve conduction velocities were normal. The follow-up ranged from 12 to 105 months (average, 58 months). During surgery in 6 of the patients, the occluded vessel was resected, and a bifurcated cephalic or basilic vein graft was reversed and anastomosed to the ulnar proper digital artery or fourth common palmar web artery and to the remaining arch.

Results.—At follow-up, 7 of 8 grafts were patent, with excellent results in 4 cases, improvement in 3 cases, and no improvement in the patient in whom thrombosis recurred. Although the series was small, the factors that evidently promoted an excellent outcome were: not smoking, a single specific traumatic event instead of repetitive trauma, and surgery within 5 months of the onset of symptoms. In 6 of the 7 patent grafts, the pulse volume recordings of formerly affected digits had returned to normal; however, 2 patients with patent grafts had residual vasospastic morbidity after ice immersion—these 2 patients were both smokers.

Conclusions.—As many as 50% of patients with ulnar artery thrombosis may be misdiagnosed initially because the symptoms of painful dysesthesias, numbness, and cold intolerance are shared by several disorders.

Noninvasive vascular tests will be positive in patients with this syndrome, and arteriography will be definitive. Provided that the thrombosis and injured intima are totally resected and the execution of the microvascular techniques is proficient, blood flow can be successfully restored to painful digits by interposition vein grafting.

▶ Vascular surgeons long ago learned the value of direct arterial reconstruction in preference to sympathectomy. It is apparent that hand surgeons are also beginning to realize the value of this procedure.

14 Miscellaneous Aneurysms

Arterial Aneurysms in Children: Clinicopathologic Classification
Sarkar R, Coran AG, Gilley RE, Lindenauer SM, Stanley JC (Univ of Michigan)
J Vasc Surg 13:47–57, 1991
14–1

Introduction.—Arterial aneurysms in children are rare, and no unified categorization of these aneurysms has been established. Knowledge of the varied clinicopathologic characteristics of arterial aneurysms in children is important in the management of such patients.

Objective.—A clinicopathologic classification of arterial aneurysms in children has been proposed based on data from 23 pediatric patients seen at the University of Michigan Medical Center between 1957 and 1989 and on previously reported data from 165 pediatric patients with arterial aneurysms.

Data Analysis.—A total of 31 arterial macroaneurysms in 23 patients (age range, 6 months to 18 years; average age, 10.2 years) were treated. The treated arteries included the aorta in 4 cases, renal in 12, superficial femoral in 4, radial in 2, ulnar in 2, hepatic in 1, gastroepiploic in 1, iliac in 1, popliteal in 1, and brachial in 1. Eleven children were asymptomatic. Of the other 12 patients, 7 presented with a mass, whereas 3 had local pain, 1 had hematemesis, and 1 had painless obstructive jaundice. The diagnosis was confirmed by arteriography or surgery. All but 1 of the children underwent surgery, and 20 survived during a mean follow-up of 3.5 years. There was 1 operative death and 1 late death 6 years after surgery.

Results.—Childhood arterial aneurysms can be categorized as true aneurysms that are associated with arterial infection, giant-cell aortoarteritis, autoimmune connective tissue disease, Kawasaki's disease, Ehlers-Danlos syndrome or Marfan's syndrome, other forms of noninflammatory medial degeneration, arterial dysplasias, congenital-idiopathic factors, and false aneurysms associated with extravascular events that cause vessel wall injury or disruption.

Summary.—The classification of arterial aneurysms in children into the proposed clinicopathologic classes should provide a better understanding of the appropriate diagnostic and therapeutic interventions for these unusual lesions.

▶ This study from an experienced and long-established vascular service is valuable in defining pediatric aneurysms. It stresses the importance of classifying each aneurysm that comes to treatment. For example, if the diagnosis is Kawasaki's disease, then the coronary arteries must be visualized. In congenital aneurysms, a proper definition of etiology affects surgical care and suggests screening of family members for aneurysms or other arteriopathy.

Antibiotic Therapy for Arterial Infection: Lessons From the Successful Treatment of a Mycotic Femoral Artery Aneurysm Without Surgical Reconstruction
Kaufman JL, Smith R, Capel GC, Shah DM, Chang BB, Leather RP (Albany VA Med Ctr; Albany Med College, New York)
Ann Vasc Surg 4:592–596, 1990   14–2

Background.—Mycotic aneurysms may result from infection of the peripheral arteries, arterial involvement in a nearby septic synthetic bypass graft, or infection of a surgical prosthesis. Primary infection of the arter-

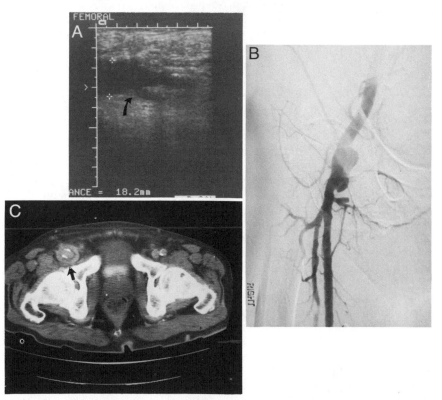

Fig 14–1.—Radiographic and vascular laboratory assessment of right femoral artery mycotic aneurysm. **A,** high-resolution ultrasonography as part of duplex scan. Longitudinal view, with anteroposterior luminal diameter marked. No thrombus is seen. Superficial femoral artery extends to right of image and profunda femoris artery origin is marked *(arrow)*. **B,** arteriographic appearance of mycotic aneurysm. **C,** CT of right femoral artery aneurysm *(arrow)*, demonstrating mural calcification and periarterial edema without abscess formation. (Courtesy of Kaufman JL, Smith R, Capel GC, et al: *Ann Vasc Surg* 4:592–596, 1990.)

ies is commonly seen as a complication of illegal intravenous drug use. Reports of a mycotic aneurysm consequent to acquired primary peripheral arterial infection are rare. Thus far, the recommended treatment for mycotic aneurysms, regardless of etiology, has been surgery. Nonsurgical treatment of a mycotic aneurysm was attempted. To date, only 2 other patients who underwent such treatment have been reported in the literature.

Case Report.—Man, 68, with type II diabetes, was admitted with symptoms of congestive heart failure. He had a history of both coronary artery disease and congestive heart failure. The patient had a urinary tract infection caused by *Staphylococcus aureus* that spread rapidly to the blood. Nafcillin was administered intravenously during the next 2 weeks. Although symptoms of fever and congestive heart failure abated, right inguinal pain, *aureua*-filled blisters, and necrotic signs developed in the right foot. Arteriography, CT scan, and ultrasound (Fig 14–1) verified the suspected right femoral aneurysm. Surgical treatment was delayed for 2 additional weeks because of the patient's poor cardiac state and newly discovered hypothyroidism. During this period of continuing nafcillin therapy, the groin symptoms resolved and the aneurysm stabilized. The total duration of parenteral nafcillin therapy was 7 weeks. The patient elected not to have surgery and has remained symptom free for 2 years.

Discussion.—This mycotic aneurysm was unusual because the infection was caused by an organism very susceptible to antibiotic therapy and was located in a site relatively easy to monitor. As more resistant organisms begin to appear in more rupture-prone thoracic or abdominal locations, both the hazard of ongoing sepsis and the breakdown of the arterial wall with catastrophic hemorrhage may mandate a surgical approach. A 6-week course of antibiotics appears to be a practical treatment for lingering endovascular infections of various etiologies.

▶ As indicated, antibiotic treatment of infectious aneurysms is a supplementary, rather than a definitive treatment.

Brachiocephalic Aneurysm: The Case for Early Recognition and Repair
Bower TC, Pairolero PC, Hallett JW Jr, Toomey BJ, Gloviczki P, Cherry KJ Jr (Mayo Clinic and Found)
Ann Vasc Surg 5:125–132, 1991   14–3

Background.—The presence of an aneurysm in the brachiocephalic arteries is a rare occurrence. The brachiocephalic aneurysm (BCA) can cause various symptoms and can lead to thrombosis, rupture, or embolization, which often requires surgery. In the past, surgical treatment focused on ligation of the aneurysm, which had a mortality rate of 30%–80%. The experience in treating 73 BCA patients between August 1950 and April 1990 was reviewed.

Methods.— All patients with BCAs who attended the clinic during the 40-year span were reviewed. The diagnosis was based on physical examination, chest roentgenogram, CT, and surgery.

Findings.— Of the 73 patients with BCA, 33 were women and 40 were men (mean age, 50.5 years). Figure 14–2 indicates the locations of the BCAs in this patient group. Neurological difficulties such as stroke and transient ischemic attacks occurred in 33 patients (43.8%). Arm claudication was found in 8 patients (11%). A group of patients (46.6%) had a palpable mass, whereas 15 (20.5%) demonstrated neurological deficits and 10 (13.7%) had lower pulse rates. Three of the patients (4.1%) experienced rupture of their subclavian artery aneurysms. Of the 73 patients, 40 (54.8%) had potentially life or limb-threatening problems. Hypertension and stroke appeared to be the most common risk factors for BCA. Nine of the patients had had a previous myocardial infarction. In addition, atherosclerosis was a very common problem, occurring in 21 patients (29%). Innominate artery aneurysms with a mean diameter of 4.5 cm were found in 6 patients. Whereas a total of 38 patients had BCA in a subclavian artery, 25 had the aneurysm in the carotid artery, and 1

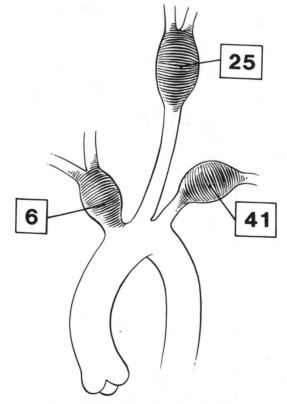

Fig 14–2.—Locations of brachiocephalic aneurysms in 73 patients (1 vertebral aneurysm not illustrated). (Courtesy of Bower TC, Pairolero PC, Hallett JW Jr, et al: *Ann Vasc Surg* 5:125–132, 1991.)

had the aneurysm in a vertebral artery. Six deaths occurred within 30 days, 3 in patients undergoing emergency procedures. The risk of death was significantly greater in emergency patients and in those undergoing a concomitant operation.

Conclusions.—These findings indicate that the occurrence of an aneurysm of the brachiocephalic arteries is a rare event. When the aneurysms do appear, they are symptomatic and can cause life- or limb-threatening problems. Elective isolated repair of the aneurysm is the recommended procedure to ensure the best possible results.

▶ This study describes a large experience with a rare group of conditions. The abstract shows the importance of publishing the papers from the Peripheral Vascular Surgery Society meeting, and the editors of *Annals of Vascular Surgery* are to be commended for doing so.

Current Trends in the Diagnosis and Treatment of Hepatic Artery Aneurysms
Blue JM, Burney DP (Moses H Cone Mem Hosp, Greensboro, NC)
South Med J 83:966–969, 1990   14–4

Background.—Aneurysms of the hepatic artery are rare, constituting 20% of all splanchnic artery aneurysms. The increased use of CT, angiography, and abdominal ultrasonography in the diagnosis of vague and unusual abdominal complaints has led to the increased antemortem diag-

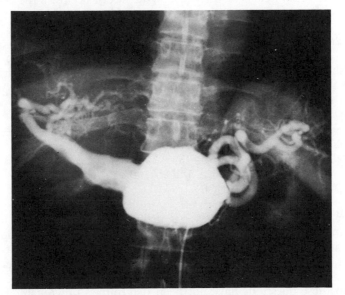

Fig 14–3.—Abdominal angiogram with contrast material in celiac artery demonstrates 8.5-cm common hepatic artery aneurysm extending to bifurcation of the right and left hepatic arteries. (Courtesy of Blue JM, Burney DP: *South Med J* 83:966–969, 1990.)

nosis of these lesions. When left untreated, hepatic aneurysms may lead to rupture and exsanguinating hemorrhage.

Case 1.—Man, 45, in Bogota, Colombia, was admitted with acute pancreatitis. Findings on abdominal CT and ultrasonography were interpreted as pancreatic pseudocyst. The patient came to the United States for a second opinion. Repeated CT and ultrasonography of the abdomen showed similar findings. However, abdominal angiography revealed an 8.5-cm aneurysm of the common hepatic artery extending to the bifurcation of the right and left hepatic arteries (Fig 14–3). At operation, the splenic and celiac arteries were ligated at their origins, the aneurysm was opened, and the aneurysmal wall was resected partially. A segment of the autogenous saphenous vein was used as a graft from the aorta to the distal hepatic artery. The distal anastomosis was sutured to a button of the aneurysmal wall, which contained the bifurcation of the right and left hepatic arteries. Histological examination of the excised aneurysmal wall revealed atherosclerosis. The postoperative course was uneventful.

Case 2.—Woman, 63, who had undergone 7 previous laparotomies for duodenal ulcer plication and hemigastrectomy with incidental splenectomy, complained of persistent lower abdominal pain without other abdominal symptoms. An abdominal CT scan suggested a hepatic artery aneurysm, and abdominal angiography confirmed the diagnosis. Aneurysmal dilatation started at the origin of the common hepatic artery, and the right and left hepatic arteries and gastroduodenal artery originated from the aneurysmal sac. The aneurysm was resected and the autogenous saphenous vein was used as an interpositional graft. The gastroduodenal artery was reimplanted into the vein graft with end-to-side anastomosis. Histological examination revealed cystic medial necrosis. The postoperative course was uneventful.

Conclusion.—Because of the well-documented natural history of progressive enlargement and eventual rupture, the aneurysms of the hepatic artery should be corrected surgically when the diagnosis is confirmed by angiography. In high-risk patients, the selective embolization of intrahepatic or subhepatic aneurysms may be a suitable alternative.

Surgical Treatment of Intestinal Artery Aneurysms

Geelkerken RH, van Bockel JH, de Roos WK, Hermans J (Univ Hosp Leiden, The Netherlands; Red Cross Hosp, The Hague)
Eur J Vasc Surg 4:563–567, 1990   14–5

Background.—Although intestinal artery aneurysms usually have an asymptomatic course, ruptures associated with a high mortality do occur. When an asymptomatic lesion is found, the physician must decide whether it should be treated surgically and which surgical technique should be used. Because this type of aneurysm is relatively rare, the answers to these questions have not been determined previously. The outcome in 15 patients treated surgically was evaluated.

Patients.—A group of 10 men and 5 women (average age, 54 years) were admitted to the study institution between 1966 and 1986. Of the 15 patients, 4 were asymptomatic, 7 were treated as an emergency, and 4 presented with shock. In the asymptomatic patients, the intestinal artery aneurysm was diagnosed during angiographic evaluation of an aortic aneurysm. The emergency patients all had acute abdominal pain.

Treatment.—A group of 7 patients underwent resection with arterial reconstruction, whereas 8 had ligation of the aneurysm. The postoperative mortality was 27% overall, but it was 43% in those patients who were treated as emergencies. There was no relationship between mortality and the amount of intraoperative blood loss. The 11 patients who had survived surgery all had an uneventful postoperative course. A histological examination revealed the etiology of the aneurysm in 13 cases. The most common causes were arteriosclerosis (5 patients), Ehlers Danlos syndrome (2 patients), and trauma (2 patients).

Conclusion.—Rupture, which occurs in as many as 13% of intestinal artery aneurysms, has a mortality rate of approximately 75% in some series. Arterial reconstruction is the recommended surgery; ligation is the second choice. Biplane abdominal angiography is required for visualization of the lesions. No variables predictive of rupture were discovered in this series, but the chance of rupture is acknowledged to be increased in pregnant and multiparous women.

▶ Most visceral artery aneurysms can be treated by ligation and excision. In the past, the diagnosis has been made after the occurrence of abdominal apoplexy. The present and future applications of vascular imaging allow elective treatment and arterial reconstruction when necessary.

The actual cause of rupture of splenic artery aneurysms during pregnancy is not known. It is unlikely that increased vascular volume and increased cardiac output are causative; however, fragmentation of the media and the internal elastic lamina must certainly be important clues.

Rupture of an Aneurysm of the Splenic Artery and Pregnancy: A Case Report
Czekelius P, Deichert L, Gesenhues Th, Schulz K-D (Philipps Univ, Marburg, Germany)
Eur J Obstet Gynecol Reprod Biol 38:229–232, 1990   14–6

Background.—Rupture of a splenic artery aneurysm during pregnancy is a rare problem, and little is known about its symptomatology, course, and treatment.

Case Report.—Woman, 30, was a primagravida who underwent treatment for hyperemesis gravidarum; she was also fitted for a McDonald cerclage for cervical incompetence. Pyelonephritis and labor pains that occurred during week 30 of the pregnancy were also treated successfully. Betamethasone was given to promote fetal pulmonary maturity during weeks 30 and 32. The patient complained of upper abdominal pain and responded to treatment for mild gastritis. Three days later she was admitted 1½ hours after collapsing at home with violent abdominal pain. The patient was in hypovolemic shock with unmeasurable blood pressure and only isolated fetal heartbeats. Immediate laparotomy and uterotomy were done; the severely hypoxic infant was resuscitated. There were 3 L of partially coagulated blood in the peritoneum. This coagulated blood came from a loculus of blood found in the greater curvature of the stomach, inside the omental bursa. The blood did not escape into the peritoneal cavity, and a perforated gastric ulcer was suspected. After stabilization of blood pressure, disseminated intravascular coagulation set in, followed shortly by cardiac arrest; the patient died. The infant died the same day; she had signs of progressive cerebral edema and trisomy 21 was diagnosed. At autopsy the mother was found to have a fusiform aneurysm of the splenic artery that was 1 cm in diameter and that extended tortuously for 4 cm from the hilus. The vessel wall showed a primary malformation in which no intima or media had been formed. A subendocardial infarct of the ventricular myocardium was also found, and erosive gastritis was confirmed.

Discussion.—The mortality rate of splenic artery aneurysm rupture during pregnancy is 69.4% for the mother and 90.8% for the fetus. Prophylactic surgery can reduce maternal mortality to .5% if the aneurysm is recognized early. Prodromal symptoms (constant pain in the left epigastrum, that sometimes radiates into the shoulder) are seen in 25% of patients. The pain may subside and flare again, with life-threatening symptoms.

Splenic Artery Aneurysm Rupture
Mines D (Hosp of the Univ of Pennsylvania)
Am J Emerg Med 9:74–76, 1991   14–7

Background.—The diagnosis of a ruptured splenic artery aneurysm (SAA) may be problematic because SAAs are usually rare and asymptomatic, and because the effects of SAA rupture resemble more common maladies.

Case 1.—Man, 46, with a recent history of heavy drinking and reflux gastritis, was seen twice in 24 hours with pain radiating from the left upper quadrant after vomiting. Gastritis was diagnosed and antibiotics were prescribed; the patient's pain diminished. At follow-up 36 hours later, the pain had lessened (except with motion), ultrasound revealed free peritoneal fluid; a gastrointestinal series was negative for the suspected perforated ulcer; hemoglobin had decreased; and bloody fluid was recovered from the abdominal puncture. Exploratory laparotomy showed bleeding from the splenic hilum. A splenectomy was performed and the patient recovered. A 1-cm aneurysm was found at the first bifurcation of the splenic artery.

Case 2.—Man, 43, who was diabetic and an intravenous drug abuser, had intense thoracic back pain and shortness of breath that began after he injected cocaine. His manner was agitated and pugnacious, and he appeared to be very ill, pale, and diaphoretic. An ECK showed sinus tachycardia with nonspecific ST-T wave changes. Despite treatment, the patient rapidly became hypotensive, unresponsive, and acidotic. Thoracic aortic dissection was suspected, but the patient died before surgery could begin. Autopsy showed a ruptured 5-cm atherosclerotic aneurysm of the splenic artery.

Discussion.—The typical SAA patient is 2–5 times more likely to be female than male, is often aged 30–50 years, and is multiparous. Ruptures, which occur during pregnancy or peripartum, are usually fatal to both mother and fetus. An SAA is generally caused by atherosclerosis and arterial wall degeneration, but it may also result from pancreatitis, septic emboli, or trauma. Because it is uncommon for an SAA to produce symptoms, it is usually discovered incidentally, either when the upper left quadrant in an abdominal radiograph shows typical "egg-shell" calcifications (in about 75% of cases), or when rupture occurs. In the latter case, patients report that the pain begins suddenly in the upper left quadrant and then spreads to the back, left flank, or shoulder. Patients may vomit, have abdominal tenderness and distention, and show signs of hypovolemic shock. Rupture may occur freely into the peritoneal cavity, which results in rapid hemodynamic failure. It may also occur into the lesser sac, in which case compression may slow bleeding transiently and diminish pain. If a ruptured SAA is suspected, an immediate surgical consultation is imperative. Although the presence of left upper quadrant calcification on roentgenogram and the presence of unanticipated fluid on abdominal ultrasound both support diagnosis of an SAA, only arteriography (time permitting) permits an exclusive diagnosis. This is the first report of possible cocaine-induced rupture of a visceral aneurysm.

▶ A very important cause of SAA, portal hypertension, was not mentioned in this abstract. This is a condition that does occur in men, unlike spontaneous SAAs that occur in women.

Transcatheter Treatment of Splenic Artery Aneurysms (SAA): Report of Two Cases

Tarazov PG, Polysalov VN, Ryzhkov VK (Ministry of Publical Health, Leningrad)
J Cardiovasc Surg 32:128–131, 1991   14–8

Introduction.—About half of all splanchnic artery aneurysms are splenic artery aneurysms (SAA). Rupture of the SAA occurs in about 10% of cases and is associated with high mortality.

Case 1.—Woman, 54, received a diagnosis of cirrhosis complicated by portal hypertension and hypersplenism; the patient was leukopenic. Celiac angiography demonstrated a large saccular aneurysm of the main splenic artery trunk. The main splenic artery trunk was embolized just proximal to the aneurysm with 3 modified Gianturco coils. The left upper quadrant pain resolved after 3 weeks, and the hypersplenism was partially corrected. A normal-sized spleen was present 8 months later, when aortography failed to fill the aneurysm.

Case 2.—Woman, 43, received a diagnosis of cirrhosis, portal hypertension, and hypersplenism. She also had a large aneurysm of the main splenic artery and multiple small intrasplenic aneurysms. The main arterial trunk was embolized with 3 coils to reduce, rather than eliminate, the splenic blood flow. Two coils were later added to complete the occlusion, and the patient recovered uneventfully. The hypersplenism resolved.

Conclusions.—Splenic artery embolization may be preferable to surgery. Transcatheter embolization proved safe in the present patients, and it did not damage the pancreas. When the spleen is grossly enlarged, a staged procedure is safer than immediate occlusion.

▶ Splenic infarction both with and without abscess formation has been reported after splenic artery embolization.

True Profunda Femoris Aneurysms: Are They More Dangerous Than Other Atherosclerotic Aneurysms of the Femoropopliteal Segment?
Tait WF, Vohra RK, Carr HMH, Thomson GJL, Walker MG (Manchester Royal Infirmary, England)
Ann Vasc Surg 5:92–95, 1991   14–9

Background.—True aneurysms of the profunda femoris artery are rare. The clinical features and complications associated with 3 such aneurysms were compared with those of common femoral and popliteal artery aneurysms.

Case Report.—Man, 76, had asymptomatic swelling of the right groin at a follow-up visit for ongoing peripheral vascular disease. He had presented with bilateral common femoral and popliteal aneurysms 4 years earlier. Arteriography of the groin showed a 3-cm aneurysm of the proximal right profunda femoris artery and a 2.2-cm aneurysm in a more distal location. Occlusion of the right superfi-

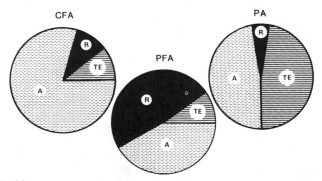

Fig 14–4.—Most common modes of presentation of aneurysms affecting the femoropopliteal segment. There were 262 aneurysms of the common femoral artery, 19 of the profunda femoris artery, and 270 of the popliteal artery. *A* indicates asymptomatic or minor local symptoms; *R*, rupture or rapid enlargement; *TE*, thrombosis or thromboembolism. (Courtesy of Tait WF, Vohra RK, Carr HMH, et al: *Ann Vasc Surg* 5:92–95, 1991.)

cial femoral artery was noted. The aneurysms were resected 5 months later, and they were replaced with a Dacron graft that remained patent.

Discussion.—Profunda femoris aneurysms account for only .5% of peripheral atherosclerotic aneurysms. The patients tend to be older men, and they often have other peripheral aneurysms. Treatment is usually successful. The condition may be difficult to diagnose because of its deep location, and because initial thromboembolism or rupture is rare (Fig 14–4). This diagnosis should be considered in all patients with groin aneurysm.

▶ Profunda femoris aneurysms appear to be a part of the generalized condition of arterial dilation and elongation (aneurysmosis), rather than isolated conditions.

Conservative Management of Asymptomatic Popliteal Aneurysm
Bowyer RC, Cawthorn SJ, Walker WJ, Giddings AEB (Royal Surrey County Hosp, Guildford, England)
Br J Surg 77:1132–1135, 1990   14–10

Background.—The optimal treatment for asymptomatic popliteal aneurysms remains controversial. In 1981, a policy of conservative management was adopted at 1 center because, if thromboembolic complications occur, the limb may be saved by thrombolysis. The results of this treatment were followed in 9 patients who had thromboembolic complications from popliteal aneurysms.

Methods.—Patients who presented with "white leg" within the first few hours of occlusion were treated by conventional catheter embolectomy. All of the patients underwent full diagnostic arteriography from the contralateral groin. If single-shot arteriography using nonionic contrast medium showed lysis, then the catheter was advanced. If the patient failed to improve, the infusion was continued and the reassessment was delayed for up to 14 hours. A 1,000-unit bolus of heparin was given at the end of treatment and heparin was given intra-arterially for 4 hours–5 hours. The catheter was then withdrawn and early elective surgery was performed if possible.

Results.—In the 6 patients who were treated within 72 hours of occlusion, 70% to 100% lysis was achieved. The average infusion time in this group was 32 hours. Among the patients treated 10 days or longer after thrombosis, none had significant lysis after streptokinase treatment. Of the 6 patients who had lysis, 3 were treated with elective reconstruction and 2 were treated with anticoagulation; 1 died of Mendelson's syndrome. In all 5 successfully treated limbs, vascular patency was maintained. There was no limb loss among the patients who underwent late treatment.

Conclusions.—Thrombosed popliteal aneurysms should be treated with thrombolysis. The complication rate for asymptomatic aneurysms is low, and thrombolytic therapy is safe and effective. Surgical treatment is no longer necessary for asymptomatic popliteal aneurysms.

▶ This article and abstract present an extremely conservative viewpoint that totally neglects the shredding distal embolic phenomena that accompany many popliteal aneurysms. Such distal plugging of the outflow vessels can make limb salvage extremely complicated when the popliteal aneurysm thromboses.

Popliteal Artery Aneurysms: Long-Term Follow-up of Aneurysmal Disease and Results of Surgical Treatment
Dawson I, van Bockel JH, Brand R, Terpstra JL (Univ Hosp Leiden, The Netherlands)
J Vasc Surg 13:398–407, 1991   14–11

Introduction.—Popliteal artery aneurysms have been associated with thromboembolic complications, a risk of new aneurysms occurring, and a decreased life-expectancy. The long-term results of popliteal aneurysms were reviewed in a series of 50 consecutively treated patients.

Patients.—Between 1958 and 1985, 50 men were treated at 1 center for arteriosclerotic popliteal aneurysms. The mean age at diagnosis was 65

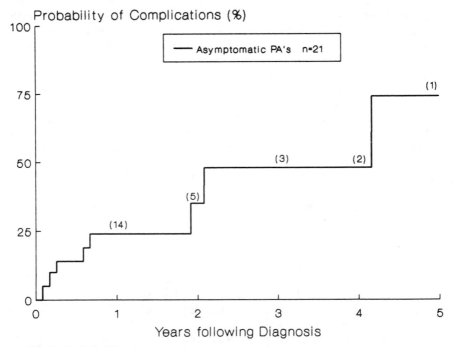

Fig 14–5.—Probability of nonsurgically treated asymptomatic popliteal artery aneurysms *(PAs)* to be associated with complications during follow-up, demonstrated by the life-table method. Numbers of limbs at risk are shown at each interval. (Courtesy of Dawson I, van Bockel JH, Brand R, et al: *J Vasc Surg* 13:398–407, 1991.)

years. A total of 21 patients had a contralateral popliteal aneurysm at the time of presentation.

Treatment.—Of the 71 aneurysms, 46 were treated initially by surgery. Of the remaining popliteal aneurysms that were not treated by surgery, 21 were asymptomatic and 4 were found in patients judged not to be medically fit for surgery. Eleven of the patients who were conservatively treated subsequently underwent surgery because of either complications or a risk of complications. In most of the cases (84%), the operative procedure consisted of bypass surgery with exclusion of the aneurysm.

Outcome.—Of the 21 asymptomatic, conservatively treated patients, 12 had complications, most within 2 years. During a mean follow-up of 5 years, 23 new aneurysms were diagnosed in 16 patients. The probability of new aneurysm formation (6% at 1 year) rose to 49% at 10 years (Fig 14–5). In patients who underwent reconstruction of a popliteal aneurysm, graft patency and foot salvage were 64% and 95% at 10 years, respectively. However, the overall survival was poor. At a mean follow-up of 5 years, 33 patients (66%) had died.

Implications.—The presence of multiple isolated aneurysms at the initial examination had the most significant influence on patient survival, even though most of the deaths resulted from myocardial infarction and not from complications of these aneurysms. Surgical reconstruction is recommended for all asymptomatic, as well as symptomatic, popliteal aneurysms. Those patients with multiple aneurysms should undergo regular, life-long follow-up.

▶ This presentation stresses complications of popliteal aneurysms that were observed for a long period of time. It correctly suggests that, whenever possible, patients should be selected carefully for reconstructive popliteal artery surgery.

Thrombosed Popliteal Aneurysm: A Problem to the Interventional Radiologist
Arlart Von IP, Gerlach A, Fürnrohr H (Katharinenhospitals, Stuttgart, Germany)
Fortschr Röntgenstr 152:430–433, 1990   14–12

Introductions.—The femoropopliteal junction is the most common location for the occurrence of arteriosclerosis and arterial occlusion. Approximately two thirds of all cases of femoropopliteal artery occlusion are caused by arteriosclerosis. However, obstructive adventitial cystic disease and entrapment syndrome can also cause occlusion of the popliteal artery. A completely thrombosed aneurysm of the popliteal artery may clinically and angiographically mimic vascular occlusion. The correct preoperative diagnosis of a blocked popliteal artery is very important because it prevents inappropriate interventional radiological therapy when vascular surgery for the aneurysm is indicated.

Experience.—During a 2-year period, more than 80 patients underwent recanalization of an occluded femoropopliteal artery via percutane-

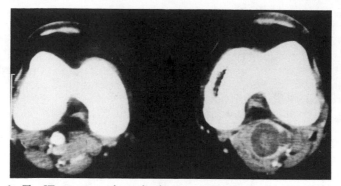

Fig 14–6.—The CT appearance of a popliteal aneurysm. A normally perfused popliteal artery (**left**) and a thrombosed aneurysm with fresh thrombus material in the center (**right**). (Courtesy of Arlart Von IP, Gerlach A, Fürnrohr H: *Fortschr Röntgenstr* 152:430–433; 1990.)

ous balloon angioplasty or fibrinolysis. Two patients had an unrecognized aneurysm of the popliteal artery and were treated incorrectly with urokinase that led to thrombosis and complete occlusion of the involved vessel. Sonography or CT is now performed routinely before interventional radiological recanalization of a popliteal artery obstruction is undertaken.

Results.—Of the 26 patients with angiographical evidence of unilateral popliteal occlusion, 11 had evidence of a thrombosed aneurysm on con-

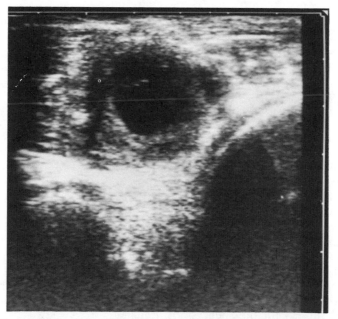

Fig 14–7.—Sonography of a large, centrally perfused popliteal aneurysm with thrombus adherent to the wall on cross section. (Courtesy of Arlart Von IP, Gerlach A, Fürnrohr H: *Fortschr Röntgenstr* 152:430–433, 1990.)

trast CT. Seven patients had a unilateral aneurysm; 4 patients had bilateral aneurysms (Fig 14–6). Real time sonography confirmed a unilateral thrombosed aneurysm in 10 of these 11 patients and a partially thrombosed contralateral aneurysm in all 4 patients with bilateral findings on contrast CT (Fig 14–7). Of these 11 patients, 6 (55%) were then found to have additional aneurysmal disease of the infrarenal abdominal aorta, the pelvic artery, and the femoral artery.

Conclusion.—Real time sonography and CT with contrast medium are useful in the differential diagnosis of aneurysmal obstruction of the popliteal artery.

▶ Lower extremity acute arterial occlusions can be treated by lytic therapy. This therapy uncovers the cause of the arterial occlusion and allows specific surgical intervention to correct the problem. The authors' experience suggests that ultrasonography of the popliteal fossa may accompany lytic therapy and uncover the cause of the arterial occlusion, even without successful thrombolysis.

Popliteal Aneurysms Identified by Intra-Arterial Streptokinase: A Changing Pattern of Presentation
Lancashire MJR, Torrie EPH, Galland RB (Royal Berkshire Hosp, London)
Br J Surg 77:1388–1390, 1990   14–13

Introduction.—Approximately one third of patients with popliteal aneurysm have an acutely ischemic leg caused by thrombosis or distal embolization, whereas another 5% to 41% have claudication, and the remaining patients are asymptomatic. However, claudication caused by popliteal aneurysm may be more prevalent than was recognized previously. This is because silent chronic thrombosis may cause symptoms of claudication that are indistinguishable from those resulting from atherosclerotic occlusion.

Patients.—During a 14-month period, 40 patients underwent intra-arterial streptokinase therapy for acute and chronic arterial occlusion; 5 had thrombosed popliteal aneurysms. In 4 of these patients, treatment was for claudication. A popliteal aneurysm was palpable before treatment in only 1 patient. The diagnosis was suspected based on the initial intravenous digital subtraction angiogram in another 2 patients. Intra-arterial streptokinase infusion successfully lysed the thrombus in all 5 patients; the patients subsequently underwent successful ligation and bypass procedures.

Conclusion.—Popliteal aneurysm may well be underdiagnosed as a cause of chronic leg ischemia. The more widespread use of intraarterial streptokinase infusion might well result in more diagnoses of occluded popliteal aneurysms in patients who were thought to have ischemia from occlusive arteriosclerotic disease.

▶ As indicated in Abstract 14–13, ultrasonography of the popliteal fossa contributes greatly to diagnosis when patients are being treated for acute popliteal artery occlusion.

15 Acute Ischemia

Upper Limb Embolus: A Timely Diagnosis
Davies MG, O'Malley K, Feeley M, Colgan MP, Moore DJ, Shanik G (St James's Hosp, Dublin)
Ann Vasc Surg 5:85–87, 1991   15–1

Background.—Upper limb embolus is less common than embolus of the lower limbs, and it must be treated aggressively to achieve successful results. Data were reviewed on 36 patients who underwent surgery for embolic occlusion of the upper limb vessels during a 10-year period.

Patients.—The symptoms included absence of radial pulse, coldness, pallor, resting pain, paresthesia, paralysis, and digital gangrene. Of the 36 patients, 8 had a history of previous embolic events; none of these events were to the arm vessels. Surgical embolectomy revealed brachial bifurcation, and adequate backflow was achieved with transverse arteriotomy with a Foley catheter.

Results.—Radial or ulnar pulses were restored in 34 patients. At 5 years the patency rate was 94% and the limb salvage rate was 97%. The postoperative complications included hematomas in 2 patients, seromas in 2, respiratory tract infections in 2, and wound infections in 3. Those patients treated within 24 hours of symptom onset did not have any major complications, whereas in 4 of the 13 patients treated after 24 hours, there was claudication in 1 patient, amputation of the 5 digits of 1 hand in 1, ischemic contracture in 1, and an above-elbow amputation in 1.

Conclusion.—The source of embolization was cardiac in most of these patients, and anticoagulant therapy was required for an indefinite period of time. Anticoagulants were also administered to patients in whom a source for embolization was undetermined. None of the patients experienced another embolic event during follow-up. Prompt diagnosis and surgical intervention is imperative for a successful outcome.

▶ The treatment of acute occlusion of the upper limb arteries by embolectomy is uniquely favorable. Patency is restored more easily in the upper limb arteries than in the lower limb arteries, and the mortality of embolectomy is considerably lower.

Aortic Dissection Presenting as Acute Leg Ischaemia
Raby N, Giles J, Walters H (Dulwich Hosp, London; King's College Hosp, London)
Clin Radiol 42:116–117, 1990   15–2

Introduction.—Aortic dissection presenting primarily with acute leg ischemia is a rare occurrence. The diagnosis was delayed in 2 instances, and the patients died.

Case Report.—Woman, 58, was admitted with acute onset of pain in the right leg. The leg was cold, white, and without pulses. The patient also complained of a dull aching pain in the chest and abdomen. After a diagnosis of acute right common iliac occlusion was made, an embolectomy was attempted under local anesthesia. However, no clot was retrieved. An arteriogram showed what appeared to be a thrombus within the right common iliac artery. It also showed distal aortic irregularity that was consistent with atheroma. However, the renal arteries were not seen, and the significance of the spiral lucencies in the left superficial femoral artery was not appreciated. The patient was treated with heparin after the right leg improved clinically. When the patient had neck and facial swelling the following day, an arch aortogram was performed. An extensive dissection of the thoracic aorta was confirmed, and the woman died an hour later.

Conclusion.—The absence of severe chest pain can delay diagnosis of an aortic dissection. These 2 cases illustrate the pitfalls of performing angiography of the lower extremities when dissection is manifested predominantly by acute leg ischemia. The signs that should be sought on films include varying degrees of compression of the lower aortic lumen, spiral linear lucencies within the lumen of the large vessels, and occlusion of the branches of the main vessels.

▶ The discovery of arterial dissection during what is expected to be a routine embolectomy is catastrophic.

Treatment of Patients With Aortic Dissection Presenting With Peripheral Vascular Complications
Fann JI, Sarris GE, Mitchell RS, Shumway NE, Stinson EB, Oyer PE, Miller DC (Stanford Univ)
Ann Surg 212:705–713, 1990   15–3

Introduction.—There is controversy over the optimal therapeutic approach for patients with aortic dissection complicated by peripheral vascular problems. An aggressive approach directed primarily at the repair of the dissected thoracic aorta was assessed.
Patients.—Between 1963 and 1987, 272 consecutive patients underwent surgery for spontaneous aortic dissection. Two types of dissection were distinguished: type A involved the ascending aorta, and type B did not. Those dissections in which the symptoms had occurred less than 14 days earlier were defined as acute, whereas those in which the symptoms had appeared more than 14 days earlier were defined as chronic. The patient group was predominantly male (196 patients) and had a mean age of 57 years. Of the patients, 85 had sustained 1 or more peripheral vascular complications (Fig 15–1).

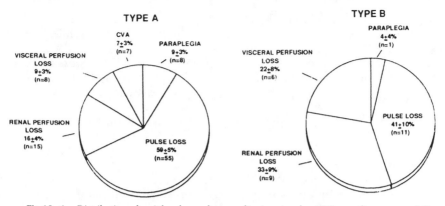

Fig 15–1.—Distribution of peripheral vascular complications (total = 120) according to type of dissection in the 85 patients who had 1 or more peripheral vascular problems. (Courtesy of Fann JI, Sarris GE, Mitchell RS, et al: *Ann Surg* 212:705–713, 1990.)

Operative Technique and Outcome.—Patients with type A dissections were approached through a median sternotomy. Those in the type B group underwent a left posterolateral thoracotomy. The overall hospital mortality rate was 25%. The mortality rate in patients with acute type A dissections (25%) was not significantly different from that in patients with chronic type A dissections (20%). In the type B group, the chronic dissections had a significantly higher operative mortality rate (40%) than the acute dissections (18%).

Implications.—The presence of peripheral vascular complications did not affect the overall operative mortality significantly. However, multivariate analysis revealed that impaired renal perfusion was a significant independent predictor of increased operative mortality risk. After repair of the thoracic aorta, the outcome was less favorable in patients with paraplegia and impaired visceral perfusion. Prompt surgical repair of the aorta will obviate the need for most peripheral revascularization procedures.

▶ The incidence of peripheral vascular complications associated with aortic dissection is clearly significant. However, it appears that 9 of every 10 such patients do not require urgent care of the peripheral vascular complication.

Intra-arterial Thrombolytic Therapy in the Management of Acute and Chronic Limb Ischaemia
Barr H, Lancashire MJR, Torrie EPH, Galland RB (Royal Berkshire Hosp, Reading, Berkshire, England)
Br J Surg 78:284–287, 1991   15–4

Background.—Acute nontraumatic lower limb ischemia is usually caused by arterial embolism or atherosclerotic vessel thrombosis. Death occurs in approximately 25% of patients, whereas another 20% to 40%

require major amputation. Therefore, the use of intra-arterial thrombolysis was assessed in patients with acute thromboembolic arterial disease and critically ischemic but viable limbs.

Patients.—A group of 54 patients with 56 ischemic limbs were treated between 1988 and 1990. There were 17 women and 37 men, aged 44–71 years. Of the 54 patients, 24 had symptoms within 1 week of the acute episode; 10, within 4 weeks; and the remainder, up to 10 weeks afterward. Five of these patients had ulceration and digital gangrene. The initial treatment consisted of low-dose intra-arterial thrombolytic therapy with streptokinase (10,000 units/hour^{-1}) or plasminogen activator (.5 mg/hour^{-1}).

Outcomes.—Complete thrombolysis was attained in 90% of the patients who had symptoms within 1 week of the acute episode and in 50% who had symptoms after 1 week. After successful lysis in 36 patients, 7 had successful bypass surgery; 13, percutaneous angioplasty; 13, no further treatment; 2, repeat thrombolysis; and 1, amputation. Treatment failure was associated with major amputation in 40% of patients. One patient died of hemorrhage and another died of stroke; both deaths were a result of thrombolytic treatment. Hematoma at the site of cannulation of the vessel was the most common complication.

Conclusions.—Although intra-arterial thrombolytic therapy can be very useful in the treatment of acute and chronic limb ischemia, potentially serious complications do occur. Therefore, patients should be selected carefully.

▶ Lytic therapy for acute arterial occlusions can successfully define the cause of the arterial occlusion in most cases. Therefore, intervention can be directed specifically at the cause of the problem. However, lytic therapy should not be considered the definitive and final solution to the problem.

Pulsed-Spray Thrombolysis of Arterial and Bypass Graft Occlusions
Valji K, Roberts AC, Davis GB, Bookstein JJ (Univ of California, San Diego; VA Med Ctr, La Jolla, Calif)
AJR 156:617–621, 1991   15–5

Background.—The excellent technical results of treating occlusions of the native arteries and of using hemodialysis and bypass grafts with pulsed-spray thrombolysis (PST) and urokinase have previously been reported. The short- and long-term clinical outcomes of PST were assessed in a large group of patients.

Methods.—The PST technique was used to lyse clots in 23 native arteries and in 25 bypass grafts; it was immediately followed by transluminal angioplasty (TLA) for the treatment of underlying stenoses in 21 of the arteries and in 24 of the grafts. For PST, the blocked vessel was accessed through an ipsilateral femoral puncture, and the clot was measured by traversing it with a guidewire. Pulsed-spray thrombolysis was not attempted if the wire would not transit the whole occlusion; this resulted in rejection of 26% of the initial 31 candidates with arterial occlusions. The therapeutic catheter was customized by punching side holes every 8 mm for a length that would span the clot. The catheter was then inserted, and 150,000 IU of concentrated urokinase were injected forcefully at a rate of 2.2-mL pulses/minute for 15 to 20 minutes. Urokinase was continued at a lower rate or concentration until the forward flow was rapid and only scattered 2- to 3-cm clots remained. Unless larger residual clots persisted, patients were heparinized only during the actual procedure.

Results.—Rapid initial clot dissolution was achieved by PST in an average of 65 minutes in all 23 native arteries and in an average of 93 minutes in 24 of the 25 bypass grafts. Recanalization accompanied by improved distal pulses and reduced symptoms was attained in 74% of the arterial occlusions and in 92% of the graft occlusions. Successful recanalization without adjunctive surgery was achieved in 65% of the arteries, 60% of the synthetic grafts, and 50% of the bypass grafts. The mean patency was 14.6 months, 4.3 months, and 3 months, respectively. There were major complications in 2 of the patients (4%) and minor complications in 11 (23%).

Discussion.—A single PST session resulted in extremely rapid and consistent clot dissolution; this reduced the time for intensive care monitoring, patient discomfort, and need for periodic angiography. The direct injection of urokinase into the occlusion permitted the use of a lower total dose of 400,000 IU—500,000 IU, compared with the total dose of 1,000,000 IU that is commonly used for other infusion techniques; this, plus the brief duration of heparin administration, probably explain the low incidence of hemorrhage. The new data from this group indicate that the beneficial results of PST alone are evanescent, and that PST combined with TLA produces poor long-term patency of saphenous vein grafts. However, the combined therapies are considered a good alternative to standard thrombolytic therapy for native arterial occlusions because the hazards from PST are minimal.

▶ The advances in endovascular repair are reported frequently in nonsurgical journals. Bookstein's ingenious thrombolytic method appears to improve the results of lytic therapy; this, in turn, allows definitive correction of the underlying problem.

16 Grafts and Graft Complications

End-to-Side Aortoprosthetic Anastomoses: Long-Term Computed Tomography Assessment
Mikati A, Marache P, Watel A, Warembourg H Jr, Roux J-P, Noblet D, Soots G
(Hôpital Cardiologique, Lille, France)
Ann Vasc Surg 4:584–591, 1990

16–1

Background.—A high incidence of thrombosis at the aortoprosthetic anastomosis has been observed during reoperations for bilateral thrombotic occlusion of the limbs of aortobifemoral bypasses. As a result, CT studies were made of a group of patients who had an aortofemoral bifurcation prosthesis implanted for 5 years or longer.

Patients.—A group of 52 men without current vascular symptoms underwent abdominal CT of graft status 5 years to 10 years after inititial surgery. The average age at surgery was 52 years. The men were former smokers. A total of 50 aortobifemoral bifurcated grafts and 2 aortoiliac grafts made of knitted double Cooley velour (44 cases), Cooley II single knit (7 cases), or Microvel (1 case) had been implanted end-to-side on the aorta. The current anteroposterior diameters at the plane of the infraanastomotic aorta, aortoprosthetic anastomosis, and limbs and stem of the graft were measured with CT. Those unilateral or bilateral saccular, lateralized expansions that were greater than 3 mm–9 mm were considered anastomotic false aneurysms if they appeared at the aortoprosthetic junction in CT.

Results.—There was thrombosis of the aorta distal to the graft in 92% of the patients, and partial thrombosis of the anastomosis (varied in size, site, and form) occurred in 40%. Although all of the patients were without symptoms, 15% had false aneurysms (Fig 16–1). The degree of dilation of the stem and limbs of the graft depended on the material used. With Microvel, the dilation values were 100% in the stem and 150% in the limbs; with double Cooley, 61% and 65%; and with single Cooley II, 36% and 28%. The amount of dilation appeared to stabilize by 5 years postsurgery.

Discussion.—Dilation of nearly all types of graft materials has been described previously, and it may increase substantially in hypertensive patients. The rate of asymptomatic aneurysms observed in this study is double the rate of symptomatic aneurysms generally reported. A CT scan may detect such anomalies better than aortography. The high rate of false aneurysms may be related to the amount of anteroposterior dilation. Many anastomoses show greater dilation in CT than can be accounted

259

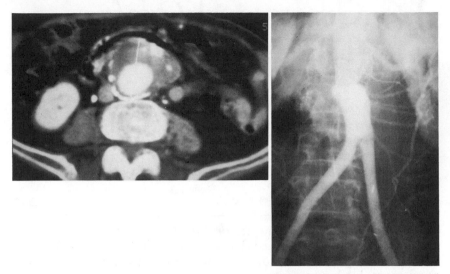

Fig 16–1.—False aneurysm of aorta occurred to left with marked dilation of prosthetic portion of anastomosis. (Courtesy of Mikati A, Marache P, Watel A, et al: *Ann Vasc Surg* 4:584–591, 1990.)

for by a "patch effect" resulting from the geometry of the side-to-end anastomosis. In this study, the observed increment could have been caused by a breakdown of the aortoprosthetic union, aneurysmal dilation of the aortic part of the anastomosis, or dilation of the prosthetic portion. A prospective study of the risks of side-to-end aortoprosthetic anastomoses would be useful.

► This important study reveals a greater incidence of graft dilation or anastomotic dilation in end-to-side anastomoses. In end-of-graft-to-side-of-femoral-artery anastomoses, the geometry of the anastomoses increases wall tension according to the law of LaPlace. Perhaps the same occurs in aortic anastomoses.

Long-Term Results of Thrombectomy for Late Occlusions of Aortofemoral Bypass
Frisch N, Bour P, Berg P, Fiévé G, Frisch R (Hôpital Central, Nancy, France)
Ann Vasc Surg 5:16–20, 1991   16–2

Background.—Several surgical treatments may be used for late prosthetic graft thrombosis. Retrograde thrombectomy may be done in combination with treatment of eventual runoff artery lesions. The long-term results of this regimen have been assessed in 62 episodes of aortofemoral bypass thrombosis occurring in 50 patients during a 5-year period.

Methods.—Eight patients had aortofemoral and 42 had aortobifemoral bypass thrombosis. There were 47 men and 3 women (mean age, 58 years). A total of 64% had thrombosis during the first 48 months (Fig 16–2). All of the patients underwent retrograde thrombectomy through

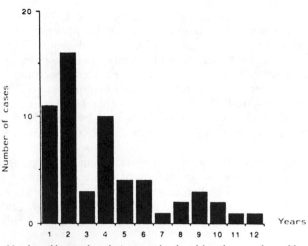

Fig 16–2.—Number of late graft occlusions as related to delay after aortofemoral bypass. (Courtesy of Frisch N, Bour P, Berg P, et al: *Ann Vasc Surg* 5:16–20, 1991.)

the distal anastomosis using a balloon catheter or, when the internal shell was bulky or friable, Vollmar's rings. Extra-anatomical bypass or complete graft replacement was done if thrombectomy failed. In 55 of the episodes, angioplasty, repeat distal anastomosis, or femoropopliteal bypass of the native runoff artery was performed. The patency of the bypass was evaluated yearly by clinical and sonographical evaluation for a mean follow-up of 47 months.

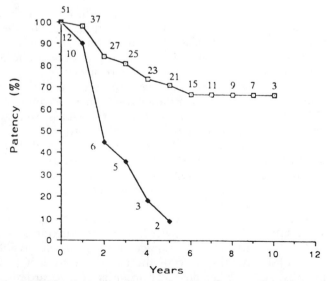

Fig 16–3.—Actuarial patency curve after graft thrombectomy in overall population *(open squares)* and in subgroup of patients having had repeat thrombectomies *(filled squares)*. (Courtesy of Frisch N, Bour P, Berg P, et al: *Ann Vasc Surg* 5:16–20, 1991.)

Results.— In the immediate postoperative period, 3 patients died and 2 required above-knee amputations. Two of the patients who underwent thrombectomy had contralateral embolism and required embolectomy. Of the 51 cases in which thrombectomy was possible, 39 remained patent; in the other 12 patients, either repeat thrombectomy or a new bypass was performed. The patency in this group was 97.8% at 1 year, 81.7% at 3 years, and 71.3% at 5 years (Fig 16–3). In the 11 cases in which thrombectomy was impossible, a new bypass was done. The patency in this group was 100% at 1 year, 75% at 3 years, and 50% at 5 years.

Conclusions.— Combined operative treatment with retrograde thrombectomy and treatment of anomalies of the native runoff arteries can yield long-term patency in patients with late thrombosis after aortofemoral bypass. Both the mortality and the morbidity are low. Endoprosthetic maneuvers must be done carefully to avoid contralateral embolism.

▶ Although this study extols the virtues of thrombectomy in the treatment of graft limb occlusion, one could look at the data and make a strong case for bypass as the best form of treatment.

Descending Thoracic Aorta as an Inflow Source for Late Occlusive Failures Following Aortoiliac Reconstruction
Branchereau A, Espinoza H, Rudondy P, Magnan P-E, Reboul J (Hôpital Sainte-Marguerite, Marseille, France)
*Ann Vasc Surg 5:*8– 15, 1991   16–3

Background.— The descending thoracic aorta-to-femoral artery bypass may be a safer and more effective procedure than the axillofemoral bypass, particularly for the repeat vascularization of the lower limbs. A group of 10 procedures performed for late failures of aortoiliofemoral reconstruction during a 5½-year period were reviewed.

Patients.— A total 19 lower limbs were revascularized in 10 men with a mean age of 60 years. Of the 5 patients who had aortobiliac or aortobifemoral bypass occlusion, 2 had aortofemoral bypass occlusion, 1 had a noninfected false aneurysm of an infrarenal side-to-side aortoprosthetic anastomosis, 1 had axillofemoral bypass occlusion, and 1 had aortobifemoral prosthetic graft degradation. The mean delay between the initial reconstruction and the revascularization was 69 months. Bifurcated grafts were inserted in 8 cases, an aortoprosthetic tube graft in 1, and an aortopopliteal tube graft in 1 (Fig 16–4).

Results.— There was 1 death caused by multiple organ failure at 23 days postoperatively. Secondary lower limb reconstruction was successful in 3 patients. The survival times ranged from 3 months to 48 months, with a mean of 14 months. Two of the patients were lost to follow-up after 3 months, and another died at 6 months of myocardial infarction; his bypass was patent at that time. There were 2 cases of graft thrombosis; 1 occurred at 5 months and was treated by thrombectomy, and 1 oc-

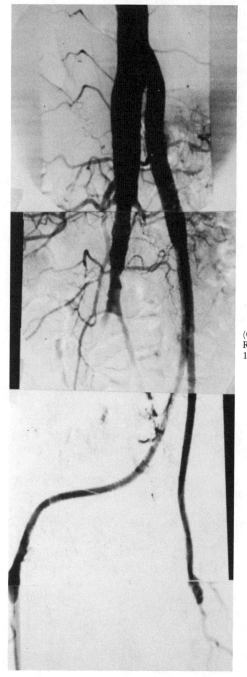

Fig 16–4.—Postoperative arteriogram. (Courtesy of Branchereau A, Espinoza H, Rudondy P, et al: *Ann Vasc Surg* 5:8–15, 1991.)

curred at 15 months and was treated by in situ thrombolysis. Both grafts remained patent, the first at 12 months and the second at 21 months. In the remaining 4 patients, the grafts were patent at 12 months to 48 months postoperatively. The primary patency rate was 55.5%, and the secondary patency rate was 100%.

Conclusions.—Descending thoracic aorta-to-femoral artery bypass is a relatively easy means of constructing extra-anatomical aortofemoral or aortobifemoral bypasses in patients who have late failure of aortoiliofemoral reconstruction. It also offers good hemodynamics of the lower limbs and avoids having to reenter the abdomen. Early morbidity and mortality are low, but when they do occur it is essentially because this operation is performed for debilitated patients with complex arterial problems.

▶ Although the indications for thoracofemoral reconstructions are few, the technique is extremely important to the vascular center that receives complex late failures after aortic grafting. It is also important to those patients who need aortic reconstruction yet have a hostile abdomen. The long-term results of such grafting are far superior to the results associated with axillopopliteal grafts.

Femorofemoral Crossover Bypass for Noninfective Complications of Aortoiliac Surgery
François F, Picard E, Nicaud P, Albat B, Thévenet A (Service de Chirurgie Thoracique et Cardio-Vasculaire, Montpellier, France)
Ann Vasc Surg 5:46–49, 1991   16–4

Background.—When a thrombosed prosthetic or vascular conduit cannot be cleared by thrombectomy, femorofemoral crossover bypass is a viable alternative to direct repeated aortic surgery. The data were reviewed on 39 femorofemoral crossover bypasses that were performed between 1973 and 1989 to treat unilateral noninfective complications of aortoiliac surgery.

Patients.—Femorofemoral bypass was performed for prosthetic occlusion in 35 patients, for a thrombosed false aneurysm in 2, and for degradation of the iliac artery in 2.

Results.—Below-knee or forefoot amputations were necessary in 2 patients. There were no intraoperative deaths. The primary patency was 87% at 1 year, 68.2% at 3 years, and 59.7% at 5 years. After successful reoperation, secondary patency was 89.6% at 1 year, 86.6% at 3 years, and 78.4% at 5 years (Fig 16–5).

Conclusion.—In the absence of associated aortic pathology, femorofemoral crossover bypass offered technical simplicity, satisfactory results, and extended benefits derived from the direct aortoiliac surgery. Future studies should examine the respective values of thrombectomy, crossover bypass, and direct repeated reconstruction for the treatment of unilateral prosthetic occlusions in a larger series of patients.

▶ As suggested by Abstract 16–3, bypass reconstruction after aortofemoral graft limb occlusion proves to be eminently satisfactory.

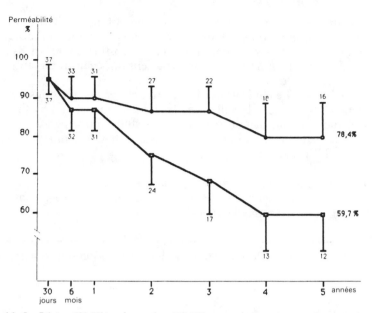

Fig 16–5.—Primary (59.7%) and secondary (78.4%) patency rates at 5 years. (Courtesy of François F, Picard E, Nicaud P, et al: *Ann Vasc Surg* 5:46–49, 1991.)

Inadequacy of Saphenous Vein Grafts for Cross-Femoral Venous Bypass
Lalka SG, Lash JM, Unthank JL, Lalka VK, Cikrit DF, Sawchuk AP, Dalsing MC
(Indiana Univ School of Medicine, Indianapolis)
J Vasc Surg 13:622–630, 1991   16–5

Background.—Cross-femoral venous bypass (CFB) grafting is a popular treatment for unilateral iliofemoral venous occlusion. The CFB is usually constructed from the contralateral saphenous vein transposed to the obstructed limb. However, such saphenous vein CFB grafts may provide inadequate relief of symptoms because of the high resistance of the small saphenous vein conduit. A mathematical model of unilateral iliac vein obstruction was used to establish a theoretic basis for choosing saphenous vein or larger diameter prosthetic CFB grafts for the relief of obstructive venous hypertension.

Methods.—Femoral vein resting and postexercise peak flows, as well as femoral vein and saphenous vein diameters, were measured in 18 healthy volunteers. These measurements were used to estimate the pressure gradient across CFBs of saphenous vein or 4-m, 6-m, 8-m, 10-cm, and 12-mm prosthetic conduits, in the presence of a venous collateral network of varying cross section.

Results.—The upper limits for normal pressure were set at 4 mm Hg for resting flows and 6 mm Hg after exercise. The mean saphenous vein diameter was approximately 4 mm, which was only about 36% of the femoral vein diameter. When the saphenous veins were used as the theoretical grafts in this model, two thirds of the volunteers had more than 80% of the flow carried by collateral circulation to maintain the standard pressure gradient after grafting. However, a prosthetic CFB of 8 mm or more in diameter eliminated venous hypertension, even in the absence of collateral venous flow.

Conclusion.—The clinical decision to use either a saphenous vein or a prosthetic CFB graft can be enhanced by measurements and by the use of a model such as that demonstrated in this study. Postoperative femoral pressure measurements are essential to establish the hemodynamic efficacy of a CFB procedure.

▶ In the peripheral circulation, there are only 2 situations in which a prosthetic graft is superior to an autogenous vein graft. The femorofemoral reconstruction is 1 of them. Can you name the other?

Reoperations for Late Complications Following Abdominal Aortic Operation
Haiart DC, Callam MJ, Murie JA, Ruckley CV, Jenkins AMcL (The Royal Infirmary, Edinburgh)
Br J Surg 78:204–206, 1991   16–6

Introduction.—Although the 5-year patency rate for aortoiliofemoral reconstruction is 85%, subsequent complications, including infection, false aneurysm, thrombosis, enteric erosion, and graft-enteric fistulae reduce the 15-year survival rate to 30%. The complications increase with each new surgical intervention. The complication outcomes of patients who required reoperation after aortic surgery were reviewed.

Methods.—Between 1979 and 1989, 50 consecutive patients who previously received aortic grafts or aortoiliac endarterectomy underwent reoperation. The mean patent age was 57 years, and the interval between the initial and subsequent procedure was an average of 50 months (range 2 months–220 months). A group of 35 patients had occlusive disease initially, whereas the remainder had asymptomatic, symptomatic, or ruptured aneurysms.

Results.—Reoperation was required for thrombosis in 27 (77%) of the 35 patients with occlusive disease; it was also required for fistulae or false aneurysm in the remaining patients. Of those patients who originally had aneurysms, 47% later had a false aneurysm and 40% had an enteric fistula. After reoperation, 8% of the patients died within 30 days; an additional 22% died in the first year, 50% at 3 years, and 63% within 5 years.

Discussion.—The initial pathology was significantly predictive of the type of late complication; patients who were operated on for aneurysms had late complications, whereas 77% of those who had primary occlusive disease later needed reoperation for graft thrombosis. The reoperation rate for thrombosis was quadruple that for aneurysm. The prognosis is poor after reoperation for late complications of either type; the need for revisional surgery may be reduced if the run-off is maximized during the original surgery for occlusive disease and if the suture lines are meticulously covered with extra tissue when aneurysms are repaired.

Diagnosis, Treatment and Prevention of Aorto-Enteric Fistulas
Goldstone J, Cunningham CC (Univ of California, San Francisco)
Acta Chir Scand 555:165–172, 1990   16–7

Introduction.—Aortoenteric fistula usually results from infection of a prosthetic aortic graft, but it can occur as a primary process when an aortic aneurysm erodes and ruptures into the bowel. Aortoenteric fistulas were found in 37.5% of 141 patients with infected aortic grafts.

Diagnosis.—Fewer than a third of the cases are diagnosed preoperatively, although as many as two thirds of patients may have suggestive clinical findings. The presence of overt sepsis raises the risk of a fistula in a patient with an infected aortic graft. A variety of bleeding patterns are seen, and gastrointestinal bleeding may be absent. Upper gastrointestinal endoscopy is an important diagnostic feature. The next most useful test is CT or MR imaging; ultrasonography has proved less useful. Angiography is necessary to properly plan reconstruction.

Management.—Surgical treatment of an aortoenteric fistula is based on controlling hemorrhage and sepsis, totally excising an infected graft, repairing the fistula, and ensuring revascularization of the lower extremities. Autogenous material is necessary when repair or reconstruction takes place in an infected field. Extra-anatomical bypass is often done first, followed immediately by transabdominal removal of the infected graft. The risk of late infection mandates long-term follow-up.

Prevention.—Most grafts are contaminated at the time they are implanted, although later hematogenous seeding is also a possibility. In this study, aortoenteric fistulas were more prevalent before viable tissue was interposed routinely between the graft and the overlying bowel.

▶ This study is included simply because it summarizes a very large experience with infected aortic grafts and provides guidelines for an approach to these problems. However, the actual prevention of aortoenteric fistulas is not clarified entirely satisfactorily.

***In-Situ* Replacement and Extra-Anatomic Bypass for the Treatment of Infected Abdominal Aortic Grafts**
Jacobs MJHM, Reul GJ, Gregoric I, Cooley DA (Texas Heart Inst-St Luke's Episcopal Hosp, Houston)
Eur J Vasc Surg 5:83–86, 1991   16–8

Objective.—For infected prosthetic abdominal aortic grafts, a combination of complete excision of the infected graft and extra-anatomical bypass is currently the therapy of choice. The operative results of 21 patients with infected abdominal aortic grafts treated by in-situ prosthetic graft replacement and extra-anatomical bypass were reviewed.

Patient Management.—A group of 12 patients had a primary perigraft infection; 9 had an infected graft secondary to an aortoenteric fistula (AEF). The infected graft was replaced with a new aortic prosthesis in 18 patients, and an axillobifemoral bypass was performed after graft excision in 3.

Results.—Among the 18 patients who had in situ replacement, 12 (including 2 with AEF) had grafts that were not incorporated into the surrounding tissue; they also had negative blood and perigraft cultures, indicating low-grade infection. All patients were alive at a mean follow-up period of 8 years, but 2 had required above-knee amputation for progressive atherosclerotic occlusive disease and 1 had undergone an axillobifemoral bypass because of reinfection. For the remaining 6 graft replacement patients (including 5 with AEF) the graft infection was severe, with perigraft fluid and blood cultures positive for 1 or more bacteria. Five patients died of sepsis within 1 month after graft replacement, and the sixth patient underwent axillobifemoral bypass because of reinfection. All 3 of the patients who underwent axillobifemoral bypass had severe graft infections and positive blood and perigraft cultures; however, all were alive at a mean follow-up period of 4.5 years.

Summary.—In patients with infected prosthetic aortic grafts, the severity of the infection influences the surgical outcome. Patients with a low-grade infection and negative blood and perigraft cultures will benefit from graft resection and in-situ replacement with a new prosthesis, whereas patients with severe graft infection with positive perigraft cultures and sepsis are better managed by excision of the infected graft and an extra-anatomical bypass.

▶ Although this study is controversial, it does provide information about a very large experience with in situ replacement of infected aortic grafts. When blood cultures are positive, the in situ replacement is unsatisfactory.

Secondary Aortoduodenal Fistulas: Value of Initial Axillofemoral Bypass
Bergeron P, Espinoza H, Rudondy P, Ferdani M, Martin J, Jausseran J-M, Courbier R (Foundation Hôpital Saint Joseph, Marseille, France)
Ann Vasc Surg 5:4–7, 1991   16–9

Background.—There is controversy over the best treatment for secondary aortoduodenal fistulas, which carry a very high mortality. The value of routine initial axillofemoral bypass before approaching the fistula was assessed.

Methods.—A group of 20 patients had operative treatment for secondary aortoduodenal fistulas during a nearly 20-year period. When the diagnosis was certain and emergency control of bleeding was not needed, initial axillofemoral bypass was done before ablation of the infected aortic prosthetic graft. When the diagnosis was uncertain or emergency laparotomy was needed to control bleeding, the routine changed during the course of the experience. In the first 10 years, the aortic graft was repaired directly or ablated, after which secondary axillofemoral bypass was done. In the past 10 years, bleeding was first controlled as necessary, axillofemoral bypass was done, and the aortic graft was then ablated. The results were evaluated at 6 months to 9 years.

Results.—Of the 13 patients who underwent initial axillofemoral bypass, 2 died in the immediate postoperative period, compared with 6 of the 7 patients who had direct surgery or initial ablation of the aortic graft. Of the remaining 12 patients, 3 died of hemorrhage from the aortic stump at 4 months, 12 months, and 14 months postoperatively. A new aortic graft was inserted in 2 patients; the abdominal aorta graft was replaced in 1, and the ascending thoracic aortobifemoral bypass graft was replaced in the other patient as a result of secondary thrombosis of the axillofemoral bypass. In the axillofemoral bypass group, the survival was 81% at a mean follow-up of 48 months.

Conclusions.—In patients with secondary aortoduodenal fistulas, performing axillofemoral bypass before repair of the aortic graft improves prognosis significantly. Although aortic stump infection may still occur and lead to recurrent aortoduodenal fistula, the risk of infection or secondary axillofemoral bypass occlusion is minimal. The prosthesis need not always be replaced.

▶ The removal of the infected graft is less important than strong nutritional support and the reversal of immunoincompetence.

Treatment of Postoperative Infection of Ascending Aorta and Transverse Aortic Arch, Including Use of Viable Omentum and Muscle Flaps
Coselli JS, Crawford ES, Williams TW Jr, Bradshaw MW, Wiemer DR, Harris RL, Safi HJ (Baylor College of Medicine, Methodist Hosp, Houston)
Ann Thorac Surg 50:868–881, 1990   16–10

Background.—Because the wound resulting from reconstruction of the ascending aorta (AA) and the transverse aortic arch (TAA) communicates directly with the skin, complications that would be trivial at other sites have grave consequences for the patient. In the 1% to 6% of patients in whom abdominal aortic and peripheral arterial operative sites become infected, an external bypass graft, resection of the infected graft, and 1 month to 6 months of antibiotic therapy produce a survival rate of 50% to 90%. However, because this approach is not suitable for infections of the AA and the TAA, the results of in situ surgery and suppressive antibiotic therapy for life were evaluated in such cases.

Methods.—The study population included 40 patients (average age, 55 years) who had infections in or near the surgical site 1 week to 5.5 years after graft replacement of the AA, TAA, or aortic arch. The infections caused complications such as aortic-right ventricular fistulas, aortobronchial fistulas, aortocutaneous fistulas, mediastinal abscess, infection of a

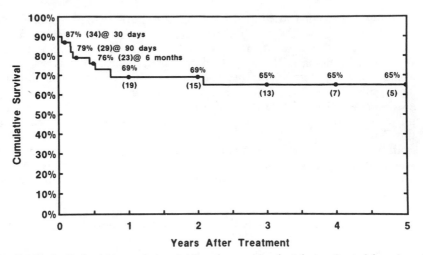

Fig 16–6.—Kaplan-Meier survival probability after operation for infection. Survival from time of treatment is shown for 40 patients. (Courtesy of Coselli JS, Crawford ES, Williams TW Jr, et al: *Ann Thorac Surg* 50:868–881, 1990.)

false aneurysm, rupture of a suture line, insufficiency of the aortic valve, antibiotic resistance, and problems with the chest wall. These complications were treated medically or by appropriate surgical methods including resuture, debridement, graft or valve-graft replacements, and patch-graft closure of false aneurysms. An important feature was the use of local living tissue, distant muscle flaps, and omentum to fill in dead space in the mediastinum. All of the surgical patients had intravenous antibiotic therapy for 4–6 weeks; they were then continued on oral suppressive antibiotics for life. The patients were followed up from 3 months to 6.5 years.

Results.—Although 5 of the patients died of complications during surgery and 2 more died in the subsequent 2 months, 29 surgically treated and 4 medically treated patients (a total of 83%) survived the early postoperative period; 70% were still alive during the follow-up period (Fig 16–6). None of the late deaths resulted from recurrent infection, a hazard avoided by all surgically treated patients.

Discussion.—The lifelong postoperative use of antibiotics was the most important principle in the concepts used in treating these patients. As long as the grafts were functional and patent in the absence of erosion or false aneurysm they were not removed. Simple false aneurysms and ruptured suture lines could be handled by debridement, patch grafts, or simple suture. In situ operations with lifelong suppressive antibiotic therapy are an appropriate intervention for infection of AA and TAA grafts.

▶ The details and diagrams in the original publication will be of great value to surgeons faced with these complex problems.

Post-Operative Vascular Infections: A Pathognomonic CT Scan Finding
Etienne G, Kassab M, Saliou C, Kessi H, Becquemin JP, Melliere D (Hôpital
Henri Mondor, Créteil, France)
J Chir (Paris) 127:589–591, 1990   16–11

Introduction.—Postoperative infection after a vascular repair requires
urgent treatment because spreading of the infectious process will endanger
the graft and its anastomoses. This complication is all the more serious because of its high risk of amputation and death. However, an urgent diagnosis is often difficult to establish. The presence of gas on a CT scan is a well
known but rare pathognomonical sign of infection. In 1 case the diagnosis
of postoperative vascular infection was made on CT findings alone.

Case Report.—Woman, 83, obese, underwent femoropopliteal grafting with a
saphenous vein because of arteriopathy of the lower extremities with pain and
decubitus. Cefamandole was given prophylactically at anesthesia induction and
for 48 hours thereafter. Three months later, the patient had a painful swelling in
the thigh of the treated leg. She was afebrile and had neither anemia nor leuko-
cytosis. All of the blood cultures were negative. Although a vascular infection
was suspected, the absence of any clinical sign was confounding. Because of the
potential danger associated with postoperative vascular infection, the patient underwent CT, which revealed a soft tissue cavity on the inner surface of the thigh
that was filled with gas and fluid. Puncture of the cavity under CT guidance retrieved a serous fluid that was sterile on direct microscopic examination. Even
though bacteriological testing showed no evidence of infection, the presence of
gas in the soft tissue favored emergency surgical exploration. A large abscess was
discovered at operation. The graft underneath the abscess was covered with gran-
ulation tissue. A culture taken from this site confirmed the presence of *Clostrid-
ium perfringens*. The patient was treated with amoxicillin, clavulanic acid, and
metronidazole. The wound healed completely in 3 months, and the graft remained patent at follow-up 1 year later.

Conclusion.—The sole finding of gas on CT scans is sufficient indication to warrant urgent surgical exploration. In this case the CT finding of
intracavitary gas allowed prompt, appropriate treatment; potential amputation was avoided.

▶ Although the radiographical sign described here may be familiar to many vascular surgeons, the opportunity it gives for perigraft fluid aspiration and culture
may not be familar. As in many other vascular conditions, early intervention is
of paramount importance in such a case.

**Evaluation of Three Techniques for Documenting *Staphylococcus Epider-
midis* Vascular Prosthetic Graft Infections**
Peter AO, Spangler S, Martin LF (Penn State Univ)
Am Surg 57:80–85, 1991   16–12

Background.—Although the incidence of infection in prosthetic vascular grafts has improved for high-virulence organisms, it has not improved for low-virulence organisms such as *Staphylococcus epidermidis,* which are the most common organisms cultured from these grafts. These infections are notoriously difficult to detect. A group of dogs was studied to determine whether nuclear MR (NMR) imaging or systemic norepinephrine (NE) kinetics were more reliable than standard angiograms.

Methods.—Twelve dogs were randomized into infected and control groups. A knitted Dacron vascular prosthetic graft was used to replace a 5-cm section of the infrarenal aorta in each animal. In the infected group, the grafts were contaminated with *S epidermidis* by soaking in an infected broth. For each animal, the NE production and clearance rates were calculated using ^{3}H-NE infusion and the steady-state radionuclide tracer method. These measurements were repeated 1 week after operation, and standard angiograms and NMR examinations were done.

Results.—Both groups showed similar angiographical results. Of the 6 infected dogs, 3 had disruption of the proximal anastomosis that was missed by angiogram. Although localized areas of high signal intensity, which suggested abscess, were not seen in any of the control dogs on NMR imaging, they were seen in 5 of the 6 infected dogs. The remaining animal had a disrupted anastomosis. Both groups of dogs had initially similar NE values; however, the NE spillover rates increased significantly after placement of the infected grafts.

Conclusions.—Norepinephrine kinetics appears to be able to detect vascular graft infection in animals before angiograms show any such evidence. Although NMR imaging is superior to angiography, its sensitivity is only 83%. When graft abnormalities are suspected, a section should be taken for culture.

▶ This very interesting experimental study explores the nonstandard methods of identification of graft infection. The conclusion of the abstract dovetails with Abstract 6–13.

Sonication Provides Maximal Recovery of *Staphylococcus Epidermidis* From Slime-Coated Vascular Prosthetics

Wengrovitz M, Spangler S, Martin LF (Pennsylvania State Univ)
Am Surg 57:161–164, 1991   16–13

Background.—Although *Staphylococcus epidermidis* is the most commonly cultured organism from infected prosthetic vascular grafts, these infections may be difficult to detect. Sonication of graft material has been proposed as a method of enhancing bacterial recovery. Vortexing and standard culture techniques of ultrasonic oscillation were compared to determine which method allowed recovery of the most bacteria from infected graft materials.

Methods.—A total of 192 segments of polytetrafluoroethylene (PFTE) and Dacron graft material were immersed in bacterial solutions of 4 different concentrations. Slime-producing strains of *S epidermidis* and *Escherichia coli* were used. Bacterial recovery was compared using direct plating, vortexing, or sonication. In the first method, the segments were placed directly onto the agar; in the other, 2 segments were placed in trypticase soy broth before sonication or vortexing before being plated onto agar.

Results.—At concentrations of 10 colony-forming unit (CFU)/mL, 10^2 CFU/mL and 10^4 CFU/mL of *S epidermidis*, direct plating was significantly less effective in recovering bacteria than either of the other 2 methods. This was true for both PFTE and Dacron graft segments. At 20^2 CFU/mL and 10^4 CFU/mL of *S epidermidis*, sonication was superior to vortexing in recovering bacteria. Because it adhered poorly to the graft segments, *E coli* could be recovered only at concentrations of 10^8 CFU/mL, and there was no significant difference between method or graft type.

Conclusions.—Sonication appears to be the best method for recovering *S epidermidis* from infected prosthetic grafts. Even at low concentrations, sonication does not seem to lead to false negative results. Grafts need not be excised in patients whose cultures are negative after sonication.

▶ This laboratory study corroborates a previous clinical study (1) that stressed the importance of sonication of the prosthetic material if *S. epidermidis* is to be recovered in culture.

Reference

1. Tollefson DF, et al: *Arch Surg* 122:38, 1987.

Femoral Noninfected Anastomotic Aneurysms: A Report of 56 Cases
Agrifoglio G, Costantini A, Lorenzi G, Agus GB, Castelli PM, Zaretti D (Univ of Milan, Italy; Univ of Pavia, Italy)
J Cardiovasc Surg 31:453–456, 1990   16–14

Background.—Although anastomotic aneurysms are not common complications of vascular surgery, they are associated with significant morbidity. Between 1975 and 1988, 56 femoral noninfected false anastomotic aneurysms (FAAs) occurred in 49 patients, 6 of whom had bilateral FAAs.

Patients.—The 59 FAAs represented 2.3% of all femoral anastomoses performed as part of aortofemoral or extra-anatomical bypass grafts during the 13-year period. The mean interval from the primary revascularization procedure to appearance of the aneurysm was 66 months (range, 12 months to 156 months), and only 1 aneurysm subsequently recurred. The majority of FAAs (78.6%) were asymptomatic. The others were complicated by acute expansion (5.3%) or thrombosis (16.1%). Aneurysm formation was caused by degeneration of the host arterial wall in

89.2%, graft failure in 5.4%, and breakage of the suture line in 5.4%. Hypertension was present in 30% of the patients.

Management.—All of the FAAs were treated surgically, except for 1 small asymptomatic aneurysm. The reconstructive procedure consisted of endoaneurysmectomy and interposition of a new end-to-end graft in 48, implantation of a fabric patch in 2, and prosthesis resuturing in 5. There was no operative mortality, and only 1 thrombosis occurred postoperatively.

Summary.—The structural weakness of the host artery was confirmed as a causative factor in the FAAs. Because of their propensity to have serious complications and their low operative mortality rate, FAAs should be repaired as soon as possible.

▶ The treatment of anastomotic false aneurysms has proven easier than finding the cause of the problem. The cause may be related to the invocation of LaPlace's law, as was suggested in Abstract 16–1.

Etiology of Prosthetic Anastomotic False Aneurysms: Pathologic and Structural Evaluation in 26 Cases

Downs AR, Guzman R, Formichi M, Courbier R, Jausseran JM, Branchereau A, Juhan C, Chakfe N, King M, Guidoin R (Laval Univ, Quebec; Univ of Manitoba, Winnipeg; Hôpital St-Joseph, Marseille, France; Groupe hospitalier de la Timone, Marseille; Hôpital Nord, Marseille)
Can J Surg 34:53–58, 1991   16–15

Introduction.—Anastomotic false aneurysms (AFAs), a relatively common late complication of grafting, can result from a number of causes. Among the recognized etiological factors are suture dissolution or fracture, graft-related defects, and elements related to the host artery or arterial-prosthetic junction. A group of 26 textile graft specimens removed because of AFA were evaluated in an attempt to further understand the formation of AFAs.

Methods.—Each graft specimen was examined morphologically, histologically, and by scanning electron microscope (SEM). At the time of graft implantation, the 26 patients (23 men and 3 women) had an average age of 56.2 years. Of the patients, 23 had been treated for aortic occlusive disease and 3 had been treated for an abdominal aortic aneurysm.

Findings.—Most of the aneurysms (21 of 26) appeared between 5 and 10 years after implantation of the graft. Monofilament suture was used in 17 cases and multifilament braided suture was used in 5; suture material was not identified in 4 specimens. No suture-related failures leading to AFA were discovered. Fraying was common (9 cases), but was not the cause of AFA formation (Fig 16–7). Fiber degradation occurred in 3 patients and probably contributed to AFA formation in 2 of these cases. In 20 patients, SEM demonstrated the presence of a discrete bacteremic colonization. However, no infection was detected clinically.

Conclusion.—Chemical degradation of the fibers, a possible contributing factor in 3 cases of AFA formation, may have been secondary to lipid

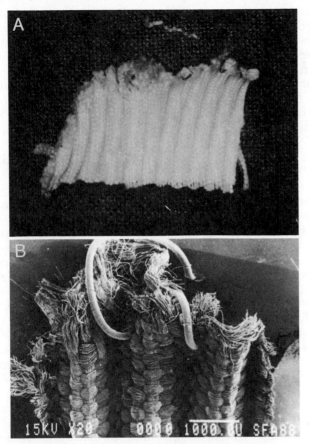

Fig 16–7.—**A,** cleaned graft specimen demonstrating fraying at edges of woven graft; **B,** scanning electron micrograph of frayed edges of graft. Original magnification, ×20. (Courtesy of Downs AR, Guzman R, Formichi M, et al: *Can J Surg* 34:53–58, 1991.)

infiltration. Although the role of bacteria is not well defined, they may contribute to degeneration of the arterial wall and the formation of AFA.

▶ The findings of this study correlate with the findings in Abstract 16–13, suggesting that *Staphylococcus epidermidis* may be an important etiological agent in the causation of anastomotic false aneurysms.

Vascular Anastomoses With Absorbable Suture Material: An Experimental Study
Schmitz-Rixen T, Storck M, Erasmi H, Schmiegelow P, Horsch S (Univ of Cologne, Germany; Klinik of the City of Karlsruhe, Germany; Klinik of Porz on the Rhine, Cologne, Germany)
Ann Vasc Surg 5:257–264, 1991   16–16

Introduction.—Vascular surgeons traditionally use nonabsorbable suture materials. Although the safety of absorbable sutures for vascular procedures has been demonstrated, their use has not gained wide acceptance. The suitability of a new synthetic, absorbable, monofilament suture material was assessed for use in vascular surgery.

Description.—The new suture is a copolymer made of trimethylene carbonate (PTC) and glycolic acid. The material decomposes in body tissue by hydrolysis. Previous animal studies have shown that PTC has a retention time in the body of up to 180 days, and that its tensile strength drops to 59% of its original value after 28 days.

Methods.—A group of 12 dogs was used in the study. Twelve abdominal aortic patch grafts and 10 femoral artery patch grafts, all of bovine heterograft material, were implanted and sutured with 6/0 PTC. In addition, 24 simple end-to-end anastomoses were made in the carotid artery and 5 in the iliac artery; all were sutured with PTC. A total of 14 iliofemoral bypass implants using 5 mm of expanded polytetrafluoroethylene (PTFE) prostheses were also performed. For comparison, 24 carotid artery anastomoses, 5 iliac artery anastomoses, and 14 iliofemoral bypass implants were performed contralaterally using nonabsorbable 6/0 polypropylene (PPP). All of the anastomoses and bypass implants were documented by arteriography and histology. Grafts from 6 dogs were harvested in the first 10 months of follow-up. The other 6 dogs were killed from 15 months to 20 months after grafting.

Results.—No suture material-related complications occurred. Healing occurred without increased incidence of false aneurysms, disruptions, or leaks in artery-to-artery or graft-to-artery anastomoses. The PTC and PPP sutures had comparable patency rates. Polytrimethylene carbonate sutures caused less inflammation and less scar tissue formation than the PPP sutures. After 4–7 months, PTC was completely absorbed by hydrolytic decomposition. Thereafter, an almost complete regeneration was observed in all layers of the vessel wall. Both PTC and PPP were histologically equivalent in the early months.

Conclusion.—The implantation of alloplastic and heterologous material using absorbable PTC sutures was successful, with histologic demonstration of a complication-free healing process. However, further experimental studies are needed before this material can be tested for vascular surgical procedures in humans.

▶ Although it is unlikely that absorbable suture material can be used routinely in arterial reconstruction in man, the excellent healing obtained in the experimental model suggests the possibility of its use in autogenous tissue reconstructions.

17 Vascular Trauma

Non-Invasive Vascular Tests Reliably Exclude Occult Arterial Trauma in Injured Extremities
Johansen K, Lynch K, Paun M, Copass M (Harborview Med Ctr, Seattle)
J Trauma 31:515–522, 1991   17–1

Background.—Although contrast arteriography accurately rules out occult arterial injuries in traumatized extremities, it is invasive, expensive, and time consuming. In a preliminary study, Doppler arterial pressure index (API) (calculated by dividing the systolic AP in the injured extremity by the AP in an uninvolved arm) of less than .90 had a sensitivity of 95% and a specificity of 97% for major arterial injury. To determine whether noninvasive tests could be substituted for arteriography, a series of patients with extremity trauma had arteriography only when the API was less than .90.

Methods.—A total of 100 injuries in 96 patients was studied; those patients with obvious signs of arterial injury were excluded. All of the patients had Doppler arterial pressure measurement and calculation of API, and those with an API less than .90 had immediate contrast arteriography. Patients with an API greater than .90 underwent management of other injuries, serial Doppler API determinations, and, in 64 cases, duplex sonography. There were 84 penetrating and 16 blunt injuries.

Results.—An API less than .90 was seen in 17 limbs; of these, arteriography was positive in 16. Vascular repair was carried out in 7 patients. In the remaining 83 limbs with an API greater than .90 (including those limbs that underwent duplex scanning), only 5 minor arterial lesions were found. "Exclusion" arteriograms decreased from 14% to 5.2% of all angiographic studies performed. The net savings during the 6.5-month study period was estimated to be $65,175.

Conclusions.—Noninvasive vascular tests appear to reliably exclude occult arterial damage in patients with extremity trauma. Such injuries should be screened by Doppler arterial pressure measurements, and arteriography should be performed only when the API is less than .90. This method of exclusion is accurate, safe, and inexpensive.

▶ Although the API will certainly detect artery occlusions, it may fail to detect pseudoaneurysms of arteriovenous fistulae.

Duplex Scanning for Arterial Trauma
Meissner M, Paun M, Johansen K (Harborview Med Ctr, Seattle)
Am J Surg 161:552–555, 1991   17–2

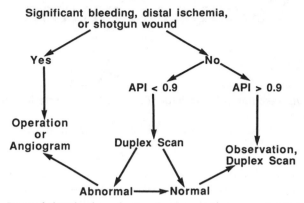

Fig 17–1.—Proposed algorithm for evaluation of patients with trauma potentially harboring a vascular injury. (Courtesy of Meissner M, Paun M, Johansen K: *Am J Surg* 161:552–555, 1991.)

Introduction.—Blunt or penetrating trauma without overt hemorrhage or distal ischemia is commonly investigated by arteriography to exclude occult arterial trauma. However, the reliability of arteriography in this setting has recently been questioned because most arteriograms are either normal or show minor abnormalities that do not require surgical intervention. Noninvasive duplex sonography was assessed as a screening tool for arterial injuries.

Patients.—During a 4-year period, 89 patients with a mean age of 29.5 years underwent duplex sonography scanning for 93 known or suspected arterial injuries to the extremities or the cervicothoracic region. Of these scans, 60 were done solely for wound proximity to nearby vascular structures; 19 scans were obtained because of suspected vascular injuries; and 12 scans were done for postoperative follow-up. One patient underwent duplex scanning for serial evaluation of an unoperated lesion.

Results.—Of the 60 scans performed for wound proximity alone, 4 (6.7%) were abnormal. Of the 19 (68%) scans done for clinical indications, 13 (68%) were abnormal. Six of the 12 (50%) scans performed for postoperative follow-up were also abnormal; however, no new injuries were discovered. Although a group of 4 patients (4.3%) with normal duplex studies had abnormal angiograms, none of these patients had major arterial injuries. There were no false positive studies.

Conclusion.—Duplex sonography is a rapid, noninvasive, inexpensive, and portable diagnostic modality that reliably diagnoses and localizes the sites of arterial disruption. The proposed noninvasive vascular diagnostic algorithm for evaluating patients who may harbor a potential traumatic vascular injury limits contrast arteriography to patients who have either an abnormal physical examination or an abnormal Doppler arterial pressure index (Fig 17–1).

▶ The use of duplex scanning to detect arterial injuries may substitute for arteriography, but it remains a very technician-dependent technique.

Ischemia in Acute Traumatic Instability of the Knee Joint
Pedrotti M, Ris H-B, Stirnemann P (Inselspital, Bern, Switzerland)
Chirurg 61:792–796, 1990   17–3

Introduction.—Acute traumatic instability of the knee is a common injury, but associated arterial trauma is rare. Unrecognized blunt trauma to the popliteal vessels may lead to later loss of function and even amputation. The records of all patients who were operated on for acute knee instability during a 12-year period were reviewed retrospectively.

Patients.—Of the 202 patients evaluated, 11 had an associated vascular injury. Of these 11 patients, 3 had an open injury, and 1 of the 3 also had a large soft-tissue defect. All of the patients had peripheral neurological deficits over the dorsum of the foot. Three patients had paresis of the peroneus, and 1 patient received a clinical diagnosis of compartment syndrome on admission. Foot pulses were absent in all patients. Four patients had complete ischemic syndrome in the foot, and 7 patients had a partial ischemic syndrome with a slight temperature difference when

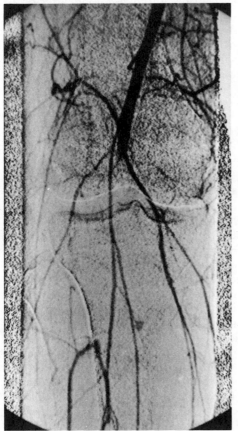

Fig 17–2.—Contrast medium stopped by subtotal ischemia in the supragenual popliteal artery; the distal connecting segment can be seen at the level of the exit of the anterior tibial artery above the collaterals. (Courtesy of Pedrotti M, Ris H-B, Stirnemann P: *Chirurg* 61:792–796, 1990.)

compared with the normal foot. The mean interval between injury and revascularization was 17.4 hours. A group of 9 patients underwent preoperative angiography; 2 had peroperative angiography. In all of the patients, the injected contrast medium stopped at the level of the knee joint, from 10 cm above to 4 cm below the knee fold (Fig 17–2).

Findings.—In 2 patients, the popliteal artery was completely disrupted at the level of the knee fold. Of these patients, 1 had a disrupted vein at the same level; the other patient had an ipsilateral iliofemoral thrombosis of an intact vein wall. A total of 9 patients had an intact adventitia with a semicircular to circular tear of the inner arterial layer. The veins at the level of the arterial injury were not involved in these 9 patients. All of the patients underwent vascular repair with autologous vein without shunting; 3 patients also had a fasciotomy of the lower leg at the same time. All patients received anticoagulants for several days after operation. No cases of postoperative ischemia occurred, and none of the patients required reoperation or amputation. There were no infections; however, 1 patient had necrosis of the medial gastrocnemius belly that had to be resected. Another patient had nonfatal pulmonary embolism. The patient with compartment syndrome underwent fasciotomy 48 hours after revascularization.

Conclusion.—Early diagnosis, revascularization with debridement of the damaged arterial wall, a tension-free reconstruction, and the liberal use of fasciotomy improve limb salvage in patients with acute traumatic instability of the knee and associated vascular injury.

▶ The YEAR BOOKS have repeatedly stressed the importance of popliteal artery injury in patients with an unstable knee. However, the diagnosis is continually missed, the injury is treated late, and multiple fasciotomies are often required for prolonged ischemia.

Axillary Artery Rupture Complicating Anterior Dislocation of the Shoulder: Case Report
Mustonen PK, Kouri KJ, Oksala IE (Kuopio Univ Central Hosp, Kuopio, Finland)
Acta Chir Scand 156:643–645, 1990   17–4

Introduction.—Although vascular complications associated with anterior dislocation of the shoulder are rare, they occur more often in atherosclerotic, elderly people. Injury may arise either at the time of dislocation or at reduction, especially if previous dislocations have resulted in periarterial scar formation. Of 330 shoulder dislocations treated during a 5-year period, 2 patients had vascular complications.

Case Report.—Woman, 74, was treated for anterior dislocation of the right shoulder 9 hours after a fall. The woman lost consciousness soon after reduction, her right hand became pale, and a hematoma of the shoulder region enlarged. When angiography revealed total occlusion of the right axillary artery, surgery was performed at once. The rupture was found to be partial, beginning in the C

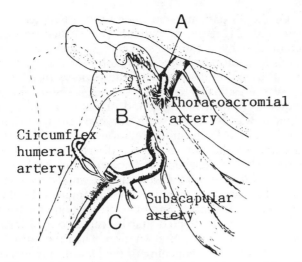

Fig 17–3.—Diagram of the normal and dislocated humerus and the parts of the axillary artery most susceptible to the injury. (Courtesy of Mustonen PK, Kouri KJ, Oksala IE: *Acta Chir Scand* 156:643–645, 1990.)

segment (Fig 17–3). Although the rupture was repaired, the distal pulses that were palpable immediately after surgery could no longer be felt the next morning. Part of the axillary artery was resected, and a vein graft was sutured between the cut ends in a second operation. At 5-year follow-up, the woman had strong distal pulses and no evidence of neurological or vascular deficit.

Conclusion.—The most vulnerable parts of the axillary artery are those near the branching vessels. When vascular injury is suspected after anterior dislocation of the shoulder, immediate operation by a vascular surgeon offers the best results. Bleeding complications that occur after reduction can be fatal. Resection of the ruptured part of the artery and an interposition graft are preferable to correction with fixating sutures.

▶ Although injuries to the adjacent vasculature are rare after dislocation of the shoulder, they do occur and are relatively easy to detect (if looked for).

Traumatic Rupture of the Aorta—Critical Decisions for Trauma Surgeons
Townsend RN, Colella JJ, Diamond DL (Allegheny Gen Hosp, Pittsburgh)
J Trauma 30:1169–1174, 1990   17–5

Background.—Both the diagnosis and the initial stabilization of patients with traumatic rupture of the aorta (TRA) are done by trauma surgeons. Patients with TRA pose special problems in resuscitative management and appropriate operative sequence, and they often have additional life-threatening injuries. A group of 54 patients with TRA treated at a level I trauma center was reviewed to determine the initial resuscitation, diagnostic sequence, and operative decision-making.

Results.—Of the 38 patients who underwent attempted aortic repair, 27 (75%) survived; 21 of the 27 patients (78%) died during phases of treatment controlled by a trauma surgeon. In the prehospital setting, pneumatic antishock garments were not helpful for these patients. During awake, unanesthetized intubation, 3 of the patients died of fatal aortic rupture that was presumably caused by acute rises in blood pressure. Neither hypotension nor a rise in blood pressure caused by blood and fluid replacement was correlated with survival. Delayed diagnosis was most frequently caused by misinterpretations of the initial chest x-ray, but delayed diagnosis did not contribute directly to any of the deaths. Fourteen patients had both abdominal injuries and TRA. Of these patients, 6 died, including 4 who died with potentially reparable injuries.

Discussion.—Patients with combined system injuries should be treated by preventing free aortic rupture and by control of other sources of blood loss. The abdomen may be treated first by rapid-control laparotomy to control major blood loss and contamination. Then the aortic injury may be addressed, followed by a reopening of the laparotomy incision and definitive repair of the abdominal injuries.

Conclusions.—The primary determinant of survival in patients with TRA is initial resuscitation. Patients with TRA may have a complete recovery if they survive long enough for the aortic repair to be attempted.

▶ This study stresses arteriography as the diagnostic modality of choice in traumatic rupture of the aorta. Newer developments are discussed in the abstracts that follow.

Medical Management of Acute Traumatic Rupture of the Aorta
Walker WA, Pate JW (Univ of Tennessee, Memphis)
Ann Thorac Surg 50:965–967, 1990   17–6

Introduction.—Acute traumatic disruption of the thoracic aorta usually requires urgent surgical repair, but some patients are not candidates for immediate surgical reconstruction. When the aortic injury is initially stable and the patient has associated life-threatening injuries that require immediate attention, a combination of pharmacological intervention to reduce the systolic blood pressure and cardiac shear forces may serve as a temporizing maneuver to prevent free rupture until surgical aortic repair can be performed more safely.

Patients.—A total of 79 patients with sustained acute traumatic aortic rupture underwent surgery. Because of associated severe injuries, 3 of these patients were stabilized medically until aortic repair could be performed. All 3 patients underwent emergent aortography. The initial pharmacological regimen consisted of intravenous administration of sodium nitroprusside to reduce the systolic blood pressure and propranolol hydrochloride to reduce the cardiac impulse. Both continuous arterial pressure monitoring and pulmonary artery catheterization to monitor cardiac output were part of the regimen. Patients underwent aortic repair when it was clinically warranted. No free aortic rupture occurred when the patients underwent aggressive medical therapy.

Conclusion.—The pharmacological treatment of acute traumatic disruption of the thoracic aorta is a viable approach to the management of patients with concomitant severe injuries that preclude immediate safe and successful aortic reconstruction.

▶ Although resuscitation is the key to success in treating traumatic aortic rupture, pharmacological management should be considered in every case.

Computed Tomography in the Evaluation of the Aorta in Patients Sustaining Blunt Chest Trauma
McLean TR, Olinger GN, Thorsen MK (Med College of Wisconsin; Houston VA Ctr; Baylor College of Medicine)
J Trauma 31:254–256, 1991   17–7

Introduction.—Traumatic aortic rupture (TAR) after blunt chest trauma is a rapidly lethal condition. However, because of improved transportation of critically injured patients, an increasing number of patients with potential TAR are arriving at the hospital alive. Aortography is the gold standard for evaluating both the aorta and the great vessels after major blunt chest trauma, but because of its potential for complications, there is controversy over which patients should be chosen to undergo angiography. Although CT is used with increasing frequency to evaluate blunt chest trauma, its accuracy for TAR has not been confirmed. The diagnostic accuracy of CT was assessed retrospectively in patients with potential TAR.

Patients.—During a 25-month period, 17 patients (mean age, 34.9 years) who had sustained blunt chest trauma underwent both chest CT and aortography to evaluate the aorta for TAR. A group of 50 patients with blunt chest trauma had aortography only. A mediastinal hematoma seen on CT was considered suspicious for TAR. Loss of the normal aortic contour was considered diagnostic for TAR.

Findings.—Of the 17 patients who underwent both examinations, 5 (29.4%) had TAR by aortography. All 5 patients had chest radiographs that were suspicious for aortic disruption. Two of the 5 patients with TAR had a normal aorta on the chest CT scan, 3 had findings that were diagnostic of disruption. Of the 12 patients without TAR, 8 had a suspicion of TAR on their chest radiograph, whereas 4 had normal chest radiographs. In addition, 8 of these 12 patients had normal chest CT scans and 4 had findings suspicious of TAR. Compared with aortography, CT scanning of the chest had a specificity of 23%, a sensitivity of 83%, and an overall accuracy of 53% for the diagnosis of TAR.

Conclusions.—When the mechanism of injury, the patient's physical condition, and the initial chest radiograph strongly suggest the possibility of aortic disruption, the patient should be taken immediately to angiography. Computed tomography should be considered only when the patient is stable and the clinical probability of aortic disruption is low.

▶ Computed tomography is useful for evaluating the aorta, the mediastinum, pleura, pulmonary parenchyma, and the diaphragm. Because some aortic tears are quite localized, the hazard of missing the aortic injury as a result of slice thickness is quite real.

Value of CT in Determining the Need for Angiography When Findings of Mediastinal Hemorrhage on Chest Radiographs Are Equivocal
Richardson P, Mirvis SE, Scorpio R, Dunham CM (Univ of Maryland Med Systems; Maryland Inst for Emergency Med Services Systems, Baltimore)
AJR 156:273–279, 1991   17–8

Background.—The results of a previous prospective study indicated that thoracic CT was useful in averting unnecessary thoracic arteriography when findings of mediastinal hemorrhage on chest radiographs were ambiguous in patients with acute decelerating thoracic trauma. A larger-scale continuation of that study was performed.

Methods.—During a 2-year period, 1,287 patients with blunt force trauma to the thorax were evaluated. Thoracic angiograms were done

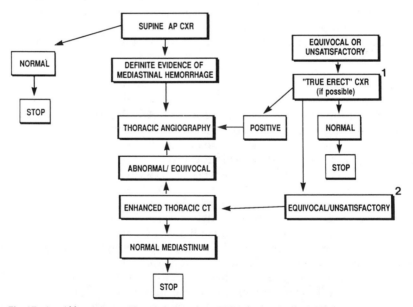

Fig 17–4.—*Abbreviations: AP*, anteroposterior; *CXR*, chest radiograph. Suggested algorithm for evaluation of patients sustaining significant blunt decelerating thoracic trauma. If chest radiograph obtained with patient supine only is possible *(1)*, choice of angiography or dynamic enhanced CT should be based on clinical level of suspicion for injury. When chest radiograph of erect patient is equivocal or unsatisfactory *(2)*, choice of angiography or CT may be influenced by the level of clinical suspicion for injury. (Courtesy of Richardson P, Mirvis SE, Scorpio R, et al: *AJR* 156:273–279, 1991.)

immediately on those patients with clearly abnormal mediastina, whereas 90 patients with equivocally abnormal chest x-rays but moderate or strong signs of injury to the major thoracic vessels received dynamic enhanced thoracic CT (Fig 17–4).

Results.—Of the patients who received thoracic CT, 70% had no evidence of hemorrhage of the mediastinum or aorta, and arteriography was not done. None of these patients evidenced delayed anomalies. In the 7% of patients who had either equivocal or uninterpretable CT scans, the subsequent angiograms were normal. Of the 16 patients with evidence of mediastinal hemorrhage on thoracic CT scan, 11 had normal thoracic arteriograms, and 4 evidenced injury to the great vessels. The CT scan often clarified the ambiguity of the original chest x-ray.

Discussion.—The introduction of thoracic CT significantly decreased the number of thoracic arteriograms performed for blunt impact trauma during this 2-year study, compared with the earlier 2-year study period. Although supine chest radiographs provide the only available view in thoracic trauma patients, they are often inadequate or misleading. Dynamic thoracic CT is useful and accurate in clarifying ambiguous results, and in averting costly and invasive arteriograms.

▶ Although CT is useful as an ancillary screening test after chest radiographs have been viewed, it does not totally replace aortography.

Thoracic Aortic Trauma: Role of Dynamic CT

Madayag MA, Kirshenbaum KJ, Nadimpalli SR, Fantus RJ, Cavallino RP, Crystal GJ (Illinois Masonic Med Ctr, Chicago)
Radiology 179:853–855, 1991   17–9

Introduction.—The early diagnosis of traumatic rupture of the aorta (TRA) in patients with significant blunt chest trauma is crucial to survival. Aortography is commonly performed whenever plain chest radiography suggests aortic injury. However, this approach generates many negative aortograms. Moreover, the reliability of chest radiographical criteria in assessing the need for aortography has been questioned. Two protocols were designed to prospectively study the efficacy of chest radiography and dynamic CT in screening for TRA in patients with blunt chest trauma.

Methods.—Protocol 1 involved obtaining a supine chest radiograph from each patient on admission to the emergency room. Those patients with abnormal chest radiographs immediately underwent aortography, whereas those patients with normal chest radiographs immediately underwent dynamic CT of the thorax. The patients with abnormal CT findings underwent aortography. If the CT scan was not suggestive of TRA, a follow-up chest radiograph was obtained either 4 hours later or according to clinical judgment. An aortography was performed if the follow-up chest radiograph was abnormal. Protocol 2 was identical to protocol 1, except that the patients underwent elective aortography within 24 hours of admission even if they had normal findings at both chest radiography and CT.

Patients.—During a 2-year period, 164 patients were admitted with significant blunt chest trauma; 114 were studied in protocol 1 and 50 were studied in protocol 2. Of the 114 patients in protocol 1, 31 underwent aortography. Of these 31 patients, 3 received a diagnosis of TRA and underwent surgery; 2 had abnormal findings on the chest radiograph and 1 had abnormal CT findings. The 83 patients who did not undergo aortography had both normal chest radiographs and normal CT scans; they were treated without surgery. None of these patients had any aortic abnormalities at follow-up chest radiography performed 6 months later. All of the patients in protocol 2 had normal chest radiographs and normal CT scans. Elective aortography performed within 24 hours in these patients was negative for TRA in all cases.

Conclusion.—The algorithm designed to screen patients with blunt chest trauma for TRA had a 100% sensitivity and a 100% negative predictive value. Unnecessary aortography was decreased by 73%.

▶ This report is useful because it confirms the findings of the previous studies.

Transesophageal Echocardiography in Acute Aortic Transection
Galvin IF, Black IW, Lee CL, Horton DA (The Prince Henry Hosp, Little Bay, Australia)
Ann Thorac Surg 51:310–311, 1991   17–10

Background.—Some individuals survive acute aortic transection because of containment of the mediastinal hematoma. Aortography has been the standard method for confirming the diagnosis of aortic transec-

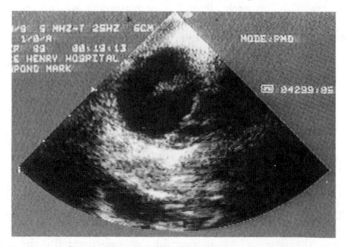

Fig 17–5.—Transesophageal echocardiography of descending aortic transection. A thick and highly mobile flap is best appreciated on real time scanning. (Courtesy of Galvin IF, Black IW, Lee CL, et al: *Ann Thorac Surg* 51:310–311, 1991.)

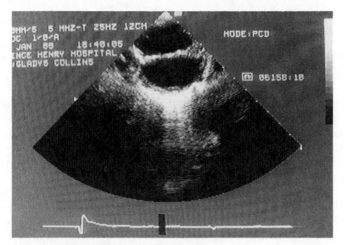

Fig 17–6.—Transesophageal echocardiography of a type B acute aortic dissection showing a fixed double-lumen arrangement. (Courtesy of Galvin IF, Black IW, Lee CL, et al: *Ann Thorac Surg* 51:310–311, 1991.)

tion, but CT has been used increasingly for such injuries. Transesophageal echocardiography (TEE) has been used in the detection of aortic dissection and other related conditions. An emergency patient underwent TEE within minutes of hospital admission and had surgery immediately thereafter.

Case Report.—Man, 22, who had been in a motorcycle accident, arrived at the hospital with multiple injuries and in shock. He was immediately intubated and hand ventilated. A large amount of abdominal swelling was observed, and no femoral pulses were present. Immediate TEE was performed in the intensive care unit with a 5-MHz phased array transesophageal transducer. An aortic tear was observed just distal to the beginning of the left subclavian artery (Fig 17–5). A freely moving flap was found over a short length of the aorta, and it differed from the more fixed double lumen of an aortic dissection (Fig 17–6). The site and localized condition of this flap suggested an aortic transection. Heart imaging demonstrated no pericardial fluid or cardiac injury. The entire TEE required only 10 minutes. The patient then had surgery to repair the aortic transection with a Dacron tube graft. The patient stabilized after surgery, recovered consciousness, and regained the movement of both lower limbs. Hepatorenal dysfunction occurred later, and the patient died of hepatic coma 43 days after surgery.

Conclusions.—The TEE procedure provided a rapid definitive diagnosis of aortic transection. The procedure may be helpful in diagnosing other forms of aortic injury, and it should be used after chest roentgenography in patients with suspected aortic injury.

▶ Transesophageal echocardiography continues to surface as an important method of detecting abnormalities of the thoracic aorta.

Anatomic and Clinical Factors Associated With Complications of Transfemoral Arteriography

Lilly MP, Reichman W, Sarazen AA Jr, Carney WI Jr (Brown Univ; Rhode Island Hosp, Providence)
Ann Vasc Surg 4:264–269, 1990   17–11

Background.—In patients who have complications of transfemoral arteriography, there is a high prevalence of arterial puncture in vessels other than the common femoral artery. Complications that required surgery occurred in 47 of 10,589 procedures reviewed during a 4-year period. The role of anatomical and clinical factors in the development of complications was assessed.

Findings.—In nearly 40% of these 47 cases, the arterial puncture was not in the common femoral artery; acute bleeding was more likely to be found. The risk of complications was higher after cardiac catheterization than after peripheral arteriography. The risk was also slightly higher in women and in older patients. Anticoagulation after the procedure was not a factor in bleeding complications. Both obese and nonobese patients showed the same distribution of puncture sites. The outcomes of the complications included 3 deaths, 1 extremity that required major amputation, and 7 extremities with persistent problems.

Conclusion.—Overall, transfemoral arteriography is a safe procedure with a low risk of serious complications. However, serious morbidity is significant when complications do occur. Those complications of transfemoral arteriography that required surgery occurred most often in patients who underwent cardiac catheterization and in patients who had punctures outside the common femoral artery. The factors that had less impact on patient risk were age, sex, body habitus, and anticoagulation.

▶ Iatrogenic arterial injury is epidemic, and its associated morbidity is considerable. Deaths occur after hemorrhage and hypotension in patients who require surgical repair.

Iliofemoral Arterial Complications of Balloon Angioplasty for Systemic Obstructions in Infants and Children

Burrows PE, Benson LN, Williams WG, Trusler GA, Coles J, Smallhorn JF, Freedom RM (Hosp for Sick Children; Variety Club Cardiovascular Lab, Toronto)
Circulation 82:1697–1704, 1990   17–12

Introduction.—Infants and children, especially those weighing less than 15 kg, are at risk for complications of the iliac and femoral arteries after diagnostic catheter procedures. The incidence, nature, and outcome of acute iliofemoral arterial complications resulting from balloon angioplasty were investigated in infants and children with aortic stenosis and coarctation restenosis.

Methods.—A group of 64 consecutive patients (mean age, 6.4 years; mean weight, 24.6 kg) was reviewed retrospectively. Balloon dilation an-

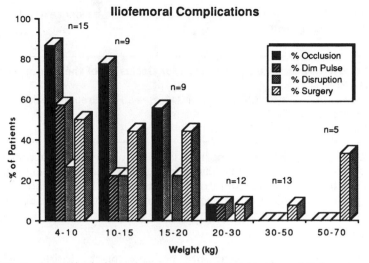

Fig 17–7.—Bar graph of relations between patient weight and incidence of iliofemoral complications; surgical treatment and early outcome of acute iliofemoral arterial complications are illustrated. *Percent Occlusion* indicates patients with arterial thrombosis and disruption; *Percent Dim Pulse*, patients with absent or diminished lower extremity pulses at the time of hospital discharge. (Courtesy of Burrows PE, Benson LN, Williams WG, et al: *Circulation* 82:1697–1704, 1990.)

gioplasty or balloon valvotomy was performed with 8F and 9F catheters without an arterial sheath. Heparin was given intravenously if pulses were not palpable after removal of the catheter. Intravenous thrombolytic therapy was instituted if the pedal pulses were not palpable after 24 hours of heparin. A poor response to these therapies led to surgical exploration, thrombectomy, and repair.

Results.—A total of 45.3% of the patients had an acute iliofemoral arterial complication, whereas thrombosis occurred in 18, complete disruption in 5, incomplete disruption in 3, and an arterial tear in 3. Of these patients, 18 underwent surgical exploration and repair. Medical and surgical treatment was effective in only 62% of the patients with complications; 11 had absent or diminished pedal pulses at the time of hospital discharge.

Conclusions.—The treatment of systemic obstructions with large high-profile balloon catheters results in a high incidence of traumatic complications of the iliofemoral arteries. Children who weigh less than 20 kg are at increased risk of such complications (Fig 17–7). Those infants who weigh less than 12 kg should probably not undergo surgical treatment of iliofemoral thrombosis in the absence of continued bleeding.

▶ As vascular consultants, we are often asked to help out when children sustain arterial trauma. Such trauma is not the same as vascular injury in adults. Witness the fact that surgical repair was disappointing in those infants who weighed less than 12.5 kg. Some pediatric cardiologists have a wait-and-see attitude about arterial thrombosis in infants and young children; however, some reports on this subject indicate a significant incidence of decreased lower extremity growth.

Limb Growth After Late Bypass Graft for Occlusion of the Femoral Artery: A Case Report

Rubinstein RA Jr, Taylor LM Jr, Porter JM, Beals RK (Oregon Health Sciences Univ, Portland)
J Bone Joint Surg 72-A:935–937, 1990   17–13

Introduction.—Failure of normal limb growth after reduction of the blood supply to an extremity has been well documented. Some interventions, such as open or percutaneous catheterization of the femoral artery, may produce occlusions and decreased limb growth. A late arterial bypass ameliorated an inequality in limb length resulting from vascular insufficiency.

Case Report.—Boy, 11 years, had occlusion of the left femoral artery that was caused by percutaneous catheterization performed at the age of 5½ weeks. Atropy of the left leg was evident at 44 months of age; the left leg was 1 cm shorter than the right leg. The child had poor exercise tolerance. To increase the chance of success, graft surgery was delayed until age 11, by which time the tibia was 2.8 cm shorter on the affected side. The left ankle brachial index, as determined in noninvasive vascular studies, was .6, compared to 1.2 on the normal side. The predicted deficit at skeletal maturity was 4 cm (Fig 17–8). An autogenous saphenous vein femorofemoral bypass immediately improved hemodynamics; the ankle-brachial indices were 1.1 on each side. The maintenance of adequate circulation was verified annually in noninvasive studies, and the limb-length discrepancy diminished slowly until only a 1-cm difference remained between the limbs at age 17, when skeletal maturation was achieved.

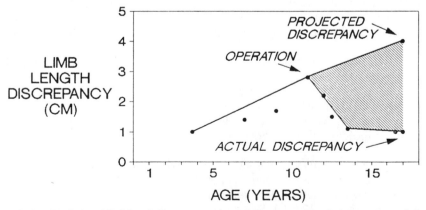

Fig 17–8.—Projected limb-length discrepancy and actual discrepancy. The *shaded area* shows skeletal growth attributed to grafting. (Courtesy of Rubinstein RA Jr, Taylor LM Jr, Porter JM Jr, et al: *J Bone Joint Surg* 72-A:935–937, 1990.)

Conclusions.—Increased growth of a limb has been documented after hypervascularity caused by fracture, osteomyelitis, sympathectomy, and arteriovenous malformations. The assessment of limb-length differences in children should include an evaluation of the circulation to the limb. If circulation is seriously impaired and the patient has decreased endurance for exercise, then surgical intervention to improve the blood supply may result in enhanced growth.

▶ As indicated in Abstract 17–12, there is controversy over the treatment of iatrogenic arterial occlusion in infants. It is valuable to know that late improvement of the blood supply may lead to increased growth of the affected limb.

Iatrogenic Subclavian Artery Pseudoaneurysms: Case Reports
Brzowski BK, Mills JL, Beckett WC (Lackland Air Force Base, Tex)
J Trauma 30:616–618, 1990   17–14

Background.—Iatrogenic arterial injuries are increasing with the frequent use of invasive monitoring and diagnostic vascular catheterization techniques. Iatrogenic subclavian pseudoaneurysms that occurred in the subclavian artery of 2 patients were assessed.

Patients.—During attempted subclavian vein cannulation using Seldinger's technique, subclavian artery pseudoaneurysms occurred in 2 men (53 and 21 years of age) after inadvertent placement of an introducer sheath into the artery (Fig 17–9). Both patients were in hypovolemic shock at the time of subclavian vein cannulation. Angiography confirmed the diagnosis. Both patients had successful primary arterial repair.

Implications.—Although they are quite rare, iatrogenic pseudoaneurysms of the subclavian artery may become more common with the in-

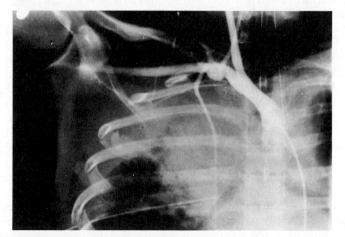

Fig 17–9.—Man, aged 21 years. Selective innominate injection defines a proximal right subclavian artery pseudoaneurysm. (Courtesy of Brzowski BK, Mills JL, Beckett WC: *J Trauma* 30:616–618, 1990.)

creasing use of invasive monitoring and diagnostic techniques. Cannulation of the subclavian vein with large-bore catheters should be avoided in hypovolemic patients. If iatrogenic arterial injury is suspected, diagnostic angiography should be undertaken to define the location of the injury and to guide the operative approach. The injury should be repaired primarily to prevent subsequent thrombosis, rupture, or embolization.

▶ As with iatrogenic femoral injury, trauma to the subclavian artery seems to be epidemic. Such trauma may require proximal control through a sternotomy.

Technical Report: The Complications of High Brachial Artery Puncture
Baudouin CJ, Belli A-M, Peck RJ, Cumberland DC (Royal Hallamshire Hosp; Northern Gen Hosps, Sheffield, England)
Clin Radiol 42:277–280, 1990   17–15

Introduction.—Femoral artery puncture is generally accepted as the access route of choice to the arterial system. However, an alternate access route must be used when femoral puncture is not available. Percutaneous high brachial puncture has been described as a safe alternative. The complications of angiography with high brachial artery puncture were reviewed.

Patients.—During a 2-year period, 51 patients underwent 52 angiographic examinations via high brachial puncture. Follow-up data were available for 49 procedures in 48 patients (age range, 40–82 years). The indications for high brachial artery puncture included a lack of palpable femoral artery pulses (30 patients) and a failed attempt at femoral artery catheterization (14 patients). The brachial artery was punctured midway between the axilla and the elbow.

Findings.—High brachial puncture was initially successful in 43 patients. A group of 12 patients had hematomas, 5 of which were graded large. Four patients had diminished or absent radial pulses at the end of the examination. Of these 4 patients, 3 had no associated ischemia, and their pulses returned spontaneously within 24 hours. The brachial and radial pulses remained chronically reduced in 1 patient. The fourth patient had ischemia caused by acute occlusion of the brachial artery. A catheter was advanced from the right femoral artery to the left subclavian artery, and the occlusion was dilated with an angioplasty balloon. There were no long-term complications. Two other patients had transient paresthesia in the distribution of the median nerve that resolved spontaneously within a few hours.

Conclusion.—The complication rate of high brachial artery puncture compares reasonably with the rate of other reported alternatives to femoral artery puncture. The technique is useful when femoral artery puncture is not possible and digital subtraction angiography is not available.

▶ This abstract stresses ischemia as a complication of brachial artery puncture. Of even more importance is the possibility of permanent neurological injury resulting from pressure neuropathy in situations of expanding hematoma. This is 1 of the true surgical emergencies and must be recognized as such.

Iatrogenic and Noniatrogenic Arterial Trauma: A Comparative Study
Lazarides MK, Arvanitis DP, Liatas AC, Dayantas JN (Athens Gen Hosp, Greece)
Eur J Surg 157:17–20, 1991   17–16

Background.—Diagnostic and therapeutic procedures can cause iatrogenic arterial trauma. The incidence of such trauma has increased in recent years because of the frequent use of cardiac catheterization and angiography and the increasingly radical surgeries available to remove lesions. Although it is well defined, the published incidence of iatrogenic trauma (as related to the number of arterial injuries) varies from 1.4% to 76%. A 6-year study of iatrogenic trauma evaluated a group of patients undergong vascular procedures.

Patients.—Between 1984 and 1989, 22 patients underwent surgery for iatrogenic injury (group A). The mean age of this group of 9 females and 13 males was 56 years. The records of 43 other patients treated for noniatrogenic arterial trauma during the same period (group B) were also evaluated. The mean age of this group of 3 females and 40 males was 35 years. Two vascular surgeons reviewed each of the 22 iatrogenic cases independently and then rated them on a 0–4 scale (0 indicated obvious fault; 4 indicated unavoidable injury).

Outcome.—The incidence of iatrogenic injury increased from 12% in 1984 to 58% in 1989 (Fig 17–10). Iatrogenic arterial trauma was related to vascular puncture, usually during catheterization or surgery. The average score for the appropriateness of the technique in the individual cases given by each of the reviewers was 2.4 and 2.2, respectively. In the noniatrogenic trauma group, injury was associated with blunt trauma (motor vehicle accident or falls) in 24 patients, stab wounds in 12, and gunshot wounds in 6. The kinds of vascular repair used did not differ significantly between the 2 groups. No significant differences were found for the incidences of the formation of arteriovenous fistula, false aneurysm, or ischemia. However, significantly more patients in the noniatrogenic injury group had hemorrhage. The incidence of associated injuries was significantly lower in iatrogenic group A than in noniatrogenic group B. The 3 deaths in group A resulted from circulatory and renal failure or from massive pulmonary embolism. The 4 deaths in group B were associated with septic shock and disseminated intravascular coagulation and with bleeding after the repair of an abdominal aortic trauma. Eleven of the group B patients (26%) and none of the patients in group A sustained permanent disability.

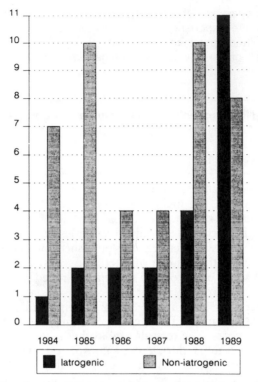

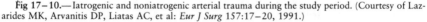

Fig 17–10.—Iatrogenic and noniatrogenic arterial trauma during the study period. (Courtesy of Lazarides MK, Arvanitis DP, Liatas AC, et al: *Eur J Surg* 157:17–20, 1991.)

Conclusions.—The fairly low score for the appropriateness of surgical technique demonstrates that some of the iatrogenic injuries could have potentially been avoided in these patients. Two factors have been implicated in iatrogenic injury: those that are physician-related (inefficient anatomical dissection, traumatic or faulty technique, or inadequate knowledge) and those that are patient-related (tumor, irradiation, inflammation, reoperation, and anatomical variation). The incidence of iatrogenic arterial injuries can be reduced by understanding all these causes.

▶ Although one would not expect there to be any similarities between iatrogenic and noniatrogenic arterial trauma, this study suggests that there are many similarities.

Iatrogenic Femoral Pseudoaneurysm and Arteriovenous Fistula: Nonsurgical Treatment
Wery D, Delcour C, Golzarian J, Azancot M, Grand C, Struyven J (Hôpital Erasme, Brussels)
J Radiol 72:91–94, 1991   17–17

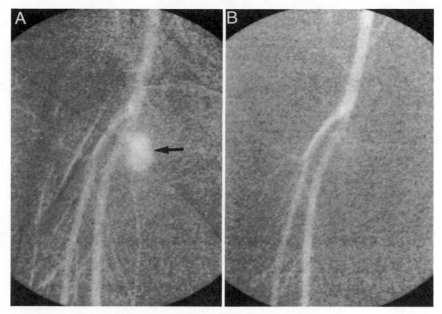

Fig 17–11.—A, intravenous digital subtraction angiography showing a pseudoaneurysm at the origin of the superficial femoral artery *(arrow)*; **B,** control examination after 45 minutes of percutaneous manual compression showing the complete disappearance of the lesion. (Courtesy of Wery D, Delcour C, Golzarian J, et al: *J Radiol* 72:91–94, 1991.)

Introduction.—Arteriovenous (AV) fistulas and pseudoaneurysms are rare complications of femoral artery catheterization. Both the use of large-diameter catheters and puncture that is performed too far from the inguinal crease increase the risk of local complications. These iatrogenic lesions have traditionally been treated surgically. However, the increased use of interventional radiology techniques and the associated increase in iatrogenic complications calls for effective noninvasive treatment. Locally applied manual compression has been successful in treatment of these complications.

Patients.—During a 6-month period, 7 patients received a diagnosis of a femoral pseudoaneurysm and 3 received a diagnosis of a femoral AV fistula subsequent to undergoing interventional radiology procedures. Of these patients, 4 had coronary angioplasty with a 9-F catheter, 3 had diagnostic angiography with a 7-F catheter, and 3 had left and right cardiac catheterization with a 7-F and a 5-F catheter. All of the patients were given 75 mg of dipyridamol 3 times daily and 300 mg of aspirin once a day. The diagnoses were confirmed by intravenous digital subtraction angiography (DSA). All 10 patients were treated by percutaneous manual compression at the puncture site. The average duration of compression was 45 minutes. The efficacy of the maneuver was assessed by intravenous DSA (Fig 17–11).

Results.—After simple manual compression, the lesion had disappeared in 7 of the 10 patients. The 3 patients in whom manual compression was unsuccessful underwent coronary angioplasty. Two of these 3 patients were given heparin anticoagulation therapy for 12 hours after angioplasty. The third patient had a pseudoaneurysm larger than 3 cm in diameter and required operation. After a mean follow-up of 3 months, none of the patients treated by manual compression alone had a recurrence of their lesions.

Conclusion.—Surgical treatment of an iatrogenic femoral pseudoaneurysm or an AV fistula confers additional trauma to patients and considerably prolongs their hospital stay. Manual compression at the puncture site successfully eliminated all 3 AV fistulas and 4 of the 7 pseudoaneurysms in this series, thus avoiding operation in 7 of the 10 patients. Locally applied manual compression is currently the treatment of first intention at this institution. Care should be taken to exert local pressure so that peripheral pulses are diminished but not eliminated.

▶ In light of the abstract that follows, this study of nondirected manual compression of the suspected iatrogenic femoral artery injury is very interesting.

Postangiographic Femoral Artery Injuries: Nonsurgical Repair With US-Guided Compression
Fellmeth BD, Roberts AC, Bookstein JJ, Freischlag JA, Forsythe JR, Buckner NK, Hye RJ (Univ of California and San Diego Med Ctr, San Diego; Mercy Gen Hosp, Sacramento, Calif)
Radiology 178:671–675, 1991   17–18

Background.—With the increasing use of larger percutaneous instruments and heparin, there has been at least a tenfold increase in the frequency of femoral artery pseudoaneurysms or arteriovenous fistulas.

Management.—For postangiographic femoral artery injuries, ultrasound-guided compression repair (UGCR) was evaluated as a possible new imaging-guided interventional procedure. With the transducer perfectly vertical, the groin is scanned for the narrow track of flow that connects the arterial lumen to the blind cavity (pseudoaneurysm) or the vein (arteriovenous fistula). A straight downward force is applied with the transducer until the flow through the track is eliminated (Fig 17–12). This position is maintained for 10 minutes, after which compression is slowly released. The compression cycles are repeated until all abnormal flow ceases or operator or patient fatigue ensues.

Patients.—Color Doppler flow imaging showed 35 pseudoaneurysms and 4 arteriovenous fistulas in patients evaluated for enlarging hematomas and/or groin bruits 1–14 days after catheter removal. Compression therapy was not performed in 10 patients because of spontaneous thrombosis, infection, skin ischemia, or excessive discomfort. The other 29 patients underwent effective UGCR, and the lesion was eliminated in 27 during a mean compression time of 30.2 minutes. One patient

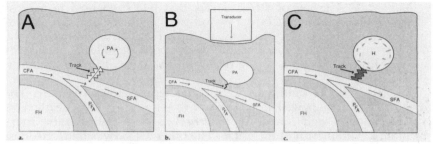

Fig 17–12.—Schematic representation of events during ultrasound-guided compression repair (UGCR) of a pseudoaneurysm. **A,** longitudinal view of postcatheterization femoral pseudoaneurysm. The common femoral artery *(CFA)* bifurcates into the superficial femoral artery *(SFA)* and profunda femoris artery *(PFA)* just below the femoral head *(FH)*. A persisting defect is present on the anterior surface of the lower common femoral artery or upper superficial femoral artery where the catheter pierced the vessel. The pseudoaneurysm *(PA)* cavity is connected to the defect by a narrow track of variable length. **B,** color flow transducer is appropriately positioned over the center of the track, and downward manual force has caused the walls of the track to appose, arresting flow into (systole) and out of (diastole) the pseudoaneurysm cavity. Ultrasound-guided compression repair is in progress. **C,** compression has been released, and a hemostatic plug of thrombus has closed the artery defect and track. The pseudoaneurysm is now a simple hematoma *(H)* that will resorb spontaneously. (Courtesy of Fellmeth BD, Roberts AC, Bookstein JJ, et al: *Radiology* 178:671–675, 1991.)

underwent surgery for an infected hematoma. The overall success rate was 90% for the 29 patients in whom UGCR was technically feasible. Some patients reported moderate discomfort during the procedure, but there were no complications. The follow-up color or flow scans at 24–72 hours were obtained in 27 patients and at 1 month–15 months in 19 patients. There were no recurrences and all of the patients were asymptomatic.

Conclusion.—For uncomplicated, catheterization-related femoral artery injuries, UGCR is a safe and technically simple procedure. It should be attempted in all patients without contraindications, excluding those with long-standing injuries. Nonsurgical repair of catheter-related femoral injuries with UGCR holds promise as a cost-effective, first line treatment.

▶ Directed compression closure of iatrogenic arterial injury decreases the morbidity of the injury considerably and will prove increasingly valuable to physicians and patients alike.

Cholecystectomy and Hepatic Artery Injuries
Halasz NA (Univ of California, San Diego)
Arch Surg 126:137–138, 1991   17–19

Background.—Injury of the hepatic artery, particularly the right artery, is a major danger of cholecystectomy. A normal liver was found in a cadaver that had undergone cholecystectomy 31 years before death, the right hepatic artery had been ligated. The incidence of this error and its significance were investigated.

Methods.—A group of 507 cadavers that had been used in a gross anatomy course during a 20-year period were investigated. If an individual had undergone cholecystectomy, the hilum was dissected to show the vascular anatomy. The abnormalities were recorded, and the individual's medical history was reviewed to determine the date of the operation, if possible.

Results.—Of the cadavers, 71 had undergone cholecystectomy. The date of operation ranged from 6 years to 41 years before death. Five vascular injuries were found. There were 3 cases of right hepatic artery ligation, 2 within 1 cm of the origin. The other artery was bifurcated just distal to the beginning of the gastroduodenal branch. One individual had a replaced right hepatic artery originating from the superior mesenteric artery; it had been interrupted in the hilum about 3 cm above the entry of the cystic duct. Most of this artery was patent because the right gastric artery originated from it 2 cm below the ligation. In the remaining case, the artery was bifurcated near its origin, with the posterior branch clipped along with the cystic duct stump. There was no atrophy or gross abnormality, nor were there any histological differences from the left lobe. The operation had been done 7 years, 16 years, and 31 years before death in the 3 patients whose date of operation could be established.

Conclusions.—The occurrence of hepatic artery injury during cholecystectomy appears to be fairly common, but the patient may survive for years without liver damage. The most likely mechanism of injury is mistaking the right hepatic artery for the cystic artery; others include catching the artery in the cystic duct clip, and hurried attempts to control hemorrhage without adequate visualization. The top-down approach, in which the gallbladder is moved from the liver bed to expose the hilar anatomy, may be a safer approach.

▶ Doing this dissection room study was an ingenious idea. It has proven to be timely in light of the fact that laparoscopic cholecystectomy is an operation from the bottom up.

Seat Belt Aorta
Randhawa MPS Jr, Menzoian JO (Boston Univ School of Medicine)
Ann Vasc Surg 4:370–377, 1990   17–20

Introduction.—Although seat belts have reduced injuries to accident victims, many types of intraabdominal injury have been associated with their use. A rare type of abdominal aortic injury may result in acute thrombosis, aneurysmal change, an intimal tear with flap formation, or distal embolization. A group of 11 cases of seat-belt associated traumatic abdominal aortic occlusion (9 previously reported and 2 new cases) was reviewed.

Case Report.—Man, 19, was a rear seat passenger wearing a lap-type belt when an auto accident occurred. The patient described pain in the abdomen and back but was hemodynamically stable. Examination revealed an abdomen that was rigid and guarded, weak femoral pulses, and a loss of sensation below T10.

Both of the legs were paralyzed. An L2-L3 fracture dislocation was found. Laparotomy revealed a transection of the rectus abdominis with 300 cc–400 cc of free blood in the peritoneal cavity. Small bowel tears were repaired before retroperitoneal exploration revealed a contused aorta containing thrombus. The intima and media were completely disrupted and distal dissection was present; a flap of degloved intima/media occupied the aortic lumen (Fig 17–13). The injured segment was replaced with a Gore-Tex graft, producing good distal pulses. Although lower limb perfusion was normal at discharge, sensorimotor function had not improved.

Aortic Injuries.—The aortic intima is most often disrupted distal to the inferior mesenteric origin. Intimal disruption may include circumferential intimal fracture with subsequent dissection, intimal laceration without occlusion or distal ischemia, or a full-thickness disruption of the intima and the media. Neurological and abdominal visceral injuries may overshadow the vascular abnormalities.

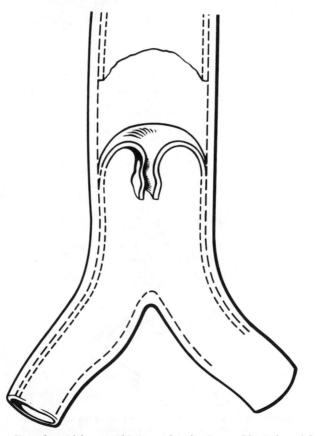

Fig 17–13.—Circumferential fracture of intima and media. Fractured layers formed flap that prolapsed on itself, thereby occluding the lumen of the aorta. (Courtesy of Randhawa MPS Jr, Menzoian JO: *Ann Vasc Surg* 4:370–377, 1990.)

Management.—Early treatment is the key prognostic factor, and the most common definitive procedure is prosthetic graft interposition. Distal pulses should be monitored after flow is restored because of the risk of peripheral embolization.

▶ Blunt trauma rarely induces abdominal aortic injury. Among the reports of such injury is 1 that describes a surfboard accident.

Operative Exposure of the Abdominal Arteries for Trauma
Fry WR, Fry RE, Fry WJ (Univ of California, Davis-East Bay; Indiana Univ Medical School, Indianapolis; St Joseph Mercy Hosp, Ann Arbor, Mich)
Arch Surg 126:289–291, 1991
17–21

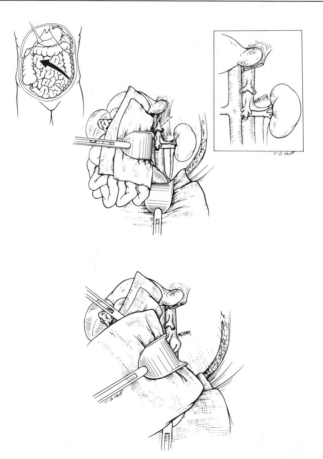

Fig 17–14.—Exposure of zone 1 abdominal arteries, including the suprarenal and supraceliac aorta, the celiac axis, the superior mesenteric artery, and the left renal artery. To expose this zone adequately, the retroperitoneal gastric fundus must be mobilized. **Top left,** *arrow* indicates incision of the peritoneal reflection; the viscera is rotated to the right. The figure enclosed in the box shows vessel exposure after division of the aortic hiatus. **Bottom,** by rotation of the left kidney, the posterolateral surface of the aorta is exposed. (Courtesy of Fry WR, Fry RE, Fry WJ: *Arch Surg* 126:289–291, 1991.)

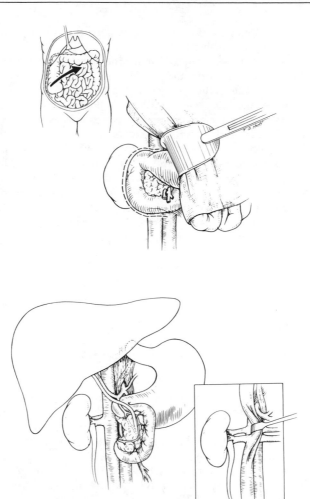

Fig 17–15.—Exposure of zone 2 abdominal arteries, including the right renal artery, the hepatic artery, the superior mesenteric artery, and the right side of the suprarenal aorta. *Arrow* indicates that the viscera is rotated to the left. (Courtesy of Fry WR, Fry RE, Fry WJ: *Arch Surg* 126:289–291, 1991.)

Background.—Trauma patients with suspected injuries to the abdominal arteries present a challenge to the vascular surgeon. Dividing the abdominal arterial tree into 4 anatomical zones provides a wide operative field and rapid, precise exposure of all major intra-abdominal arteries.

Surgical Technique: Zone 1.—Zone 1 includes the suprarenal artery, the celiac axis, the superior mesenteric artery, and the left renal artery (Fig 17–14). By dividing the peritoneal reflection over the descending colon, the splenic flexure, and the peritoneum that attaches the spleen to the diaphragm, these vessels can be exposed. By further dividing the peritoneum as it reflects over the fundus of the stomach, the spleen, stomach, and left colon can be mobilized to the midline. Extension of the laparotomy incision into the left side of the chest provides control of the thoracic artery at a higher level.

Surgical Technique: Zone 2.—Included in zone 2 are the right renal artery, the right side of the suprarenal aorta, the proximal right side of the superior mesenteric artery, and the common hepatic artery (Fig 17–15). An incision in the peritoneal reflections of the right colon and hepatic flexure allows exposure of the right renal artery. Further maneuvers expose the inferior vena cava, the right renal vein, and the origin of the left renal vein.

Surgical Technique: Zone 3.—Access to zone 3, which includes the infrarenal aorta, the inferior mesenteric artery, and the proximal common iliac arteries, can be accomplished by rotating the small bowel to the right upper quadrant.

Surgical Technique: Zone 4.—Included in zone 4 are the distal common iliac arteries and the internal and external iliac arteries. No visceral mobilization may be required to gain access to these arteries. Adequate exposure to the right iliac system may require mobilizing the cecum cephalad.

▶ It is of some interest to note that the authors of this article are a father and his 2 sons.

Penetrating Injuries of the Abdominal Aorta
Frame SB, Timberlake GA, Rush DS, McSwain NE Jr, Kerstein MD (Naval Hosp, San Diego; Univ of South Carolina; Tulane Univ)
Am Surg 56:651–654, 1990   17–22

Objective.—Despite the progress in the management of trauma patients, there has been no improvement in survival after penetrating injuries to the abdominal aorta. To define the factors that may contribute to the death of these patients, the charts of 56 consecutive patients with penetrating injuries to the abdominal aorta were reviewed.

Data Analysis.—The overall mortality was 73%. The most common cause of death was exsanguination (63%). The mechanism of injury was gun shot wound (GSW) in 82% of patients, shotgun wound (SGW) in 5%, and stab wound (SW) in 13%, with corresponding mortality of 78%, 67%, and 43%, respectively. Mortality in GSWs from a .22 caliber firearm was 0%, compared with 92% from a firearm of .38 caliber or larger. The average initial systolic blood pressure (ISBP) was 53 mm Hg, and it did not differ significantly between survivors and nonsurvivors. Only 1 of the 18 patients with an ISBP of 0 mm Hg (6%) and 3 of the 30 patients with an ISBP less than 70 mm Hg (10%) survived, compared with 46% of the patients with an ISBP greater than 70 mm Hg. Thoracotomy was performed in the emergency department in 6 patients, and 5 patients were resuscitated to reach the operating room (OR), but all subsequently died. The average time from injury to OR was 75 minutes. It was significantly longer among survivors (122 minutes) than among nonsurvivors (53 minutes), indicating that survivors showed response to resuscitative efforts. A group of 6 patients underwent thoracotomy before celiotomy for control of the thoracic aorta; 3 survived with 1 late death, for an overall survival rate of 33%. The number and location of the associated injuries did not affect survival. Most patients had injuries below the level of the superior mesenteric artery, but injury proximal to this vessel was not a negative prognostic factor.

Summary.—In patients with penetrating injuries to the abdominal aorta, the best prognostic factors appear to include response to initial resuscitation (indicating tamponade and slowing or cessation of continued blood loss) and injury caused by a knife or a .22 caliber GSW.

▶ Penetrating injuries of the abdominal aorta become complicated when resuscitation is accompanied by coagulopathy and hypothermia. Even survivors of resuscitation and aortic repair are at risk of death by sepsis.

Penetrating Iliac Vascular Injuries: Recent Experience With 233 Consecutive Patients
Burch JM, Richardson RJ, Martin RR, Mattox KL (Baylor College of Medicine; Ben Taub General Hosp, Hoston)
J Trauma 30:1450–1459, 1990   17–23

Background.—As many as 25% of the abdominal vascular injuries treated at urban trauma centers are penetrating injuries of the iliac vessels. In these cases, the control of hemorrhage is challenging because multiple vascular and combined venous and arterial injuries are typical; mortality ranges from 25% to 40%. The pathology, management, and influences on morbidity and mortality were reviewed in a group of such patients.

Patients.—A total of 206 men and 27 women (mean age, 29 years) were treated for iliac vascular injuries caused by firearm wounds (87%) or stab wounds (13%). The locations of the injuries are mapped in Figure 17–16. A total of 415 vascular lesions were found in the 233 patients evaluated; 51% had multiple injuries, 32% had arterial and venous injuries, and 8% had bilateral iliac vascular injuries.

Surgical Procedures.—Resuscitative thoracotomy was used in 29 of the 140 patients with preoperative shock, and in 12 patients in shock during surgery. The surgical techniques most commonly used for treatment of vascular injuries were lateral suture for the common iliac arteries and external iliac vein; ligation for the internal iliac vein and artery; either technique for the common iliac vein; and lateral suture, end-to-end anastomosis, or polytetrafluoroethylene graft for the common iliac vein.

Results.—Mortality in the hospital was 28%; 85% of these fatalities were caused by shock or excessive bleeding and they occurred within 48 hours of admission. All but 1 of the 41 patients who received resuscitative thoracotomy perished. Of the 125 patients with common iliac vein or inferor vena cava injuries, 2 of the 82 who were treated with repair and none of the 43 who were treated by ligation died of pulmonary embolism. Complications related to the treatment of vascular injury were found with injuries in sites other than the internal iliac arteries and veins.

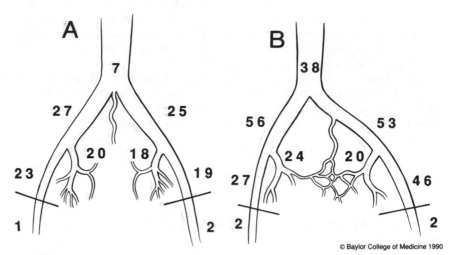

© Baylor College of Medicine 1990

Fig 17–16.—A, locations of arterial injuries. **B,** locations of venous injuries. (Courtesy of Burch JM, Richardson RJ, Martin RR, et al: *J Trauma* 30:1450–1459, 1990.)

Discussion.—It is unfortunate that better techniques are not available to prevent exsanguination, because successful management of this problem is the greatest unmet challenge in dealing with penetrating iliac vascular injuries. Although complications and late deaths may arise from the choice of treatment of arterial and vascular injuries, desperation measures (such as ligation of the common or external iliac arteries) may be unavoidable in these emergency situations. Repair of venous injuries, in contrast to ligation, produces fewer acute and chronic repercussions.

▶ Although associated injuries are important in treating patients with iliac vascular injuries, these patients have the same problem as patients with penetrating injuries of the aorta—exsanguination. An efficient emergency medical service delivers these patients for care, whereas an inefficient system allows them to die in the field.

Penetrating Trauma to the Carotid Vessels
Khoury G, Hajj H, Khoury SJ, Basil A, Speir R (American Univ of Beirut, Lebanon)
Eur J Vasc Surg 4:607–610, 1990   17–14

Background.—During a 13-year period, the American University of Beirut Medical Center treated 510 neck injuries. A total of 48 patients had 53 carotid injuries, 45.8% of which were shrapnel injuries. Bullet wounds accounted for 33% of the injuries. Whereas 39 patients had lacerations, 5 had complete disruption of the carotid vessels and 3 presented in coma. The mean patient age was 25.3 years; 44 of the patients were men. A group of 36 patients required emergency surgery. Of the 14 patients in shock, 5 had neurological deficits. The injured vessels were ligated in 6 patients. Three of these were external carotid injuries. Among the 9 patients who did not undergo initial surgery, 6 had chronic arteriovenous fistulas and 3 were in a coma.

Management.—Seven patients intubated in the emergency room were considered to have full stomachs, and they underwent crash induction with cricoesophageal compression. A group of 4 patients were intubated while they were awake because of such factors as shifted trachea, severe bleeding from the mouth, or fractured mandible. A patient who underwent elective surgery for carotid artery aneurysm required fiberoptic laryngoscopic intubation because of vocal cord paralysis. Ketamine HCl was most commonly used for induction. All but 2 of the patients had intraoperative blood transfusions.

Results.—The average time from injury to repair was 3 hours. Nine of the patients died, for an overall mortality of 18.8%; 4 died of multisystem failure, so mortality for isolated carotid injury was 10.4%. The repaired group achieved definite improvement, but hemodynamic status significantly affected mortality. At follow-up, 5 patients had persistent neurological deficits and 4 had chronic arteriovenous fistulas; 2 patients had false aneurysms.

Conclusions.—If repaired promptly within 3 hours, carotid artery injury has an acceptable mortality. Those patients who are unconscious or who present with a neurological deficit have a less optimistic prognosis. A conservative approach may lead to the late appearance of arteriovenous fistulas or false aneurysms.

▶ The medical center at the American University of Beirut has served as a battlefield hospital for the past 15 years. Their experience confirms that carotid artery injuries should be repaired even in unconscious patients and stroke patients.

Clinical and Angiographic Findings in Extremity Arterial Injuries Secondary to Dog Bites
Snyder KB, Pentecost MJ (Univ of Southern California, Los Angeles; Los Angeles County Hosp)
Ann Emerg Med 19:983–986, 1990   17–25

Introduction.—In the Los Angeles County Hospital jail ward, the annual number of patients evaluated for dog bite injuries more than doubled between May 1986 and May 1989. During this period the number of extremity angiograms increased from 2 to 42 annually, with 46 of 48 angiograms being done to evaluate injuries sustained from police dog bites.

Patients.—Of the 37 young men (average age, 27 years) who were admitted to the hospital for injuries resulting from dog bites and who also underwent angiography of the affected extremities, 35 were from a larger group of 486 prisoners who had police dog bites and who were admitted to the jail ward. Active bleeding, an enlarging hematoma, sensory or motor deficits, missing or diminished arterial pulse, or nearness of the injury to a major vessel were considered indications for angiography.

Results.—All of the patients who had angiograms had multiple puncture wounds and soft tissue damage. Although the injuries were distributed equally between the upper and lower extremities, 8 of the 10 positive arterial injuries were in an arm (the right arm in 7 cases). Occlusion occurred in 6 patients and was the most frequent vascular damage; 2 patients had partial or complete arterial transection and 2 had intimal tears. Surgical repair was required in 3 of the 10 cases.

Discussion.—Vascular injuries caused by dog bites have both blunt and penetrating components; the 21% frequency of positive angiograms in this study was similar to that in other studies of penetrating or blunt traumas. Significant injuries occurred even in those patients who met only the angiographical criterion of proximity to a major vessel. In this study, a minimum of 7.2% of the patients who had police dog bites were injured severely enough to warrant angiography; in contrast, during the same period only an estimated .44% to 1% of the patients seen in the emergency department for nonpolice dog bite injuries met the criteria for angiography. Police dog bites tend to be more damaging because these large dogs are trained to bite and hold on; the suspects frequently struggle, thus exacerbating the tissue damage.

▶ Did you know that the biting force of a sentry dog has been measured at 100 pounds to 200 pounds of pressure per square inch?

Paediatric Arterial Injury: Management Options at the Time of Injury
Mills RP, Robbs JV (Univ of Natal Med School, Congella, South Africa)
J R Coll Surg Edinb 36:13–17, 1991   17–26

Introduction.—Arterial injury in children presents serious challenges for vascular surgeons. These problems encourage the adoption of a "wait and see" protocol. The use of early obligatory surgery in the management of pediatric patients with arterial injuries was studied, and the contribution of digital subtraction angiography (DSA) was especially considered.

Patients.—All patients younger than 12 years who were managed for vascular injury were included in the study. The clinical records of 40 patients (7 girls, 33 boys) treated during a 4-year period were analyzed retrospectively. These patients were compared with 1,893 children treated for limb fractures during the same 4-year period in an orthopedic clinic. The incidence of accompanying arterial injury was approximately 2.1%. Of the 40 study patients, 11 had traumatic injury and 29 had blunt injury. The protocol for treating penetrating arterial injury after the detection of absent distal pulses in an ischemic limb was mandatory emergency surgery. In the early patients, detection of absent distal pulses was done by the direct arterial route; however, later patients underwent DSA.

Case Report.—Boy, 10 years, had a fractured left humerus and absent distal pulses. After finding no obvious arterial injury, the surgeon chose to inject contrast medium by direct arterial puncture. The resulting radiograph demonstrated an arterial spasm (Fig 17–17).

Findings.—In the penetrating injury group, 2 of the 11 patients had an arterial ligation but did not experience any disability. In the group that underwent arterial repair, all of the children had good results except for a 5-month-old boy with a congenital aortic valve stenosis. This child underwent an arteriotomy and correction of his heart lesion and, although he died 6 hours later, his death was not related to the femoral artery repair. Based upon the proscribed protocol, 14 of the 29 patients with blunt trauma had no significant organic arterial pathology at operation; an arterial spasm was diagnosed. No operative deaths occurred in this group. In those patients with arterial spasms, normal distal pulses returned between 12 hours and 24 hours after surgery. All 13 patients who

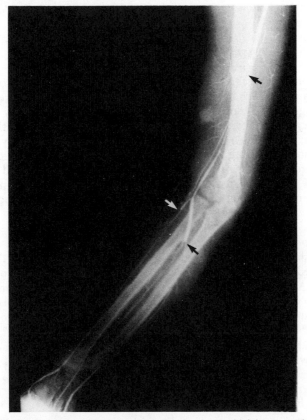

Fig 17–17.—Direct angiogram of a boy, 10 years, with a fractured left humerus. The appearances suggest arterial spasm. (Courtesy of Mills RP, Robbs JV: *J R Coll Surg Edinb* 36:13–17, 1991.)

had limb vessel repair experienced the restoration of peripheral pulses before leaving the hospital.

Conclusions.—These patients can be divided into 2 groups: those with obvious ischemic limbs and those with a viable limb without palpable pulses. The use of DSA may identify the patients with arterial spasm for whom surgery is unnecessary.

▶ There is very little information that will guide us in treating pediatric vascular trauma. Much of the literature is concerned with iatrogenic injury. Although a diagnosis of spasm is to be disparaged in an adult, the incidence of spasm is greater in children because a minimum reduction in the small-caliber vessels makes distal pulses disappear. Working on the small vessels of children requires both magnification and an extremely gentle technique in the passage of the smallest balloon embolectomy catheters.

The Use of Internal Jugular Vein as Interposition Graft for Femoral Vein Reconstruction Following Traumatic Venous Injury: A Useful Approach in Selected Cases
Woodson J, Rodriguez AA, Menzoian JO (Boston Univ School of Medicine)
Ann Vasc Surg 4:494–497, 1990   17–27

Background.—Because of the increase in violence in our society, surgeons may encounter battleground-type venous injuries that require special management. Data from the Vietnam Vascular Registry and from nonmilitary cases have documented long-term morbidity with ligation, supporting the need to prevent the late sequelae of venous hypertension by adequately repairing the original vascular trauma. Prosthetic materials may lead to high risk of infection and thrombosis when used in venous repair. Use of the internal jugular vein may expedite surgery and produce less problems in healing the reconstruction for complex common femoral vein repair.

Case Report.—Man, 18, incurred a shotgun wound to both legs and a large wound to the right lateral thigh with a right groin hematoma (Fig 17–18). Excessive bleeding from the femoral vein necessitated the oversewing of the vein's distal end. A jugular interposition graft into the femoral vein was completed. A 7 cm segment of the left internal jugular vein was employed for femoral vein repair, with an end-to-end anastomosis performed proximally and an end-to-side (functionally end-to-end) anastomosis performed distally. The natural "Y" segment of the contralateral greater saphenous vein served to reconstruct the common femoral artery, with end-to-end anastomoses to both the profunda femoris and the superficial femoral arteries. Good blood flow in the common femoral vein and artery was verified postoperatively by Doppler exam. The patient recovered and showed no limb swelling 3 months after surgery.

Implications.—Compared with ligation, femoral vein reconstruction prevents short-term venous congestion and long-term venous hyperten-

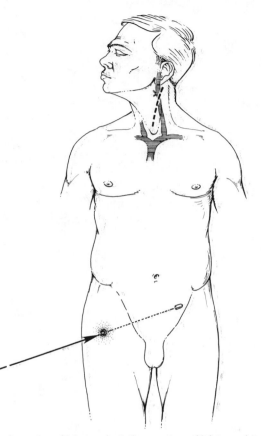

Fig 17–18.—*Arrow* shows area of injury and missile tract. Area of left internal jugular vein is also shown, with *dotted line* representing anterior sternocleidomastoid incision. (Courtesy of Woodson J, Rodriguez AA, Menzoian JO: *Ann Vasc Surg* 4:494–497, 1990.)

sion and stasis. Use of the internal jugular vein allows for adequate size match, ease of harvest, and low morbidity.

► Repair of venous injury is a controversial subject and may actually be unnecessary.

18 Portal Hypertension

Hemodynamic Events in a Prospective Randomized Trial of Propranolol Versus Placebo in the Prevention of a First Variceal Hemorrhage
Groszmann RJ, Bosch J, Grace ND, Conn HO, Garcia-Tsao G, Navasa M, Alberts J, Rodes J, Fischer R, Bermann M, Rofe S, Patrick M, Lerner E (VA Med Ctr, West Haven, Conn; Yale Univ; Hospital Clinic i Provincial, Barcelona, Spain; Faulkner and Lemuel Shattuck Hosp, Boston)
Gastroenterology 99:1401–1407, 1990   18–1

Introduction.—Propranolol is being used increasingly for the prevention of a first gastroesophageal variceal hemorrhage in cirrhotic patients. The efficacy of propranolol for preventing rebleeding from the varices is still controversial. The mechanism by which propranolol and other β-adrenergic blockers decrease the risk for variceal bleeding remains unclear.

Methods.—The hemodynamical events that occurred after the administration of propranolol or placebo were studied in 73 men and 29 women (age range, 25–72 years) with cirrhosis, portal hypertension, and endoscopically confirmed esophageal varices. Of the patients, 51 were randomly allocated to receive propranolol, whereas 51 received placebo. All of the patients underwent hepatic and systemic hemodynamical studies at baseline, and 3 months, 12 months, and 24 months thereafter.

Results.—Only 2 (4%) of the 51 patients treated with propranolol had a variceal hemorrhage, compared with 11 (22%) of the 51 patients treated with placebo. Of the 13 variceal hemorrhages, 11 occurred during the first year of the study. At baseline, both groups had similar hepatic venous pressure gradients (HVPGs). However, after 3 months of treatment, the mean HVPG had decreased from 18.1 mm Hg to 15.7 mm Hg in the propranolol-treated patients, but not in the placebo-treated patients. At subsequent evaluations, the HVPG decreased significantly from baseline values for both groups. A decrease in HVPG to 12 mm Hg or less was achieved in 14 propranolol-treated patients and 7 placebo-treated patients. None of these patients bled from esophageal varices, and their mortality rate also decreased.

Conclusion.—Because most bleeding events occurred during the first year, propranolol seems to exert its protective effect during the period associated with the largest reduction in the HVPG. A decrease in the HVPG to 12 mm Hg or less is the single most useful prognostic indicator, and this should be the goal of all pharmacologic treatment of portal hypertension.

▶ For many reasons, portal hypertension is becoming less of a surgical problem today than it was in the past. This study suggests that propranolol has the potential to improve the natural history of alcoholic liver disease.

Prediction of Variceal Hemorrhage in Cirrhosis: A Prospective Follow-Up Study
Kleber G, Sauerbruch T, Ansari H, Paumgartner G (Univ of Munich; Biometric Ctr for Therapeutic Studies, Munich, Germany)
Gastroenterology 100:1332–1337, 1991   18–2

Introduction.—The use of prophylactic measures to prevent first bleeding from varices in patients with liver cirrhosis has been questioned. A better basis for selecting high-risk patients was investigated by defining the significance of different laboratory, clinical, and endoscopic criteria.

Methods.—A group of 68 patients with alcoholic cirrhosis and a group of 41 patients with posthepatitic or cryptogenic cirrhosis, all without previous variceal bleeding, were assessed by endoscopic, clinical, and laboratory parameters. These parameters included red color sign, diameter and number of variceal columns, platelet count, presence of varices in the gastric fundus, and Child-Pugh class. The patients were followed for a mean of 21 months; first variceal bleeding or death or both were end points of the study.

Results.—There was a bleeding incidence of 29% and a mortality rate of 46%. There was a significant correlation between presence of varices in the gastric fundus, presence of red color sign, and size of the largest varix and the bleeding incidence. An alcoholic etiology for cirrhosis was also associated with bleeding incidence, but none of the above-mentioned factors correlated with mortality. Encephalopathy, ascites, and age older than 50 years were definitely associated with survival, but not with incidence of bleeding.

Discussion.—This study found several strong predictors for variceal hemorrhage in cirrhosis. The presence of concomitant varices in the gastric fundus was a strong prognostic indicator for bleeding, followed by a red color sign and a variceal diameter greater than 5 mm. Further studies with a larger number of subjects will better verify these results.

Arterioportal Fistulas: Twelve Cases
Pietri J, Remond A, Reix T, Abet D, Sevestre H, Sevestre MA (Hôpital Sud, Amiens, France)
Ann Vasc Surg 4:533–539, 1990   18–3

Background.—Although they were formerly scarce, reports of arterioportal fistulas (APF) are increasing for 2 reasons: improved detection by use of celiac-mesenteric arteriography and escalating incidences of iatrogenic fistulas after transhepatic invasive techniques. The etiology and management of APF was evaluated in 12 patients.

Patients.—During a 20-year period, 14 cases of APF were found in 12 patients. The etiology, symptoms, and treatment are summarized in the table. In 7 of the 8 cases in which APF followed liver biopsy, gastroduodenal surgery, or colon resection, the origin was considered to be iatrogenic. However, detection of the fistulas was delayed 7 days to 2 years

Clinical Findings, Etiologic Considerations and Therapy of 12 Patients
With Arterioportal Fistulas

Patient	Sex/Age	Etiology	Topography	Clinical presentation	PH	MI	HB	Treatment
1	M/30	Congenital	Hepaticoportal	DTH Encephalopathy Ascites Bruit	+	+	Normal	Left hepatectomy
	M/35	id	SMA (jejunum)	Pain Mass bruit	−	−	NA	Bowel resection
	M/42	id	SMA (cecum)	Rectal hemorrhage Bruit	NA	−	NA	None (died)
2	F/32	Congenital	Splenic	DTH Pain Mass Bruit	+	−	NA	Splenectomy
3	F/44	HB	Hepaticoportal	Hemobilia	NA	−	Cirrhosis	Embolization
4	M/48	HB	Hepaticoportal	DTH Bruit	NA	−	Cirrhosis	Embolization
5	M/49	Gastrectomy	Hepaticoportal	Pain Bruit	−	−	Hepatic congestion	Resection
6	M/39	Aneurysm	Splenic	DTH Bruit	−	−	NA	Splenectomy
7	M/62	Aneurysm	Splenic	DTH Ascites Bruit	+	+	NA	Splenectomy
8	F/46	Gastrectomy	GDA	Pain Weight loss Bruit	+	+	Hepatic congestion	Embolization
9	M/42	Gastrectomy	LGEA	Pain Bruit	−	−	Normal	Embolization
10	M/54	Right colectomy	SMA	Pain Bruit	−	−	NA	Resection
11	M/72	Left colectomy	IMA	Mass Bruit	+	−	NA	Resection
12	F/60	Left colectomy	IMA	DTH Bruit	−	+	Normal	Embolization

Abbreviations: SMA, superior mesenteric; GDA, gastroduodenal artery; LGEA, left gastroepiploic artery; IMA, inferior mesenteric artery; DTH, digestive tract hemorrhage; PH, portal hypertension (over 20 cm H_2O); MI, mesenteric ischemia; HB, hepatic biopsy; NA, not applicable.

(Courtesy of Pietri J, Remond A, Reix T, et al: *Ann Vasc Surg* 4:533–539, 1990.)

after biopsy and 5 years–11 years after surgery. All of the patients had celiomesenteric arteriograms. Although the fistulae were found mainly in the hepatic or splenic arteries, they were also found in the superior mesenteric, gastroduodenal, right inferior gastric, or inferior mesenteric arteries. Surgical removal of the fistula (with resection of associated parenchyma as needed) was performed in 8 cases; arterial transcatheter embolization using coils was the treatment of choice in the remaining 5 treated cases.

Results.—After treatment and closure of the shunt, high portal pressure was alleviated completely in the 5 patients with that symptom. Three patients with chronic mesenteric ischemia showed striking improvement; and the lesions soon healed in a patient with ischemic colitis. Hemorrhage did not recur in any patient. A total of 9 patients remained symptom free, although rebleeding occurred in the 2 patients with alcoholic cirrhosis. New fistulas were found in a patient with congenital APF.

Discussion.—Iatrogenic APF (which currently represents 50% of published cases) can be secondary to hepatic biopsy, transjugular or transhepatic catheterization, or resectional surgery of the stomach, small intestine, spleen, or colon. The most common complications are gastrointestinal hemorrhage or intestinal ischemia, and the incidence of portal hypertension may reach 50%. Many of the iatrogenic fistulas are single and distal. When the flow rate of the fistula is low and its diameter is less than 8 mm, metallic coil embolization produces excellent results. Surgery is warranted when the fistula has a high flow rate or has arisen right on a large arterial trunk. Long-term observation of these patients is appropriate because problems may recur in patients with associated liver pathology or congenital APF despite initially successful treatment.

▶ Increasing numbers of arterioportal fistulas are being discovered. The technique of closure must be individualized, and both interventional radiographical and surgical techniques are appropriate.

Current Management of the Budd-Chiari Syndrome
Klein AS, Sitzmann JV, Coleman J, Herlong FH, Cameron JL (Johns Hopkins Med Insts)
Ann Surg 212:144–149, 1990   18–4

Introduction.— The Budd-Chiari syndrome, which results from hepatic venous outflow occlusion, is rare but often fatal. Numerous surgical procedures have been proposed to decompress the congested liver by converting the portal vein into an outflow tract. A group of patients with the Budd-Chiari syndrome who were treated surgically at 1 center was studied.

Management.— A total of 26 patients were treated during a 15-year period. The median age at diagnosis was 37 years; 21 patients were women. Of the patients, 9 had polycythemia vera; 6 had estrogen therapy; 5 had a previous hepatitis A or B infection: and 4 had cirrhosis. The most common presenting feature was ascites. The hepatic function at diagnosis was only slightly abnormal. Hepatic vein catheterization confirmed the diagnosis of the Budd-Chiari syndrome in all cases. Inferior vena cavography revealed caval occlusion in 4 patients, significant caval obstruction in 13, and a normal vena cava in 9. Interpretation of the vena cavogram was useful for selecting appropriate surgical procedures. A group of 23 patients had percutaneous liver biopsy before surgery with no morbidity or mortality. Well-established cirrhosis was seen on biopsy, in 4 cases.

Results.— Thirty mesenteric-systemic venous shunts were done on all patients. In 11 of the patients, a mesocaval shunt was done. In 1 patient, conversion to a mesoatrial shunt was required as a second procedure. A mesoatrial shunt was done as the initial procedure in 15 patients. Graft thrombosis that occurred in 2 of these patients prompted 1 and 2 revisions, respectively. Of the patients, 31% died before hospital discharge after receiving a mesenteric-systemic venous shunt. The remaining 18 were discharged well with patient shunts. Follow-up ranged from 9 months to 13 years, with a median of 43 months. Five patients died between 5 months and 84 months after surgery. The 3-year actuarial survival rate was 65% and the 5-year actuarial survival rate was 59%.

Conclusion.—Untreated hepatic venous thrombosis leads to progressive liver failure and death. Most patients with the Budd-Chiari syndrome can be safely, successfully treated with an appropriate selection of mesocaval shunt, mesoatrial shunt, or orthotopic liver transplantation.

▶ This abstract describes a large series of patients with Budd-Chiari syndrome. Neither mesocaval shunting nor mesoatrial shunting is entirely satisfactory. Therefore, hepatic transplantation may ultimately surface as the best method of treating these patients.

19 Vena Cava Surgery

Safety and Efficacy of Thrombolytic Therapy for Superior Vena Cava Syndrome
Gray BH, Olin JW, Graor RA, Young JR, Bartholomew JR, Ruschhaupt WF
(Cleveland Clinic Found)
Chest 99:54–59, 1991   19–1

Background.—Isolated case reports have suggested a beneficial effect of thrombolytic therapy for superior vena cava (SVC) syndrome. A retrospective chart review was used both to assess the efficacy and safety of thrombolytic therapy in treating a large group of patients with SVC and to define the factors that are predictive of success.

Treatment.—A total of 326 patients with SVC syndrome or thrombosis of the SVC were seen between 1982 and 1990. Of these patients, 16 received thrombolytic therapy. Eleven patients received urokinase in a dose of 4,400 units/kg bolus followed by 4,400 units/kg/hour. A group of 5 patients received streptokinase in a dose of 250,000 bolus followed by 100,000 units/hour. After 24 hours, therapy was either discontinued if venography showed no thrombolysis or continued until venography demonstrated complete lysis. The mean duration of treatment was 40 hours for urokinase and 41 hours for streptokinase.

Results.—A venogram showed complete clot lysis in 9 patients (56%) (Fig 19–1). Thrombolytic therapy was effective in 8 of 11 patients with central venous catheters (73%), versus 1 of 5 patients without catheters (20%). It was also effective in 8 of 11 patients treated with urokinase (73%), compared with 1 of 5 who received streptokinase (20%). Thrombolytic therapy was successful in 7 of 8 patients with symptoms for 5 days or less (88%), compared with 2 of 8 patients with symptoms for more than 5 days (25%). Catheter function was preserved in all patients in whom thrombolytic therapy was effective. There were no significant hemorrhagic complications. Nausea and vomiting were noted in urokinase-treated patients, and a significant allergic reaction occurred in 2 patients who were treated with streptokinase.

Conclusion.—Thrombolytic therapy is effective and safe in many patients with SVC syndrome. The factors that are predictive of successful lysis include use of urokinase compared with streptokinase, presence of central venous catheters, and presence of symptoms for 5 days or less.

▶ Tuberculosis and syphilitic aortic aneurysms have been replaced by central venous catheters and pacemaker wires as causes of superior vena cava syndrome. In addition, total parenteral nutrition and the need for long-term antibiotic therapy produce a near epidemic of superior vena cava thrombosis. Medical or surgical treatment becomes mandatory when CNS disturbances, con-

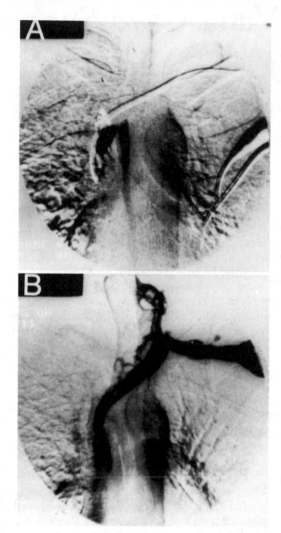

Fig 19–1.—A, venogram showing SVC obstruction prior to thrombolysis. Catheter is present in left subclavian vein and SVC. **B,** complete clot lysis after 40-hour infusion of urokinase through the indwelling catheter. The patient's symptoms resolved and the catheter access was preserved. (Courtesy of Gray BH, Olin JW, Graor RA, et al: *Chest* 99:54–59, 1991.)

junctival edema, dysphagia, or respiratory compromise occur. Early recognition of the syndrome and local delivery of the lytic agent will prove most efficacious and may even allow retention of the central venous catheter itself.

Resectable Leiomyosarcoma of Inferior Vena Cava Presenting as Carcinoma of the Pancreas: Case Report
Nordback I, Mattila J, Tarkka M (Univ of Tampere; Tampere Univ Central Hosp, Tampere, Finland)
Acta Chir Scand 156:577–580, 1990   19–2

Background.—Although the introduction of ultrasonography and CT has greatly improved the diagnosis of leiomyosarcoma of the inferior vena cava, misdiagnosis remains possible with these rare tumors. Data on a patient in whom inferior vena cava vein leiomyosarcoma manifested as carcinoma of the pancreas were reviewed.

Case Report.—Woman, 61, had epigastric symptoms. Ultrasound scan and CT suggested a mass in the head of the pancreas. Pancreatography showed filling of the pancreatic duct with contrast medium only in the head of the gland. Exploratory laparotomy revealed a 4-cm tumor attached to the inferior vena cava just distal to the renal veins; the pancreas was normal. Histological examination revealed a moderately differentiated leiomyosarcoma. The vessel wall was resected and reconstructed with a polytetrafluoroethylene patch.

Conclusion.—The diagnosis of leiomyosarcoma of the inferior vena cava can be difficult, partly because there are no specific symptoms, including a lack of vascular symptoms. With a high index of suspicion, diagnosis can be made by ultrasonography, CT, or MRI. The treatment of this rare tumor is surgical, but the prognosis remains poor.

▶ Because the prognosis of vena cava leiomyosarcomas is poor, palliative treatment with externally reinforced polytetrafluoroethylene grafts is justifiable. Perhaps more radical resections will result in a greater rate of cure in the future.

Prospective Comparison of Computed Tomography and Duplex Sonography in the Evaluation of Recently Inserted Kimray-Greenfield Filters Into the Inferior Vena Cava
Guglielmo FF, Kurtz AB, Wechsler RJ (Jefferson Med College; Thomas Jefferson Univ Hosp, Philadelphia)
Clin Imag 14:216–220, 1990   19–3

Study Plan.—A total of 25 consecutive patients seen prospectively during a 2-year period were assessed by both duplex sonography and CT to analyze the inferior vena cava for complications after Kimray-Greenfield filter (KGF) insertion. The first postoperative study was conducted within a week of surgery; the second was performed within the next week. The 14 evaluable patients had a mean age of 59 years. Oral contrast medium was used for the CT scan.

Findings.—Computed tomography was diagnostic in 86% of the patients and sonography was diagnostic in 50%. Two CT studies were indeterminate for clotting because of inadequate intravenous contrast. The presence or absence of thrombosis was diagnosed correctly in all 10 patients who underwent technically adequate CT and sonographic studies. The filter position was much better assessed by CT. Pericaval hematomas were demonstrated by CT in 2 patients whose sonographic studies were negative for hematoma. The 2 categories assessed by CT only were filter angulation (seen in 11 patients) and prong perforation (seen in 7 patients).

Conclusions.—Duplex sonography may be used primarily to assess patients with Kimray-Greenfield caval filters. If the study is not definitive, a contrast-enhanced CT examination is indicated. If any complication other than caval thrombosis is clinically suspected, then CT is the preferred study.

▶ Computed tomography study of vena cava filters shows that tilted filters occur frequently and that such tilting may allow emboli larger than 3 mm in diameter to pass through the struts. As was observed in this study, perforation of the cava by the struts is common in such a position. Furthermore, this study showed that 4 of 25 consecutive patients had intracaval thrombosis, suggesting that the patency of the filter is assured in more than 80% of patients.

Permanent Inferior Vena Caval Interruption: Indications and Techniques in 1989
Dimaria G (Hôtel-Dieu, Paris)
Sem Hôp Paris 66:2672–2674, 1990   19–4

Introduction.—The indications for interruption of the inferior vena cava (IVC) to prevent the occurrence or recurrence of pulmonary embolism (PE) are not well defined in patients with venous thrombosis of the lower extremities. Although there has been much progress in the medical and surgical treatment of venous thrombosis, it is still not possible to predict which patients are at risk for PE or which patients will have a recurrence. Criteria for the use of IVC interruption were suggested.

Management.—Inferior vena cava interruption is justified in those patients with massive PE in whom even a minor recurrence of PE would be life threatening, and in those patients with preexisting cardiac or respiratory failure who have moderately severe PE. It is also justified in patients with minor PE in whom anticoagulant or thrombolytic therapy is contraindicated (for instance, because of recent major surgery). Patients with minor PE who have already undergone embolectomy for PE are also eligible for interruption. Inferior vena cava interruption is acceptable in patients who have had several minor PE episodes and who are at risk for chronic postembolic cor pulmonale. Patients with a large, free-floating iliocaval clot whose mobilization could cause massive PE and patients with severe PE who also have heparin-induced thrombocytopenia are also eligible for IVC interruption. However, the use of IVC interruption is questionable in those patients with a history of PE who are scheduled for major surgery and in those patients with a single episode of moderately severe PE who are in good general health. Interruption is not warranted in patients with iliac venous thrombosis in which the thrombus adheres completely to the vessel wall, nor is it recommended in patients with popliteal or subpopliteal venous thrombosis, even if the thrombus is nonadherent to the vessel wall.

Methods.—Placement of an endocaval Kimray-Greenfield filter or any of its variations is the interruption procedure of choice. Because it requires general anesthesia and makes placement of a filter hazardous, the use of a pericaval Adams-de-Weese clip should be limited to those patients in whom the thrombus extends into the vena cava and to those patients who require intra-abdominal surgery.

Discussion.—Rigorous criteria for the decision to interrupt the vena cava cannot be defined, and each case should be decided individually. During the past 10 years, approximately 120 IVC interruption procedures have been performed, representing somewhat less than 10% of the number of patients treated for venous thrombosis.

▶ Now that long-term safety and a 96% protection rate against recurrent pulmonary embolism have been established for the Greenfield filter, there has been considerable interest in broadening the indications. This report does not detail the author's experience; instead, it lists a series of indications in a graded fashion from good to unwarranted. The rationale for recommending the use of a caval clip for thrombus extending into the vena cava is difficult to justify because the filter is quite safe under these circumstances either above or below the renal veins. The most significant risk would result from the general anesthesia, laparotomy, and manipulation of the cava that are required to insert a clip. Availability of the titanium Greenfield filter for percutaneous insertion using a 12-French carrier has both simplified the approach and made it more cost effective.—L.J. Greenfield, M.D.

20 Thromboembolism

Venous Stasis and Vein Lumen Changes During Surgery
Coleridge-Smith PD, Hasty JH, Scurr JH (Univ College and Middlesex School of Medicine, London)
Br J Surg 77:1055–1059, 1990 20–1

Background.—Recent studies have shown that venous distention occurs in the upper limb veins during surgery. The role of distention in subsequent deep vein thrombosis (DVT) was explored by Scurr et al. who found that postoperative DVT was prevented by the patient's wearing graduated compression stockings. Whether the deep veins of the lower extremities dilate during general anesthesia and surgery was investigated.

Findings.—High-resolution ultrasound images of the gastrocnemius and posterior tibial veins in 62 patients undergoing surgery showed no evidence of dilatation at the induction of anesthesia. By the end of the procedure, however, distention reached 22% to 28%. The gastrocnemius veins were more distended than the posterior tibial veins. In patients who received an infusion of 1 L of saline in addition to basal requirements, distention of 57% occurred, compared to 22% in the control group.

Conclusion.—The findings provide direct anatomical evidence of intraoperative venous distention and concomitant blood flow changes. Venous distention may contribute to endothelial damage, thereby promoting the formation of DVT.

▶ The meaning of this study is that there is a slowing of venous blood flow during anesthesia and an increase in residence time of blood in calf veins. As suggested by the authors, damage to the endothelium may predispose such veins to thrombosis.

Deficiencies of Coagulation-Inhibiting and Fibrinolytic Proteins in Outpatients With Deep-Vein Thrombosis
Heijboer H, Brandjes DPM, Büller HR, Sturk A, ten Cate JW (Academic Med Ctr, Amsterdam)
N Engl J Med 323:1512–1516, 1990 20–2

Background.—Recent surgery, prolonged immobilization, and the presence of malignant disease have been recognized as predisposing factors for deep vein thrombosis (DVT). Isolated deficiencies of proteins involved in the fibrinolytic system or in inhibiting coagulation may lead to a hypercoagulable state and cause recurrent venous thromboembolism. Deficiencies of antithrombin III, protein C, protein S, and plasminogen have been implicated as the cause of DVT.

Study Design.—The prevalence of protein deficiency was studied prospectively in 280 outpatients with DVT and in 140 age- and sex-matched controls without DVT.

Findings.—The prevalence of antithrombin III, protein C, protein S, or plasminogen deficiency in patients with venous thrombosis was 8.3% (23 of 277 patients), and that in the controls was 2.2% (3 of 138 patients). The positive predictive value of an isolated protein deficiency was 9% in patients with a history of venous thrombosis, 16% in patients with a family history of venous thrombosis, and 12% in patients with an episode of venous thrombosis before age 41.

Summary.—In the overwhelming majority of outpatients (91.7%), the etiology of venous thrombosis could not be explained. Only 8.3% of patients with venous thrombosis had a protein deficiency. Neither a history of recurrence, a family history, nor a juvenile onset of venous thrombosis was useful in identifying patients with protein deficiencies.

▶ Clinically, routine studies for coagulopathy in patients with DVT are singularly unrewarding. This carefully done, modern study confirms that in more than 90% of patients a search for the coagulopathy is simply not worthwhile.

Analysis of 1084 Consecutive Lower Extremities Involved With Acute Venous Thrombosis Diagnosed by Duplex Scanning
Kerr TM, Cranley JJ, Johnson JR, Lutter KS, Riechmann GC, Cranley RD, True MA, Sampson M (Good Samaritan Hosp, Cincinnati)
Surgery 108:520–527, 1990   20–3

Background.—Studies on the sites of origin and patterns of venous thrombosis in the lower extremities are based largely on postmortem examinations or invasive tests. The introduction of duplex scanning has provided a noninvasive method to define the locations, patterns, and frequency of acute venous thrombosis of the lower extremities.

Method.—In a retrospective study, 8,658 consecutive lower extremity venous duplex scans performed between 1982 and 1988 were reviewed. The incidence, location, and distribution patterns of acute deep or superficial thrombi in 1,084 lower extremities in 953 patients were studied.

Data Analysis.—The series included 485 women (mean age, 62.9) and 468 men (mean age, 58.8). There were 371 patients with right-sided thrombi, 451 with left-sided thrombi, and 131 with thrombi in both extremities. Women were uniformly older than the men, and the left leg was involved significantly more often than the right leg. Proximal vein sites accounted for 71.5% of the thrombus locations. Of the 3,169 veins involved, acute thrombi occurred most frequently in the popliteal vein, followed by the superficial femoral, posterior tibial, and common femoral veins, all 4 vessels accounting for 51.7% of the sites involved. In single-thrombus patterns, the greater saphenous, soleal, and lesser saphenous veins were commonly involved. Single thrombi were significantly more common in the below-knee deep venous system, whereas multiple thrombi favored above-knee locations. Multiple and bilateral thrombi showed many unique patterns of thrombosis.

Summary.—Data obtained from duplex scanning of the venous system of the lower extremities vary from those of previous attempts at describing the pathologic-anatomical patterns of acute venous thrombosis. The frequency, locations, and patterns of distribution of acute venous thrombi vary with age, sex, and the leg involved.

▶ Cranley's laboratory in Cincinnati has an enormous experience with duplex scanning for venous thrombosis. This report of their experience defines the frequency, location, and patterns of distribution of deep venous thrombosis definitively.

Occult Cancer in Patients With Deep Venous Thrombosis: A Systematic Approach
Monreal M, Lafoz E, Casals A, Inaraja L, Montserrat E, Callejas JM, Martorell A
(Hosp Germans Trias i Pujol, Barcelona)
Cancer 67:541–545, 1991   20–4

Background.—Patients with cancer are at increased risk for the development of deep venous thrombosis (DVT). Some reports have postulated that DVT may be a clue to occult malignancy; however, others have found that occult malignancy occurs more often in patients without identifiable risk factors for DVT. Intensive work-up were performed during admission of 113 consecutive patients with DVT in an attempt to detect possible cancer at an earlier stage.

Methods.—Each patient underwent physical examination, chest radiography, upper gastrointestinal endoscopy, CT scanning, abdominal ultrasound, and evaluation of the erythrocyte sedimentation rate, whole blood count, biochemistry, and carcinoembryonic antigen levels. If a malignancy was suspected, the patient underwent further appropriate tests. Patients were observed periodically at an outpatient clinic after discharge.

Results.—Eleven patients received a diagnosis of cancer during admission. Of these, 5 had symptoms suggestive of malignancy, but the primary complaints that led all 11 patients to seek medical treatment were referable to thrombophlebitis. In 3 patients, cancer was detected at an extremely early stage. Cancer was found more often in patients with abnormal lactic dehydrogenase levels and in those with idiopathic DVT than in those with secondary DVT. Two additional patients with idiopathic DVT had adenomatous polyps, which are thought to be colorectal cancer precursors. Abnormal carcinoembryonic antigen levels led to the diagnosis of colonic cancer on colonoscopy in 2 patients. Urinary bladder carcinoma was detected at an extremely early stage by ultrasound and CT in 2 patients. Large benign pelvic tumors were detected in 5 patients, and absent superior inferior vena cava were detected in 2.

Conclusions.—The work-ups for cancer in patients with DVT should include routine laboratory tests, evaluation of the erythrocyte sedimentation rate, lactic hydrogenase and carcinoembryonic antigen levels, chest radiography, and abdominal ultrasound or CT. These findings revealed no correlation between age, hemoglobin concentration, eosinophil count, or routine coagulation tests and cancer.

▶ One must be careful in interpretation of these findings. A search for an occult malignancy usually proves as unrewarding in patients with DVT as the search for coagulopathy has proven to be.

Phlegmasia Cerulea Dolens Associated With the Lupus Anticoagulant
Baethge BA, Payne DK (Louisiana State Univ, Shreveport)
West J Med 154:211–213, 1991   20–5

Background.—Phlegmasia cerulea dolens (PCD), a severe peripheral venous thrombosis caused by complete obstruction of the venous drainage of a limb, is often associated with hypercoagulable states.

Case Report.—Woman, 50, was admitted with sudden pain and swelling of the right leg. She had discontinued long-term warfarin sodium therapy 2 weeks earlier for previous deep venous thrombosis. The patient was morbidly obese and had marked edema of the right leg, which appeared dusky and erythematous. The right leg was 8 cm bigger at the midthigh and 6 cm bigger at the midcalf than the left leg. Her serum creatinine level was 194.5 μmol/L and blood urea nitrogen was 8.6 mmol/L of urea. Prothrombin time was 14 seconds. Her activated partial thromboplastin time (APTT) of 57 seconds corrected to 41 seconds after mixing with normal serum, confirming the presence of an inhibitor. Lupus anticoagulant was confirmed by thromboplastin dilution assay. Phlegmasia cerulea dolens was diagnosed on clinical grounds, and intravenous heparin was begun. Impedance plethysmography could not be done because of the size of the leg. Ultrasonography and CT showed massive edema and enlarged subcutaneous veins consistent with deep venous occlusion. Swelling and cyanosis continued for 36 hours until distal pulses could no longer be felt. An intravenous bolus of 250,000 units of streptokinse, followed by continuous infusion of 100,000 units per hour for 3 days reduced pain and swelling. Heparin therapy was then resumed, and the leg improved in the next 14 days. The patient continued to take warfarin therapy 1 year after discharge and had venous stasis dermatopathy and persistent edema of the leg.

Discussion.—Lupus anticoagulant leads to thrombosis by an unknown mechanism. Anticoagulation therapy is usually successful in such cases. All patients with lupus anticoagulant have a prolonged APTT, and some have prolonged prothrombin and thrombin times. Phlegmasia cerulea dolens is a potentially fatal disorder for which surgery is usually recommended if patients fail to respond to heparin within 6–12 hours. Thrombolytic therapy was used in this case because of the presence of the lupus anticoagulant. This case supports the suggestion that all patients with hypercoagulable abnormalities are at high risk of PCD.

► Throughout this YEAR BOOK, the phenomenon of venous and arterial thrombosis in association with lupus anticoagulant has been stressed. This antiphospholipid antibody is related to the anticardiolipin antibody, and its exact and important relationship to thrombosis has not been defined precisely.

Baker's Cyst Simulating Deep Vein Thrombosis
Chaudhuri R, Salari R (Guy's Hosp, London; Lewisham Hosp, London)
Clin Radiol 41:400–404, 1990   20–6

Background.—About half of the patients with suspected deep vein thrombosis (DVT) have positive findings on emergency phlebography; the remainder may be discharged without diagnosis. Similar symptoms may be produced by rupture of an enlarged gastrocnemo-semimembranous bursa, or Baker's cyst. Although occasional compression or deviation of the popliteal vein may be observed in otherwise negative phlebograms of these patients, the correct diagnosis may require arthrography. Arthrography was done in 23 patients with leg pain, swelling, and phlebograms negative for DVT.

Methods.—From a series of 388 patients who underwent phlebography for suspected DVT, lateral and frontal arthrographic studies were made after injection of contrast medium and gentle exericse in those who were negative for DVT but in whom lateral deviation of the popliteal vein was observed. Ultrasound examination of the popliteal fossa was done in 2 patients.

Results.—Of the 23 patients (aged 24–81), 18 had ruptured Baker's cysts, and 4 had no rupture or walled off rupture. In one third of the patients with Baker's cysts, upward dissection to the thigh occurred. There was 1 patient with a false positive result who had neither DVT nor Bak-

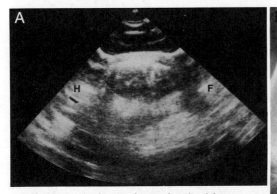

Fig 20–1.—**A,** ultrasound scan of popliteal fossa. Baker's cyst is marked (×). There is no evidence of rupture, although it contains debris (*H,* head; *F,* feet). **B,** arthrogram of the same patient showing small upward rupture. (Courtesy of Chaudhuri R, Salari R: *Clin Radiol* 41:400–404, 1990.)

er's cyst. Ultrasound revealed Baker's cysts in both patients who underwent it. Rupture was found in only 1. The other was found to have a rupture by arthrography (Fig 20–1).

Discussion.—Because the management of patients with Baker's cyst differs markedly from that for patients with DVT, the differential diagnosis is important. The anticoagulation therapy that would be used for DVT may cause hematoma and calf muscle contractures in patients with a ruptured Baker's cyst. Ultrasound is recommended as the first diagnostic test in cases of suspected DVT. If no thrombus or ruptured Baker's cyst is found, phlebography should be performed to exclude calf vein thrombosis. If a cyst is present or the popliteal vein is deviated or compressed but phlebography is negative, contrast arthrography is recommended.

▶ Careful duplex ultrasound studies make phlebography unnecessary in this condition.

Management of Deep Venous Thrombosis in the Pregnant Female
Rosenfeld JC, Estrada FP, Orr RM (St Luke's Hosp, Bethlehem, Pa)
J Cardiovasc Surg 31:678–682, 1990   20–7

Background.—Although rare, deep venous thrombosis (DVT) during pregnancy can cause significant complications in the mother and fetus. Diagnosing and treating thrombophlebitis in pregnant women presents a challenge to the treating physician, who must consider both the patient and her unborn child.

Procedure.—In a 4-year period, 7,867 deliveries were performed. In this series, 5 women were treated before delivery for DVT of the lower extremities. After the diagnosis was confirmed by ultrasonography, heparin was administered by continuous intravenous drip for 1–10 days. With the disappearance of symptoms, heparin was injected subcutaneously every 8 hours. The patients were discharged from the hospital and instructed on self-injections, which were continued until the time of active labor.

Results.—None of the patients had symptoms of pulmonary embolism, and there were no hemorrhagic or thrombocytopenic complications. All patients had a normal child. A heparin-related rash occurred in 1 patient.

Discussion.—Clinical findings often do not lead to the accurate diagnosis of DVT. Phlebography, which is the most accurate method of diagnosis, is often not recommended during pregnancy because it involves roentgenography. Isotope studies are also contraindicated in pregnant women. Noninvasive studies for diagnosis should include Doppler ultrasonography along with impedance plethysmography, phleboreography, or duplex ultrasonography. Heparin is the treatment of choice for confirmed DVT during pregnancy and can also be used prophylactically in high-risk pregnant women.

▶ This article summarizes current thinking on the management of the pregnant woman with DVT and repeats the lesson that warfarin crosses the placental barrier and causes birth defects whereas heparin does not.

Clinical Findings Associated With Acute Proximal Deep Vein Thrombosis: A Basis for Quantifying Clinical Judgment
Landefeld CS, McGuire E, Cohen AM (Case Western Reserve Univ)
Am J Med 88:382–388, 1990   20–8

Introduction.—Deep vein thrombosis (DVT) is a life-threatening condition that can be treated effectively with a timely diagnosis. However, the diagnosis of acute proximal DVT is notoriously inaccurate. Clinical epidemiologic studies using multivariate analysis have shown that combinations of clinical findings are often more useful than individual findings in estimating the probability of a particular diagnosis. An attempt was made to identify those clinical factors that would be useful in estimating the probability of acute proximal DVT.

Methods.—During a 2-year period, of 392 patients who underwent unilateral venography, 355 were examined in detail. These 219 women and 136 men had a mean age of 56 years. Standardized forms were used to collect data on 76 clinical items, most of them have been suspected as having a role in DVT. Independent clinical correlates of proximal DVT, identified by multivariate discriminant analysis in 236 randomly selected patients, were then tested in the remaining 119 patients. All venograms were interpreted by standard criteria. Interobserver agreement was evaluated in a sample of 119 venograms.

Findings.—Ninety-six patients (27%) had venographic evidence of acute DVT, 185 (52%) had normal venograms, and 74 (21%) had equivocal venographic findings. Swelling of the symptomatic leg above the knee, swelling below the knee, recent immobility, cancer, and fever were independent clinical correlates of proximal DVT. Patients with none of these 5 clinical findings were at very low risk (5%) for acute proximal DVT, patients with 1 finding were at medium risk (15%), and patients with 2 or more findings were at high risk for acute proximal DVT (42%). If venography had been performed only in patients with 1 or more of these 5 factors, proximal DVT would have been observed in 97%; 92% of the patients would have had equivocal findings, and venography would have been avoided in 26% of patients with normal venograms. Only 2 cases of proximal DVT would have been missed.

Conclusion.—Five specific findings were identified as useful in estimating the probability of acute proximal DVT in patients undergoing venography. The probability of finding acute proximal DVT on a venogram was predicted by the number of clinical factors present in an individual patient.

▶ This study makes a strong case for the obvious, i.e., the use of duplex scanning rather than phlebography in the diagnosis of DVT.

Mortality From Pulmonary Embolism in the United States: 1962 to 1984
Lilienfeld DE, Chan E, Ehland J, Godbold JH, Landrigan PJ, Marsh G (Mount Sinai School of Medicine, New York; Univ of Pittsburgh Graduate School of Public Health)
Chest 98:1067–1072, 1990   20–9

Purpose.—The effect of advances in the prevention of and therapy for pulmonary embolism (PE) in the United States was evaluated using mortality trends for PE from 1962 to 1984.

Data Analysis.—Between 1962 and 1974, age-adjusted mortality rates increased by 67% to 100% for white and nonwhite men and women. From 1975 to 1984, age-adjusted mortality rates declined by 20% to 28%. Age-specific mortality for those older than 40 years followed the pattern of the age-adjusted mortality rates, with increases in all age groups between 1962 and 1974, followed by a decline from 1975 to 1984. For all demographic groups, PE mortality rates increased with age (table). Except for the middle-aged nonwhite subjects whose mortality from PE was 50% greater than that for white subjects, PE mortality rates were similar for white and nonwhite men and women. Men had approximately 20% higher PE mortality rates than women in both white and nonwhite groups.

Discussion.—These mortality trends may reflect improved ascertainment of cases and better prevention of disease. The magnitude of the rates suggests that the indications for prophylactic anticoagulation should be expanded.

▶ Epidemiologic study of PE is difficult. From this study, we can take it as a fact that PE remains an important clinical entity. Clearly, it should be prevented whenever possible.

Incidence of Venous Thromboembolism Verified by Necropsy Over 30 Years
Lindblad B, Sternby NH, Bergqvist D (Lund Univ, Malmö, Sweden)
Br Med J 302:709–711, 1991   20–10

Objective.—The changing frequency of venous thromboembolism in the past 30 years was assessed by reviewing autopsy records longitudinally. Although medical advances might be expected to reduce the frequency of this condition, the advent of aggressive reconstructive surgery in elderly patients may statistically neutralize the benefits of such advances.

Methods.—All autopsies done in 1987 in the departments of general surgery, internal medicine, infectious disease, oncology, and orthopedics were evaluated, as were records for 1957, 1964 and 1975; those autopsies in which venous thromboembolism was found were analyzed in detail.

Results.—In 1987, autopsies were done on 76.9% of the 1,293 patients who died. A third of these had evidence of venous thrombosis. Pulmonary emboli accounted for 260 of these cases and were fatal in 93 patients, contributed to the death of 90, and were apparently unrelated to the cause of death in 77. Twenty-one emboli contributed to or caused death after operations, but autopsy did not reveal the origin of emboli in

Relative Change in Age-Specific PE Mortality Rate in the United States, 1962 to 1984, by Race and Sex

Race, Sex	Age (yr)											
	30-34	35-39	40-44	45-49	50-54	55-59	60-64	65-69	70-74	75-79	80-84	85+
White												
Men	43*	23†	25‡	35‡	14‡	37‡	36‡	21‡	32‡	36‡	50‡	56‡
Women	1‡	10‡	45‡	75‡	49‡	44‡	49‡	48‡	37‡	42‡	58‡	66‡
Non-white												
Men	44	20*	50*	4‡	29‡	50‡	48‡	16‡	19‡	31‡	103‡	65‡
Women	12‡	2‡	40‡	12†	12†	21‡	46‡	54‡	72‡	71‡	54†	79†

*P <.05 (Cochran-Armitage test).
†P <.01 (Cochran-Armitage test).
‡P <.005 (Cochran-Armitage test).
(Courtesy of Lilienfeld DE, Chan E, Ehland J, et al: *Chest* 98:1067–1072, 1990.)

106 cases. Clots were found in the deep veins of 239 patients. In the 4 years studied, results were remarkably similar, but the autopsy rate declined from more than 96% in 1975, 1964, and 1957 to 76.9% in 1987.

Conclusions.—In this general hospital population, the incidence of venous thrombosis has not changed in the past 3 decades. Prophylaxis or early mobilization has been more common in recent years, but it is possible that the positive effects of preventive measures were counterbalanced by a doubling of the medically vulnerable over-65 population during the study period. To be certain that the venous thrombosis rate has remained constant, a high necropsy rate, corrections for population age composition, and variations in aggressiveness of management according to age must be taken into account.

▶ The study reported in this abstract suggests that there is not an increased incidence of deep venous thrombosis and pulmonary embolism. Perhaps the effects of prophylaxis have been cancelled by an increased age of the hospital population.

A Population-Based Perspective of the Hospital Incidence and Case-Fatality Rates of Deep Vein Thrombosis and Pulmonary Embolism: The Worcester DVT Study
Anderson FA Jr, Wheeler HB, Goldberg RJ, Hosmer DW, Patwardhan NA, Jovanovic B, Forcier A, Dalen JE (Univ of Massachusetts, Worcester and Amherst; Univ of Arizona)
Arch Intern Med 151:933–938, 1991   20–11

Background.—There is uncertainty as to the incidence and case-fatality rates of acute deep vein thrombosis (DVT) and pulmonary embolism. A community-wide study of venous thromboembolism was done to examine the incidence and in-hospital and long-term case-fatality rates of hospitalized patients with DVT and/or pulmonary embolism.

Methods.—All patients discharged from 16 short-stay hospitals in an 18-month period with a diagnosis of acute DVT and/or pulmonary embolism were studied. Their medical records were individually reviewed and validated based on specific hospital discharge diagnoses. Sociodemographic characteristics, risk factors for venous thromboembolism, concurrent medical conditions, diagnostic methods, therapeutic interventions, and prophylaxis also were included in the analysis.

Results.—Of 151,349 acute-care discharges, 1,372 patients had a discharge diagnosis of acute DVT and/or pulmonary embolism, and a subset of 405 had their first recognized episode of venous thromboembolism. For DVT alone, the average annual incidence was 48/100,000. For pulmonary embolism with or without DVT the incidence was 23/100,000. For both conditions, incidence rates increased exponentially with age (Fig 20–2). For venous thromboembolism, the in-hospital case-fatality rate was 12%. Among discharged patients, case-fatality rates were 19% at 1 year, 25% at 2 years, and 30% at 3 years.

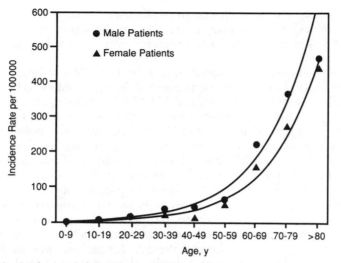

Fig 20–2.—Incidence rate of clinically recognized deep-vein thrombosis and/or pulmonary embolism per 100,000 population. The increase in rates for both male and female patients is well approximated by an exponential function of age. The modeled rate for male patients *(upper curve)* is significantly higher $(P < .05)$ than that for female patients *(lower curve)*. (Courtesy of Anderson FA Jr, Wheeler HB, Goldberg RJ, et al: *Arch Intern Med* 151:933–938, 1991.)

Conclusions.—Based on extrapolation of data from this population-based study, there are about 170,000 new cases of clinically recognized venous thromboembolism in short-stay hospital patients each year in the United States, and 99,000 hospitalizations for recurrent disease. Including clinically undetected disease, the true incidence of DVT is probably much higher than reported in this study. Mortality remains uncertain because of the low rate of autopsy.

► This study and those reviewed in previous abstracts point out the disturbing fact that true incidence rates of both DVT and pulmonary embolism are much higher than is clinically apparent.

Fatal Pulmonary Embolism Associated With Surgery: An Autopsy Study
Hauch O, Jørgensen LN, Khattar SC, Teglbjærg CS, Wåhlin AB, Rathenborg P, Wille-Jørgensen P (Univ of Copenhagen; Hillerød Central Hosp, Denmark)
Acta Chir Scand 156:747–749, 1990   20–12

Purpose.—Fatal postoperative pulmonary embolism is considered a rare complication of surgery. However, several studies have attributed up to 15% of postoperative deaths to such embolisms. The incidence of fatal postoperative pulmonary embolism was examined.

Methods.—Only deaths that occurred within 30 days of operation were classified as postoperative deaths. Based on autopsy findings, pulmonary embolisms were classified as fatal, contributory, or incidental to the death. If patients did not die of postoperative embolism, the prognosis was poor for those with malignant disease, end-stage chronic disease, cardiac or respiratory failure, severe infection or sepsis, or a life expectancy of less than 5 years. The prognosis was classified as good in all other cases.

Results.—Two major hospitals had a total of 2,609 in-hospital deaths in 1986, with autopsies being performed in 1,603 cases (61%). There were 253 postoperative deaths, and 131 (55%) of these patients were autopsied. Pulmonary embolism was classified as the primary cause of death in 74 of the 131 cases; 16 (12%) had postoperative pulmonary embolisms. The 10 men and 6 women had a median age of 72 years. Nine of the 16 patients would have had a good prognosis if pulmonary embolism had not occurred. Fatal embolism was an unexpected autopsy finding in 10 cases (63%). Only 3 of these 16 patients had received thromboembolic prophylaxis. In 13 patients pulmonary embolism was considered a contributory cause of death, but none of the patients would have had a good prognosis even without embolism, which was an unexpected finding at autopsy. After adjusting the data for patients who died outside the hospital and for unautopsied deaths, the incidence of fatal postoperative pulmonary embolism was estimated at 1.2–1.3/1,000.

Discussion.—Although fatal postoperative pulmonary embolism is relatively rare, more than half of the patients in this study would have had a good postoperative prognosis if embolism had not occurred. Thromboembolic prophylaxis in all patients older than age 40 years who undergo more than minor surgery is highly recommended.

▶ In this study, half of the pulmonary embolism fatalities occurred after gastrointestinal surgery and only 2 after orthopedic manipulations. Surprisingly, 2 deaths occurred after vascular surgical procedures. As the abstract states, only 3 of the 16 patients who died of pulmonary embolism had received prophylaxis for deep vein thrombosis.

Effects of Epidural Anesthesia on the Incidence of Deep-Vein Thrombosis After Total Knee Arthroplasty
Sharrock NE, Haas SB, Hargett MJ, Urquhart B, Insall JN, Scuderi G (Hosp for Special Surgery, New York)
J Bone Joint Surg 73-A:502–506, 1991   20–13

Background.—Postoperative deep vein thrombosis (DVT) has been reported in 40% to 88% of patients undergoing total knee arthroplasty. Epidural anesthesia may reduce the prevalence of DVT after total hip arthroplasty compared with that experienced after general anesthesia. The effect of epidural anesthesia on the rate of thrombosis after total knee arthroplasty was examined.

Methods.—The results of all total knee arthroplasties performed by 1 surgeon between September 1984 and December 1988 were reviewed retrospectively. Of the 705 knee arthroplasties conducted, 377 patients had a unilateral procedure and 164 had bilateral arthroplasty. Patients receiv-

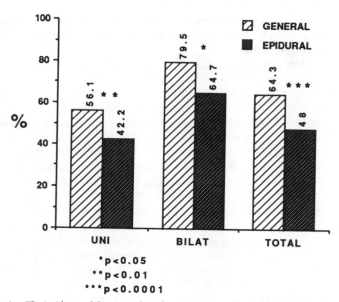

Fig 20–3.—The incidence of deep-vein thrombosis in patients who had unilateral or 1-stage bilateral total knee arthroplasty. (Courtesy of Sharrock NE, Haas SB, Hargett MJ, et al: *J Bone Joint Surg* 73-A:502–506, 1991.)

ing epidural anesthesia had an average age of 69 years; those receiving general anesthesia were, on average, 67 years old. All patients had received 650 mg of aspirin twice daily as prophylaxis against DVT. A perfusion lung scan was performed on all patients at baseline, and on the fifth, sixth, or seventh postoperative day. Lumbar epidural anesthesia consisted of 15–25 mL of .75% bupivacaine or 2% lidocaine with epinephrine. General anesthetic agents included thiopental, isoflurane, nitrous oxide, succinylcholine, and fentanyl.

Findings.—The overall rate of DVT was significantly lower in patients receiving epidural anesthesia after both the unilateral and the bilateral procedures (Fig 20–3). Deep vein thrombosis occurred in 64% of patients given general anesthesia and in 48% of those given epidural anesthesia. The greatest reduction occurred in the number of proximal thrombi. Two patients who received general anesthesia and 2 who received epidural anesthesia had symptomatic pulmonary emboli, which were confirmed on lung scans. No fatal pulmonary emboli occurred during the study period.

Conclusion.—These findings indicate that epidural anesthesia lowered the rate of DVT after total knee arthroplasty, especially for proximal thrombi, which are considered the greatest risk for embolization. The overall rate of DVT was still high in this study. Using adjuvant prophylaxis with this surgical procedure is recommended.

▶ This very interesting study of a high-risk surgical population seems to show that epidural anesthesia does decrease the incidence of DVT. The rate of DVT presumably could be lowered even further by effective prophylactic measures.

Prevention of Deep-Vein Thrombosis and Pulmonary Embolism After Total Hip Replacement: Comparison of Low-Molecular-Weight Heparin and Unfractionated Heparin

Eriksson BI, Kälebo P, Anthmyr BA, Wadenvik H, Tengborn L, Risberg B (Gothenburg Univ, Sweden)
J Bone Joint Surg 73-A:484–493, 1991   20–14

Background.—Low-molecular-weight heparin, in animal studies, has less interaction with platelets and less effect on overall ex vivo clotting than regular heparin. A prospective, randomized, double-blind study was done to compare the safety and efficacy of low-molecular-weight and standard heparin in 136 patients having total hip replacement. All were older than age 40 years.

Methods.—The patients were admitted for elective total hip replacement and randomly allocated into 2 groups. Low-molecular-weight heparin, 5,000 IU/day, was given to 67 patients and standard sodium heparin, 5,000 IU 3 times per day, to 69. Treatment began 12 hours preoperatively in the group given low-molecular-weight heparin and 2 hours preoperatively in those given standard heparin; treatment was continued for 10 days. Twelve days after surgery, 122 patients underwent bilateral ascending phlebography and 127 underwent pulmonary scintigraphy.

Results.—There were 44 cases of deep vein thrombosis among the patients undergoing bilateral ascending phlebography, affecting 30% of those given low-molecular-weight heparin and 42% of those given standard heparin. Two patients in each group were symptomatic. The difference in total rate of thrombosis was insignificant, but only 9.5% of the patients given low-molecular-weight heparin had thrombosis in the thigh, compared with 30.5% of patients given standard heparin. Among the patients undergoing pulmonary scintigraphy, there were 27 cases of pulmonary embolism, affecting 12.3% of the group given low-molecular-weight heparin and 30.6% of those given standard heparin. Only 3 patients had clinical signs of embolism. The group given low-molecular-weight heparin had significantly less total blood loss and required a lesser total amount of transfused blood.

Conclusions.—Although the overall incidence of DVT was not significantly different between low-molecular-weight and standard heparin, low-molecular-weight heparin is superior in preventing femoral thrombosis and pulmonary embolism. The use of low-molecular-weight heparin also reduces blood loss and transfused blood, thus improving safety.

▶ Many studies on the prophylactic efficacy of low-molecular-weight heparin could have been included in this issue of the YEAR BOOK. Two were chosen simply to make the point that low-molecular-weight heparins are effective and are associated with a lower risk of hemorrhagic complications than is standard heparin.

Efficacy and Tolerance of Low Molecular Weight Heparin in the Preventive Treatment of Deep Venous Thrombosis During Non-Emergent Total Hip Arthroplasty: A Multicenter Prospective Trial

Simon P, Kindermans A, Kempf JF, Postel M (Centre Hospitalier Universitaire Hautepierre, Strasbourg, France; Centre Hospitalier Universitaire Cochin, Paris)
J Chir (Paris) 127:252–257, 1990   20–15

Introduction.—The high incidence of deep vein thrombosis (DVT) associated with total hip arthroplasty has been well reported. Most French orthopedic surgeons agree on the need for some type of preventive treatment, but the optimal preventive regimen has not yet been defined. A prospective, multicenter trial was carried out to evaluate the efficacy and patient tolerance of low-molecular-weight heparin in the prevention of DVT after elective total hip arthroplasty.

Patients.—Sixty-five men and 84 women (mean age, 65.5) underwent hip replacement surgery at 1 of 13 participating centers in France. Treatment consisted of daily subcutaneous injections of CY 216, which contains 180 units of low-molecular-weight heparin per mg. Individual doses varied with body weights and surgical schedules. Heparin therapy was started 12 hours before operation and continued for 10 days afterward. Prophylactic efficacy was assessed by bilateral phlebography performed on day 10 after operation. Complete phlebographic data were available for 139 patients.

Results.—Postoperative DVT of the lower extremities developed in 18 patients (12.9%). The thrombosis was proximal in 5 (3.6%) and distal in 13 (9.3%). Three of the 18 patients had a previous history of thrombosis, 11 had risk factors for thrombosis (e.g., obesity and cigarette smoking), and 4 had unusually long operations. Only 2 patients with DVT had no predisposing risk factors. None of the patients had a pulmonary embolism, and none died. The mean perioperative blood transfusion requirement was 470 mL. Ninety-three patients did not require postoperative transfusions. The mean postoperative transfusion requirement for the remaining patients was 211 mL. Three patients (2%) experienced a major local hemorrhage requiring premature discontinuation of treatment. Thirty-five patients had only minor hemorrhagic events not requiring discontinuation, and 113 patients (76%) had no sign of hemorrhage.

Conclusion.—Single daily injections of low-molecular-weight heparin given in fixed doses based on body weight and day of operation effectively lower the incidence of postoperative DVT after total hip replacement. The low incidence of premature treatment withdrawal confirms that this preventive protocol is well tolerated.

▶ The advantages of low-molecular-weight heparin include the ability to use a single daily dose, a fixed dose, and a low incidence of hemorrhagic complications.

Prevention of Venous Thrombosis After Total Knee Arthroplasty: Comparison of Antithrombin III and Low-Dose Heparin With Dextran
Francis CW, Pellegrini VD Jr, Stulberg BN, Miller ML, Totterman S, Marder VJ (Univ of Rochester; Cleveland Clinic Found)
J Bone Joint Surg 72-A:976–982, 1990   20–16

Introduction.—Between 41% and 84% of the patients having total knee arthroplasty who do not receive prophylaxis experience venous thrombosis. Two percent to 10% of these have symptomatic pulmonary embolism. Congenital or acquired deficiency of antithrombin III (AT) is associated with a high risk of venous thrombosis, and prophylaxis with AT and heparin has been found to reduce thrombotic complications after hip arthroplastic surgery. The heparin and AT regimen was compared with dextran prophylaxis to avoid thrombotic complications after total knee replacement.

Methods.—Of 83 patients scheduled for total knee arthroplasty, 42 were randomly assigned to receive AT and heparin and 41 were given dextran. The dextran regimen consisted of a loading infusion of 10 mL/kg over 12 hours starting 2 hours preoperatively and continuing for 5.5 days at 7 mL/kg daily. For the other regimen, 3,000 IU of intravenous AT and 5,000 IU of subcutaneous heparin were given 2 hours preoperatively. Then, 2,000 IU of AT was given daily over 20 minutes, and 5,000 IU of heparin was given every 12 hours for the next 5 days. Ascending venograms, generally obtained 5–7 days postoperatively, were scored by an investigator blind to the patients' drug regimens.

Results.—Of 39 patients given AT and heparin who had interpretable venograms, 35% experienced venous thrombosis, in contrast to 80% of the 38 dextran-treated patients. This significant difference was attributable to more frequent thrombosis in the deep veins of the calf in patients who received dextran. In all but 2 cases, thrombosis was asymptomatic. Venous thrombosis developed in 5 of 9 patients who underwent bilateral operations. Thrombosis developed in all patients with a postoperative AT level less than 65% of their baseline value.

Discussion.—The combination of AT and heparin is a more effective therapy than dextran. The 80% incidence of thrombosis after the latter treatment is as high as in studies with no prophylaxis. The likelihood of thrombosis after total knee arthroplasty may be related to the postoperative level of AT.

▶ Although the administration of AT has been a fruitful avenue of investigation, it is more likely that fractionated heparin will be accepted as a means of prophylaxis in the future.

Mechanical Measures in the Prophylaxis of Postoperative Thromboembolism in Total Knee Arthroplasty
Lynch JA, Baker PL, Polly RE, Lepse PS, Wallace BE, Roudybush D, Sund K, Lynch NM (Orthopedic Assoc, Topeka)
Clin Orthop 260:24–29, 1990   20–17

Introduction.—Patients who undergo total knee arthroplasty are at high risk for deep venous thrombosis (DVT) and pulmonary embolism. Because DVT is difficult to diagnose in its early stages, DVT prophylaxis is desirable, if not mandatory. Low-molecular-weight dextran, aspirin, and warfarin effectively reduce DVT and pulmonary embolism, but they are associated with significant complications. In contrast, mechanical measures—e.g., continuous passive motion (CPM) devices and sequential pneumatic compression stockings (SPCSs)—are free of complications. The effectiveness of these prophylactic modalities was assessed.

Study Design.—Between 1972 and 1989, a total of 2,161 patients underwent total knee arthroplasty. All patients had preoperative perfusion lung scans. Ventilation lung scans were done if perfusion lung scans were positive. Bilateral lower extremity venograms and perfusion lung scans were performed on day 5 after operation. Dextran 40, heparin, aspirin, and warfarin were used for postoperative prophylaxis from 1972 to 1983, CPM was used from 1983 to 1984, and CPM and SPCSs were used from 1984 to 1986. Although CPM and SPCSs were still used from 1986 to 1989, warfarin was given to alternate patients.

Results.—In a 1972 control group of untreated patients having total knee arthroplasty, the incidence of DVT was 73% and the incidence of pulmonary embolism was 24%. Dextran 40 reduced the incidence of DVT to 57% and of pulmonary embolism to 20%, but this drug was discontinued after anaphylaxis occurred in 2 patients. Heparin had no prophylactic value, because the incidence of thromboembolic disease was similar to that in untreated controls. In addition, 4 heparin-treated patients had significant bleeding complications. Warfarin reduced the incidence of DVT to 40% and of pulmonary embolism to 16%, but there were again significant bleeding complications. Aspirin increased the incidence of DVT to 46% and of pulmonary embolism to 18%, but there were no complications. The use of CPM alone reduced the incidence of DVT to 20% and of pulmonary embolism to 6%. The addition of SPCSs further reduced the incidence of DVT to 11% and of pulmonary embolism to 6%. The addition of warfarin to the mechanical prophylactic regimen provided no additional benefit.

Conclusions.—In patients who undergo total knee arthroplasty, mechanical methods such as CPM and SPCSs effectively reduce the incidence of postoperative DVT and pulmonary embolism without any complications. The addition of warfarin to CPM and SPCSs does not augment the antithromboembolic effect of the mechanical methods.

▶ Mechanical prevention of DVT has many advantages. It is easy to monitor and causes few side effects while retaining efficacy. However, experience teaches that the cuffs are frequently absent, misapplied, or function less.

Intermittent Pneumatic Compression to Prevent Proximal Deep Venous Thrombosis During and After Total Hip Replacement: A Prospective, Randomized Study of Compression Alone, Compression and Aspirin, and Compression and Low-Dose Warfarin
Woolson ST, Watt JM (Stanford Univ)
J Bone Joint Surg 73-A:507–512, 1991   20–18

Background.—Prophylaxis against deep venous thrombosis (DVT) is important in patients having hip arthroplasty. Whether the intraoperative and postoperative use of intermittent pneumatic compression reduces the rate of DVT was examined, and the frequency of this complication was compared using 3 prophylactic measures: intermittent pneumatic compression alone, intermittent pneumatic compression and aspirin, and intermittent pnuematic compression and low-dose warfarin.

Methods.—The study sample comprised 196 patients older than 39 years who underwent 217 total hip arthroplasties. Patients started walking by the third day after operation. The procedure was done to revise a previous hip placement or endoprosthesis in 28% of cases. Patients were randomized into 3 groups: intermittent pneumatic compression alone was used in 76 instances, compression and aspirin in 72, and compression and low-dose warfarin in 69. Venography was done before discharge and an anverage of 7 days postoperatively to determine the presence of DVT.

Results.—Proximal DVT occurred in 12% of the group having compression alone, 10% of those having compression and aspirin, and 9% of those having compression and warfarin; the differences were not significant. Increased age was a significant risk factor, but revision and a history of DVT were not. The overall relative frequency of 10% was significicant lower than the 20% to 50% frequencies reported for the control groups of other studies.

Conclusions.—In total hip replacement patients, intermittent compression during and after surgery reduces the rate of proximal DVT. Combination of this prophylaxis with oral doses of aspirin or low-dose warfarin does not appear to augment this effect, although the sample size in this study was small.

▶ Intermittent calf compression reduces the incidence of DVT and, presumably, pulmonary embolism, but the addition of other means of prophylaxis does not have a synergistic or additive effect.

Late Changes in Veins After Deep Venous Thrombosis: Ultrasonographic Findings
Gaitini D, Kaftori JK, Pery M, Markel A (Technion-Israel Inst of Technology, Haifa, Israel)
Fortschr Roentgenstr 153:68–72, 1990   20–19

TABLE 1.—Correlation Between Ultrasonographical and Clinical Findings on Follow-up Examinations

No. of extremities	Ultrasonography	Postphlebitic syndrome
27	+	+
11	−	−
4	+	−
3	−	+

Abbreviations: Plus sign, positive for chronic DVT; *minus sign,* negative for DVT.
(Courtesy of Gaitini D, Kaftori JK, Pery M, et al: *Fortschr Roentgenstr* 153:68–72, 1990.)

TABLE 2.—Correlation Between Initial Site of Thrombus
and Follow-up Ultrasound Studies (45 Legs)

Original site	No.	Abnormal on follow-up	Normal on follow-up
Popliteal vein only	10	6	4
Femoral vein only	16	12	4
Popliteal and femoral veins	19	13	6
Total	45	31	14

(Courtesy of Gaitini D, Kaftori JK, Pery M, et al: *Fortschr Roentgenstr* 153:68–72, 1990.)

Purpose.—Although ultrasonography is helpful in evaluating deep venous thrombosis (DVT), its value is questionable in assessing patients with past DVT who have a swollen, painful lower extremity. In a prospective study, 43 patients were reevaluated 3–32 months after an acute episode of DVT. All of the patients had received conventional anticoagulant therapy. High-resolution and continuous-wave Doppler ultrasonography was performed.

Findings.—Ultrasonographic findings were abnormal in 31 (69%) of the 45 extremities examined; 27 of these 31 patients and 3 of 14 with normal findings were symptomatic or had signs of postphlebitic syndrome (Table 1). Abnormal veins were either narrowed with a very echogenic lumen (representing persistent occlusion) or had a relatively sonolucent lumen and thickened walls (representing recanalization). Partly occluded veins were only partly collapsible on probe compression. The continuous-wave Doppler findings were similar to those in acute DVT. The correlation between the initial site of the thrombus and follow-up findings is shown in Table 2.

Conclusions.—All patients with acute DVT should have sonography on follow-up after 6–12 months. If a baseline study is not available or the diagnosis is in doubt, contrast phlebography is indicated before anticoagulant therapy is started if new acute findings develop.

▶ Once again, duplex ultrasound has defined the pathologic anatomy of the vein after DVT, suggesting that prevention is wise both for decreasing the incidence of pulmonary embolization and for decreasing the morbidity of late venous stasis disease.

Can Fibrinolytic Agents Prevent Postthrombotic Venous Insufficiency?

Marcon JL, Bonijoly S, Favre E (Centre Hospitalier Général, Annonay, France)
Sem Hôp Paris 67:207–212, 1991   20–20

Introduction.—The goal of therapy in patients with deep venous thrombosis (DVT) is to prevent pulmonary embolism and avoid the sequelae of postthrombotic syndrome. Heparin therapy has effectively reduced the incidence of embolism in these patients from 20% without treatment to the current 5% rate. In contrast, the incidence of postthrombotic syndrome still ranges from 50% to 70%. Whether administration of fibrinolytic agents can lower the incidence of postthrombotic syndrome without drastically increasing the risk of hemorrhage was examined.

Patients.—During a 2½-year period, 34 patients with DVT of the lower extremities were treated with locally applied streptokinase; 24 were reexamined. (Four patients had died and 6 did not return for reexamination.) Phlebography was performed at baseline and after treatment. Postthrombotic venous insufficiency was monitored clinically and with impedance plethysmography and venous Doppler studies. All patients were treated with pump-released heparin but at half the dose required for maintaining effective anticoagulation. Streptokinase was usually administered at a daily dose of 500,000 IU for 3–5 days, depending on the phlebographic findings. The average follow-up was 4 years 2 months.

Outcome.—At the follow-up examination 17 patients were free of deep venous insufficiency and 7 patients (29%) had moderate venous insufficiency. None of the patients had severe venous insufficiency. The phlebographic findings at the end of treatment did not correlate with the later finding of venous insufficiency. Factors identified as predictive of residual venous insufficiency included preexisting venous disease, failure to recanalize the vessels communicating with the popliteal-femoral junction, and late recanalization that resulted in an avalvular vein, which was a source of reflux. None of the patients without these risk factors had postthrombotic insufficiency.

Conclusion.—Short-term fibrinolytic therapy effectively reduced the incidence of postthrombotic venous insufficiency in patients treated for DVT to 29%. Prompt recanalization, preferably within the first 5 days after the diagnosis, prevents valvular destruction and the occurrence of postthrombotic reflux.

▶ Although this study suggests that venous stasis changes can be reduced by lytic therapy, there is need for further and perhaps even more careful study.

Long-Term Results of Venous Thrombectomy Combined With a Temporary Arterio-Venous Fistula
Plate G, Åkesson H, Einarsson E, Ohlin P, Eklöf B (Central Hosp, Helsingborg, Sweden; Univ of Lund, Sweden; Univ of Kuwait)
Eur J Vasc Surg 4:483–489, 1990   20–21

Background.—A previous study has shown that, in acute iliofemoral venous thromboses, a flow-increasing arteriovenous fistula constructed at the groin level prevents rethrombosis of the iliofemoral segment. Further refinements in the technique of venous thrombectomy have also been encouraging. In a prospective randomized study, 58 patients with acute iliofemoral venous thrombosis were assigned to either conventional antico-

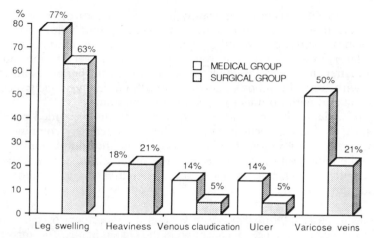

Fig 20–4.—Postthrombotic sequelae in 22 medical and 19 surgical patients 5 years after an acute iliofemoral venous thrombosis. (Courtesy of Plate G, Åkesson H, Einarsson E, et al: *Eur J Vasc Surg* 4:483–489, 1990.)

agulation or acute thrombectomy combined with a temporary arteriovenous fistula. Clinical, morphological, and physiologic evaluation was available for 41 patients at 5 years.

Outcome.—There were no significant differences in clinical results between the 19 surgical patients and the 22 medical patients, although there were slightly more asymptomatic patients (37% vs. 18%) and fewer severe postthrombotic sequelae (16% vs. 27%) in the surgical group (Fig 20–4). Radionuclide angiography showed that the iliac vein was significantly less frequently occluded in the surgical group compared with the medical group, but occlusion plethysmography revealed that

Mean Values (Ranges) for Physiological Tests Performed 5 Years
After an Acute Iliofemoral Venous Thrombosis

	Treatment Medical	Surgical	P-value Mann–Whitney U test
Occlusion plethysmography	$n = 20$	$n = 17$	
MVO (ml/min/100 ml)	45 (12–87)	61 (24–161)	N.S.
Foot volumetry	$n = 19$	$n = 14$	
EV_{rel} (ml/100 ml/min)	0.9 (0.0–1.8)	1.0 (0.0–1.9)	N.S.
Q/EV_{rel} (min^{-1})	4.7 (0.5–18.3)	3.3 (1.1–7.4)	N.S.
Foot vein pressure	$n = 18$	$n = 10$	
Pressure reduction (%)	36 (−6–78)	52 (26–81)	N.S.
Ambulatory venous pressure (mmHg)	60 (21–95)	43 (18–70)	$P < 0.05$
90% refill time (s)	13 (0–71)	14 (4–38)	N.S.

Note: Because 1 patient in each group had an EV_{rel} = 0, the Q/EV_{rel} could only be calculated for 18 and 13 patients, respectively. The Mann-Whitney U test was used for the statistical analyses.
(Courtesy of Plate G, Åkesson H, Einarsson E, et al: *Eur J Vasc Surg* 4:483–489, 1990.)

outflow capacity was not significantly better (table). Furthermore, venous reflux and muscle pump function, as assessed by foot volumetry and/or foot vein pressures, did not differ significantly between treatment groups. Ambulatory venous pressure was significantly lower in the surgical group. After thrombectomy, there was a tendency for better results in patients with fresh thrombosis and those in whom iliac vein clearance was complete and with no underlying vein compression.

Conclusion.—The small number of observations precluded providing statistical evidence of benefit with venous thrombectomy combined with a temporary arteriovenous fistula, although this procedure appears to improve the long-term outcome. Because the difference is not very striking, anticoagulation remains an acceptable alternative for acute iliofemoral venous thrombosis.

▶ Despite the long-term advocacy of venous thrombectomy by the Swedish groups, the procedure has not caught on in the United States. This report then becomes very important. It represents a definitive study in which no statistical difference could be found between the 2 treatment groups. It could be that the study contained too few patients and a difference that was actually present was missed (type two error).

Ligation of the Superficial Femoral Vein in Prevention of Pulmonary Embolism: An Old Fashion Procedure?
Louagie Y, Van Ruyssevelt P, El Hammouti F, Theys S, Janssens Th, Buche M, Schoevaerdts JC (Academic Hosp of Mont-Godinne, Yvoir, Belgium)
J Cardiovasc Surg 31:416–423, 1990   20–22

Background.—Ligation of the femoral vein (LFV) for the prevention of thromboembolism remains controversial. The records of 73 patients who underwent interruption of the superficial femoral vein (SFV) to prevent pulmonary embolism were reviewed.

Methods.—Preoperative phlebography showed a thrombus in the posterior tibial vein in 67.3% in the superficial femoral or popliteal vein in 56.6%, in the long saphenous vein in 10.6%, in the common femoral vein in 19.5%, and in the iliac vein in 2.7%. Pulmonary embolism had occurred in 76.7% and was associated with neoplasm in 13.7%. The main indication for surgery was the presence of floating thrombus in the superficial femoral or posterior tibial veins in 97.3%. Ligation of the SFV was performed in 93 limbs, and iliac or femoral thrombectomy was completed in 32.3%. The procedure was performed under local or regional anesthesia in 82.8% of patients. The average follow-up period was 3 years.

Results.—The hospital mortality rate was 1.4%. The 3-year survival rate, considering only pulmonary-embolism-related deaths, was 95.3%. Recurrent pulmonary embolism occurred in 11.1%, for a 3-year pulmonary-embolism-free rate of 90.8%. Mild symptoms related to LFV and the postthrombotic syndrome were common but tended to decrease with time. In 64 limbs, bilateral strain-gauge plethysmography was performed and the times needed to obtain a 50% ($T_{1/2}$), 75% ($T_{3/4}$), and 100% decrease in calf volume were calculated for the operated limb and compared with those for the untreated limb. At 1 month after LFV, $T_{1/2}$ and $T_{3/4}$ were similar to those of controls in 49% and 61% of patients, respectively.

Conclusion.—With LFV, there were minimal long-term effects and only mild changes in venous drainage. Ligation of the femoral vein should be used more frequently in patients with embolism determined by phlebography to be from sources below the groin level, particularly when a free-floating thrombus in the popliteal or femoral vein threatens a critically ill patient.

▶ It is unlikely that this report will have any impact on current practice.

The Greenfield Filter as the Primary Means of Therapy in Venous Thromboembolic Disease
Fink JA, Jones BT (Akron City Hosp, Oh)
Surg Gynecol Obstet 172:253–256, 1991   20–23

Introduction.—The Greenfield vena cava filter effectively prevents pulmonary embolism in patients with venous thromboembolic disease. A recent study showed that the long-term outcome after Greenfield filter placement is independent of the use of postfilter anticoagulation. The outcome in patients who had Greenfield filters placed as the only therapeutic modality was compared with that in a historical group of patients who had anticoagulation alone in the treatment of thromboembolic disease.

Patients.—During a 5-year period, 165 patients underwent Greenfield vena cava filter placement; 78 were available for long-term follow-up. Forty-two of these 78 patients had Greenfield filter placement as the primary therapeutic modality. Of these 42 patients, 15 had deep venous thrombosis (DVT) and 27 had pulmonary embolism before filter placement. Follow-up ranged from 6 to 48 months, and the mean follow-up period was 14 months.

Results.—At follow-up, 14 (33%) of the 42 patients who received Greenfield filter therapy alone had leg swelling, 2 (5%) had leg ulceration, 1 (2%) had recurrent DVT, and none had recurrent pulmonary embolism. Only 19% of the patients wore prescription support hose after discharge, and only 46% of patients in whom postphlebitic sequelae developed were compliant with their use. When the outcome in these 42 patients was compared with that in a historical control group of patients with venous thromboembolic disease who had been treated with anticoagulation alone, the incidence of postphlebitic sequelae did not differ significantly between the 2 groups. The efficacy of anticoagulation alone in the prevention of pulmonary embolism has been reported at 95% to 98%. The efficacy of Greenfield filter placement alone was better than

95%. Whereas major complications of anticoagulation occur in 2% to 15% of patients, and even more often in older patients, the overall complication rate of Greenfield filter placement was less than 10%.

Conclusion.—The Greenfield vena cava filter should be used as primary therapy in patients with venous thromboembolic disease, particularly in patients older than 65 years of age.

▶ This abstract presents an interesting point of view that seems radical but may be conservative.

Variable	No. of Patients (n = 96)	Nonsurvivors (n = 36)	Survivors (n = 60)	p Value
Sex				
Male	50 (52)	23 (46)	27 (54)	0.073
Female	46 (48)	13 (28)	33 (72)	
Date of operation				
1968–1978	19 (20)	6 (32)	13 (68)	0.42
1979–1983	45 (47)	20 (44)	25 (56)	
1984–1988	32 (33)	10 (31)	22 (69)	
Associated heart or lung disease				
Yes	11 (11)	7 (64)	4 (36)	0.061
No	85 (89)	29 (34)	56 (66)	
First clinical episode				
>15 days	21 (22)	9 (43)	12 (57)	0.57
≤15 days	75 (78)	27 (36)	48 (64)	
Shock				
Yes	78 (81)	33 (42)	45 (58)	0.043
No	18 (19)	3 (17)	15 (83)	
Cardiac arrest				
Yes	24 (25)	14 (58)	10 (42)	0.015
No	72 (75)	22 (31)	50 (69)	
Thrombolysis				
Yes	30 (31)	7 (23)	23 (77)	0.053
No	66 (69)	29 (44)	37 (56)	
Age (y) *	52 ± 14	55 ± 12	50 ± 15	0.055

Univariate Analysis of Risk Factors for Death: Clinical Variables in 96 Patients

Numbers in parentheses are percentages.
*Data are shown as the mean ± the standard deviation.
(Courtesy of Meyer G, Tamisier D, Sors H, et al: *Ann Thorac Surg* 51:232–236, 1991.)

Pulmonary Embolectomy: A 20-Year Experience at One Center

Meyer G, Tamisier D, Sors H, Stern M, Vouhé P, Makowski S, Neveux J-Y, Leca F, Even P (Laennec Hosp, Paris)
Ann Thorac Surg 51:232–236, 1991   20–24

Background.—Although thrombolysis is widely accepted as the front-line therapy for most patients with massive pulmonary embolism, it is contraindicated in some cases. Treatment failure occurs in 15% to 20% of patients; in the most severe cases, it can result in death. An experience with pulmonary embolectomy under cardiopulmonary bypass (CPB) was reviewed in an attempt to gain a better understanding of the factors predicting outcomes.

Patients.—Ninety-six consecutive patients with acute massive pulmonary embolism underwent pulmonary embolectomy under CPB at 1 center between 1968 and 1988. The surgical mortality was 37.5%. Both univariate and multivariate analyses were used to evaluate 12 clinical and hemodynamic factors.

Results.—According to multivariate analysis, cardiac arrest and associated cardiopulmonary disease predicted operative death independently. Of the 55 patients available for long-term follow-up (range, 2–144 months), 6 had died and 5 complained of persistent mild or severe exertional dyspnea (table).

Conclusions.—These findings should help clinicians to assess the preoperative risks in patients undergoing pulmonary embolectomy. In view of the long-term results, pulmonary embolectomy is still an acceptable procedure for those few patients who do not benefit from medical treatment.

▶ Thrombolytic therapy should be considered in patients with massive pulmonary embolization, but those who are hemodynamically unstable and who remain compromised must go to pulmonary embolectomy.

Subclavian Vein Thrombosis: A Continuing Challenge

Hill SL, Berry Re (Community Hosp of Roanoke Valley, Roanoke, Va; Roanoke Mem Hosp)
Surgery 108:1–9, 1990   20–25

Background.—Deep venous thrombosis of the upper extremity represents only 1% to 3% of all diagnosed deep venous thromboses, but it remains a potentially morbid entity. The records of patients with a diagnosis of subclavian vein thrombosis seen from 1982 through 1987 were reviewed to assess the frequency, causes, and treatment of subclavian vein thromboses.

Patients.—During the 6-year period, subclavian vein thrombosis was diagnosed in 40 (3.5%) of 1,158 patients with venous thrombosis. The average age of the 20 men and 20 women was 46 years. Causes of the thrombosis included intravenous catheters in 32% of patients, anatomi-

SUBCLAVIAN VENOUS THROMBOSIS

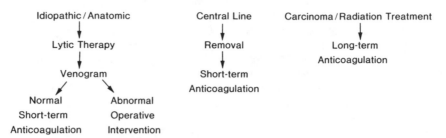

Fig 20−5.—Algorithm for treating subclavian venous thrombosis. (Courtesy of Hill SL, Berry RE: *Surgery* 108:1−9, 1990.)

cal abnormalities in 45%, and carcinoma with postoperative radiation in 22.5%. Despite the rapid increase in the use of the subclavian veins for pacemaker leads, hyperalimentation, and permanent intravenous access for chemotherapy during the period, there was no significant increase in the incidence of symptomatic subclavian vein thrombosis.

Treatment.—Treatment consisted of lytic therapy in 20% of patients, heparinization in 55%, and elevation with removal of the central line in 25%. Anatomical abnormalities with compression of the vein responded well to either heparinization or lytic therapy, but 2 patients required surgery for persistent narrowing or stricture. Patients with carcinoma or radiation responded well after removal of the central lines and coumadin therapy. Overall, all patients had a good response to treatment. None progressed to venous gangrene and only 1 (2.5%) had a documented pulmonary embolus.

Summary.—Subclavian vein thrombosis, although rare, is becoming a more recognized disease entity. This self-limited process, when treated promptly and effectively, results in minimal long-term morbidity and no mortality. Its cause is multifactorial, and treatment options and results are diverse (Fig 20−5). Medical treatment, consisting of lytic therapy, heparin, coumadin, aspirin, elevation, and removal of the central line, usually provides long-term benefit unless the thrombosis is complicated by an anatomical abnormality. Surgical options include venous thrombectomy and correction of the anatomical abnormality.

▶ Unfortunately, subclavian venous thrombosis is no longer rare. This abstract outlines conventional treatment, including removal of the central line, use of lytic therapy when necessary, and venous decompression if upper extremity stasis systems persist.

Axillary-Subclavian Vein Thrombosis: Changing Patterns of Etiology, Diagnostic, and Therapeutic Modalities
Aburahma AF, Sadler DL, Robinson PA (West Virginia Univ; Pfizer Central Research, Groton, Conn)
Am Surg 57:101−107, 1991   20−26

Introduction.—Axillary-subclavian vein thrombosis, representing 1% to 2% of deep venous thrombosis, has historically been treated conservatively with rest, limb elevation, warm compresses, and, recently, anticoagulation therapy. As many as 74% of conservatively treated patients may have some lingering disability; complications in 12% may be anything but benign—venous gangrene and pulmonary embolism being examples. A retrospective review was undertaken to identify changing patterns in the causes, diagnosis, and management of axillary-subclavian vein thrombosis. The records of patients treated in the past decade were reviewed.

Patients.—Fifty-two patients aged 18–81 years were treated for axillary-subclavian vein thrombosis; 18 patients (group A) were treated in the first half of the decade and 34 patients (group B) during the second half. All had swelling and pain in the affected arm, and all underwent venography for diagnostic substantiation. All of the patients in group A and 79% of those in group B were managed traditionally, with the addition of intravenous heparin and oral warfarin therapy; the remainder of group B had thrombolytic therapy with urokinase or streptokinase, then anticoagulation. The minimum follow-up was 1 year.

Results.—Although the percentage of patients who had effort-related or spontaneous axillary-subclavian vein thrombosis did not change over the decade, remaining at 28% to 29% in each group, there were significant changes in the proportions of axillary-subclavian vein thrombosis caused by other factors. In only 17% of group A was the etiology related to intimal injury or catheter insertion, but 47% of group B had thromboses after insertion of subclavian or internal jugular catheters for monitoring central venous pressure, for parenteral nutrition, or for chemotherapy. In group A, 55% of patients had axillary-subclavian vein thrombosis probably caused by the hypercoagulable state produced by malignancy, or venous compression by a tumor, or a variety of systemic disorders; these causes accounted for only 24% of cases in the second 5-year period. Whereas 73% of patients who received traditional therapy still had venous claudication and/or edema, 71% of those who had thrombolytic therapy were without residual symptoms.

Conclusions.—In contrast to the predominance of malignancy or systemic disease as a cause of axillary-subclavian vein thrombosis in earlier years, it is now more common for iatrogenic causes to provoke most incidents. Noninvasive techniques, especially venous duplex imaging, are the safest means to begin diagnosis; venography can be used for confirmation. Thrombolytic therapy, despite risks, was effective in the present series; it may be preferable to anticoagulants because the patients are often young men who cannot afford the potential loss of productivity that may result from use of the latter.

▶ In this study, iatrogenic causes of subclavian vein thrombosis are obvious. Although duplex ultrasound is effective in diagnosis, the use of phlebography allows instillation of lytic agents and, therefore, therapy as well as diagnosis.

Subclavian Vein Obstruction and Thoracic Outlet Syndrome: A Review of Etiology and Management

Sanders RJ, Haug C (Univ of Colorado)

Ann Vasc Surg 4:397–410, 1990

20–27

Introduction.—Subclavian vein compression in the costoclavicular space is an uncommon condition. Because it can cause venous obstruction, it is considered a form of thoracic outlet syndrome. The literature

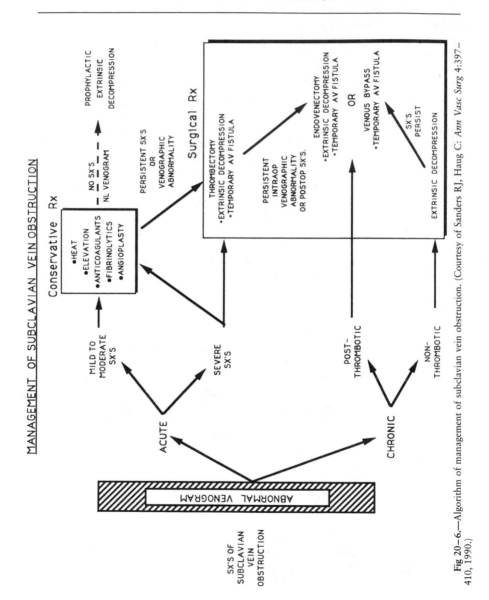

Fig 20–6.—Algorithm of management of subclavian vein obstruction. (Courtesy of Sanders RJ, Haug C: *Ann Vasc Surg* 4:397–410, 1990.)

was reviewed concerning acute and chronic axillary-subclavian vein obstruction, both thrombotic and nonthrombotic.

Symptoms and Signs.—Primary axillary-subclavian venous obstruction is probably caused by abnormal positions during extremes of activity. Typical clinical signs and symptoms include pain, swelling, cyanosis, and venous distention in the upper extremity. Symptoms are usually aggravated by exercise. Venography is considered the primary diagnostic tool, but venous duplex scanning has also been used to detect venous obstruction in the axillary-subclavian veins. Venous pressure measurement may be useful for patients with nonthrombotic obstruction.

Treatment.—The treatment options for acute mild to moderate obstruction of the axillary-subclavian vein include heat, elevation, anticoagulants, fibrinolytics, and angioplasty (Fig 20–6). Thrombectomy is recommended for patients with severe acute obstruction. For postthrombotic or nonthrombotic chronic obstruction, treatment alternatives include decompression by first-rib resection, claviculectomy, scalenectomy and soft tissue division, endovenectomy, and venous bypass.

Discussion. Although acute subclavian vein thrombosis has generally been treated with conservative measures, some degree of chronic postphlebitic symptoms of swelling and aching develops in at least half of the patients. Thus a more aggressive approach based on the newer nonoperative and operative techniques is recommended.

▶ An abstract cannot do justice to this long and complete review, which includes many drawings of technique of venous reconstruction.

Pinch-Off Syndrome: A Complication of Implantable Subclavian Venous Access Devices
Hinke DH, Zandt-Stastny DA, Goodman LR, Quebbeman EJ, Krzywda EA, Andris DA (Med College of Wisconsin; St Nicholas Hosp, Sheboygan, Wis)
Radiology 177:353–356, 1990   20–28

Background.—Implantable central venous access devices (ISVADs) placed through the subclavian vein may become obstructed as a result of catheter compression between the clavicle and first rib; this is called the pinch-off syndrome (POS). If the catheter passes through the areolar tissue in the costoclavicular space outside the subclavian vein before it pierces the vessel medially, it is more susceptible to compression by the clavicle and first rib. A properly placed catheter should traverse the costoclavicular space within the subclavian vein.

Study Design.—To minimize this complication of ISVADs, the chest radiographs of 11 patients with POS were compared with those of 22 matched asymptomatic controls and 100 consecutive routine clinic patients. Comparisons were based on a radiographic scale of catheter distortion: grade 0 indicates normal; 1, abrupt change in course with no luminal narrowing; 2, luminal narrowing; and 3, complete catheter fracture.

Findings.—Pinch-off syndrome was present in 8 of 11 patients within 3 weeks of placement, including 7 with grade 2 catheter deformation on initial chest radiographs. The other 3 patients had a delayed appearance of POS (range, 12–37 weeks). Among the control patients, grade 1 catheter deformation was present in 33% and grade 2 in only 1%. Catheter fracture or fragmentation occurred in 2 of 5 patients with grade 2 POS in whom the catheters were removed more than 3 weeks later.

Conclusions.—Pinch-off syndrome, a well-recognized complication of ISVADs, is most commonly detected shortly after placement. Grade 2 catheter deformation represents significant catheter compression and the potential for serious complications. The significance of grade 1 is uncertain because of its high prevalence in controls.

▶ This abstract stresses the very narrow space between the clavicular head and the first rib. More and more, it is clear that this is the abnormality associated with the entity of subclavian venous thrombosis.

Conventional Versus Thrombolytic Therapy in Spontaneous (Effort) Axillary-Subclavian Vein Thrombosis

AbuRahma AF, Sadler D, Stuart P, Khan MZ, Boland JP (West Virginia Univ)
Am J Surg 161:459–465, 1991   20–29

Background.—Previous therapy for spontaneous (effort) vein thrombosis has included bed rest, limb elevation, warm compresses, and anticoagulation drugs. Other treatments for this condition have comprised venous thrombectomy and thrombolytic agents. The evaluation of any of these treatments is complicated by the fact that more than 75% of the patients have clinical signs of improvement without any therapy.

Patients.—Ten patients (mean age, 35 years) with effort axillary-subclavian vein thrombosis were treated during a 36-month period. The patients were followed for up to 1 year and data obtained on reexamination. All patients initially had marked edema and pain in the involved arm, and none appeared to have an underlying cause. The first 6 patients treated (between June 1986 and April 1988) received conventional therapy. Dissatisfaction with poor results in these 6 patients prompted the use of streptokinase in the next 2 patients and urokinase in the last 2 patients. Conventional treatment consisted of intravenous heparin followed by sodium warfarin.

Results.—The table summarizes the results of venography and/or duplex ultrasonography after treatment. Patients receiving thrombolytic therapy experienced better outcomes than those treated with conventional anticoagulation agents. Three of 4 patients receiving thrombolytic therapy had complete resolution of the symptoms and the thrombus; the remaining patient experienced a partial resolution that was confirmed by venography and duplex imaging. Three of the 6 patients treated with conventional anticoagulants had no resolution of symptoms and throm-

Cases of Effort Axillary-Subclavian Vein Thrombosis (ASVT)*

No.	Age	Sex	Time†	Arm Involved	Treatment	Clinical Response‡	Status of ASVT by Venogram (v)/Duplex (d)
1	35	M	2	Right	Heparin & warfarin	No improvement	Occluded—6 months (v)
2	45	F	3	Right	Heparin & warfarin	Some improvement	Occluded—6 months (d & v)
3	27	M	4	Right	Heparin & warfarin	No improvement	Occluded—1 year (d & v)
4	36	M	6	Left	Heparin & warfarin	Some improvement	Occluded—9 months (d & v)
5	51	F	3	Right	Heparin & warfarin	No improvement	Occluded—1 year (d & v)
6	32	M	5	Left	Heparin & warfarin	Full resolution	Open—6 months (v)
7	33	M	4	Right	Streptokinase, heparin & warfarin	Total resolution	Open—1 year (d & v)
8	28	M	3	Right	Streptokinase, heparin & warfarin	Some improvement	Partial resolution 8 months (d & v)§
9	41	M	5	Right	Urokinase, heparin & warfarin	Total resolution	Open—6 months (d & v)
10	25	M	2	Right	Urokinase, heparin & warfarin	Total resolution	Open—10 months (d & v)

*Pretherapy diagnosis was made by venous duplex and venogram in all patients.
†Time of onset of symptoms to start of therapy (days).
‡Defined as no improvement if arm swelling did not change during the course of treatment, some improvement if partial resolution of the swelling or arm pain was obtained, or total resolution if the arm size returned to normal with complete relief of pain.
§All patients treated with thrombolytic therapy had total resolution of the thrombus within 2 to 3 days of treatment (confirmed by venogram/duplex) with the vein remaining open, except patient 8.
(Courtesy of AbuRahma AF, Sadler D, Stuart P, et al: *Am J Surg* 161:459–465, 1991.)

bus, whereas 1 other had complete resolution and the remaining 2 had partial resolution of the symptoms but no resolution of the thrombus.

Conclusion.—These findings support the use of thrombolytic therapy as the treatment of choice for effort vein thrombosis in healthy patients if the condition is diagnosed within 7 days of the onset of symptoms. Thrombolytic therapy is preferred to conventional treatment because of the risk of disabling complications if conservative methods are not effective and to thrombectomy because of the risks of this operation.

▶ Lytic therapy for subclavian-axillary venous thrombosis uncovers the cause of the condition and allows a decision to be made regarding treatment by surgical intervention. Balloon dilation of the residual venous stricture is rarely successful.

Selective Low-Dose Thrombolysis in Patients With an Axillary-Subclavian Vein Thrombosis
Van Leeuwen PJCM, Huisman AB, Hohmann FR (Hospital Enschede, Enschede, The Netherlands)
Eur J Vasc Surg 4:503–506, 1990   20–30

Introduction.—Conservative treatment of the relatively rare clinical entity axillary-subclavian vein thrombosis has not enjoyed great success in prevention of postphlebitic syndrome. Thrombolysis, a technique that has been successful in treatment of occlusive syndromes, was proposed as a new treatment. The thrombolytic efficacy of a low dose of selectively delivered streptokinase infusion on axillary-subclavian vein thrombosis was investigated in 6 patients, 4 men and 2 women (average age, 32 years).

Treatment.—Fluoroscopy-confirmed axillary-subclavian vein thrombosis was primary in 5 patients and secondary, around a catheter system, in 1. The dominant arm was affected in 4 patients. Symptoms of thrombosis had lasted for a mean of 9 days at the time of treatment. Under fluoroscopic control, a catheter was inserted into the thrombus; after an initial 10,000-IU bolus, 10,000 IU of streptokinase was continuously infused per hour until effective thrombolysis was achieved. The catheter was repositioned by the radiologist 2 or 3 times daily. After thrombolysis, heparin was infused, and patients were given oral coumarin derivatives. They were discharged when symptom free.

Results.—All patients responded with recanalization and good flow of contrast medium; the mean time to achieve effective thrombolysis was 44 hours, with an average total dose of 500,000 IU of streptokinase. Only in the patient who had had symptoms for 6 weeks were residual venous wall defects observed. Urokinase in a dosage of 60,000 IU/hr was used with equal success as a substitute in 1 patient who had an allergic reaction to streptokinase. The average length of hospitalization was 11 days.

Discussion.—The success of the thrombolytic method for axillary-subclavian vein thrombosis is promising, because conservative treatment of this effort-induced thrombosis results in late sequelae in 30% to 91% of primary cases. The selective treatment requires a total dose of only 500,000 IU of streptokinase, in contrast to the 1.5 million IU/hr used for systemic treatment. Two important factors in the high success rate in this study were optimization of the catheter tip location by frequent repositioning and prompt treatment of patients after onset of symptoms. Although short-term results of this therapy are excellent, data on long-term outcomes are not yet available.

21 Primary Varicosities

Primary Venous Aneurysms
Friedman SG, Krishnasastry KV, Doscher W, Deckoff SL (Cornell Univ, Manhasset, NY)
Surgery 108:92–95, 1990   21–1

Background.—Venous aneurysms are a rare finding. Whereas rupture of an arterial aneurysm can occur if timely operation is not performed, rupture of a venous aneurysm is almost unheard of. Aneurysms of the popliteal vein are the most dangerous, and early surgical intervention is always indicated. Only 12 patients with popliteal venous aneurysms have been reported in the literature.

Patients.—Two men, aged 32 years and 41 years, initially noticed a painless swelling of the left upper extremity that decreased in size when the arm was raised and became prominent when the arm was placed in a dependent position. Both patients denied trauma. One patient was a sanitation worker and the other was an x-ray technician. Both patients underwent venography, which revealed a saccular dilatation of the cephalic vein. They both underwent excision of the aneurysms and ligation of the feeding vessels. The patients returned to work within 2 weeks and did well during 8 months of follow-up.

Case Report.—Woman, 42, with a 2-year history of a painless mass of the left neck, was found to have a 1.5-cm cystic mass over the anterior border of the sternocleidomastoid muscle. Ultrasound examination revealed an aneurysm of the external jugular vein with no intraluminal thrombus or other abnormalities. The lesion remained unchanged during 3 years of observation.

Conclusion.—Venous aneurysms are rare lesions, and their cause remains unknown. This entity should be included in the differential diagnosis of a subcutaneous mass.

▶ The venous aneurysm, a curiosity, is a focal dilation of a vein. The actual cause remains unknown but may involve defective connective tissue metabolism, congenital weakness, or degenerative change. The final histologic change is a decrease in smooth muscle cells and replacement of the vein wall by fibrous connective tissue. Only when the aneurysm is in a large vein that contains loosely attached thrombus does the condition become a threat to life.

Systemic Venous Aneurysms
Yokomise H, Nakayama S, Aota M, Daitoh N, Katsura H (Natl Himeji Hosp, Hyogo, Japan)
Ann Thorac Surg 50:460–462, 1990   21–2

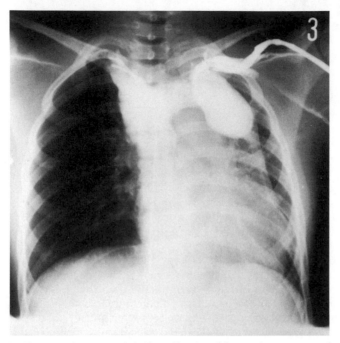

Fig 21–1.—Venous angiogram reveals fusiform dilatation of the superior vena cava and saccular dilatation of the left innominate vein. (Courtesy of Yokomise H, Nakayama S, Aota M, et al: *Ann Thorac Surg* 50:460–462, 1990.)

Background.—Nearly 10% of mass lesions in the chest are vascular in origin. Among these, systemic venous lesions are exceedingly rare: Only 17 superior vena cava (SVC) aneurysms have been reported since 1950. The advent of modern imaging techniques has made the older practice of exploratory thoracotomy unnecessary in such cases. Angiography and CT were used to advantage in the diagnosis of an SVC aneurysm combined with aneurysm of the left innominate vein.

Case Report.—Boy, 13 years, healthy and symptom free, was referred for assessment of shifting of the cardiac shadow to the left on his thoracic radiograph. The CT scan showed marked contrast medium uptake by an enlarged SVC and a left anterior mediastinal mass. Fusiform dilatation of the SVC and saccular dilatation of the left innominate vein were revealed by venous angiography (Fig 21–1). In no previous reports has the fusiform type of SVC aneurysm burst or produced thrombus, but surgical intervention was planned because the saccular aneurysm carried the risk of pulmonary embolism. This 5 × 4-cm aneurysm, into which the dilated second, third, and fourth intercostal veins drained, was resected after isolation and division of the veins. The left lung seemed hypoplastic. The enlarged SVC appeared normal and without clots, but an old clot was discovered inside the resected innominate vein aneurysm. Normal vein architecture ruled out inflammation and structural flaws. Venous angiograms 3 weeks after surgery showed no stenosis.

Discussion.—Of the 2 subtypes of SVC aneurysm, fusiform and saccular, only the saccular type appears to require surgical intervention; the prognosis for untreated fusiform aneurysms is excellent, judging from the literature. The etiology of SVC aneurysms is unknown, but it does not generally appear to be an inherent fragility of the vessel wall.

▶ Although systemic venous aneurysms are rare, it is apparent that the majority require no treatment whatsoever.

The Scanning Electron Microscope in the Pathology of Varicose Veins

Mashiah A, Rose SS, Hod I (Kaplan Hosp, Rehovot, Israel; Hebrew Univ, Jerusalem; Univ Hosp at South Manchester, England)
Isr J Med Sci 27:202–206, 1991   21–3

Introduction.—The etiology of varicose veins is still under study, but histologic and transmission electron microscope research suggests that a weak upper valve of the long saphenous vein is not the chief cause of varicose veins in the legs. Excised varicose veins, especially from the upper end of the long saphenous vein, were studied with a scanning electron microscope (SEM).

Methods.—Twenty-nine women (average age, 30 years) had undergone surgery for symptomatic varicose veins of the lower extremity. All 29 had a high ligation of the long saphenous vein at the saphenofemoral junction, removal of the upper vein, and multiple excisions of the varices. Specimens were immediately placed in 2.5% glutaraldehyde in buffered saline, and all segments were mounted alike for observation in a Jeol SEM.

Results.—All layers of the normal venous wall and the varices were easily observed, there being no alterations in the intima and adventitia. In the upper section of the saphenous vein, valve thickness, shape, and size appeared normal. The media of all varices exhibited marked thinning.

Implications.—The weakness of the venous wall in the varicose vein apparently can be localized or can occur in scattered areas. Interestingly, no changes were seen in the saphenofemoral valve itself, although all 29 patients were thought to have saphenofemoral valve incompetence. The weak vein wall theory, which proposes that valvular incompetence would affect the vein below the incompetent valve, was supported. Because varices often lie outside the long saphenous vein, the routine stripping of this vessel may not be effective and therefore is not recommended.

▶ It remains astounding that such a common condition as varicose veins could remain so poorly understood. Clearly, the condition is characterized by weakness of the vein wall, which allows dilation and elongation. The latter is the cause of the tortuosity. Varicosities develop along the main tributaries to the saphenous vein or originate from perforating veins. Secondary valvular incompetence occurs if the valve ring is affected by the weakening process. From a clinical point of view, studies such as this have confirmed that treatment of varicosities should concentrate on removal of the varix from the circulation, and that the greater saphenous vein and lesser saphenous vein should be removed only if those structures are varicose.

Reappraisal of the Oxygenation of Blood in Varicose Veins
Scott HJ, Cheatle TR, McMullin GM, Coleridge Smith PD, Scurr JH (Middlesex Hosp, London)
Br J Surg 77:934–936, 1990   21–4

Background.—The pathogenesis of varicose veins is incompletely understood. Several studies have implicated abnormal arteriovenous communications and resultant raised oxygen tension in venous leg blood as a causative factor. The oxygen tension of blood from patients with varicose veins was compared with that from normal legs. The effect of posture on these measurements also was examined.

Study Design.—The study was done in 13 patients with uncomplicated varicose veins and in 13 normal controls. In patients with varicose veins, blood samples were obtained from the cephalic vein and from a varicosity of the calf near the ankle, first after the patients lay supine for 30 minutes, and then after they stood for 30 minutes. In controls, blood samples were taken from the long saphenous vein. Blood samples were also obtained simultaneously from arm veins. Transcutaneous oxygen tension was measured continuously throughout the study.

Results.—Blood taken from varicose veins after the patients were supine for 30 minutes had a significantly higher oxygen tension than blood taken from the veins of normal controls. However, both patients and controls had higher oxygen tension in leg vein blood after lying supine than after standing for 30 minutes. Oxygen tension in arm vein blood was similar in both groups. Changes in transcutaneous oxygen tension correlated poorly with changes in oxygen tension in venous blood.

Conclusions.—Although these findings are consistent with the presence of arteriovenous shunting, the finding that normal controls also had higher oxygen tension in leg vein blood after lying supine than after standing suggests that other mechanisms must also be involved in the pathogenesis of varicose veins.

▶ Although it is acknowledged that varicose veins contain more oxygenated blood than normal veins, an explanation of this phenomenon has not been forthcoming, even though studies on this problem go back as far as 1843 and the subject has been analyzed by minds as great as Blalock's in 1929. Many studies, including those of Haimovici (1–3), have shown the presence of arteriovenous communications in patients with varicose veins. My own thought on the subject is that the capillary barrier is broached by the persistence of chronic venous hypertension, and that arteriolar oxygenated blood is dumped into the varicosities under high pressure. This, in turn, produces the abnormal warming of the skin in the region of the varicosities.

References

1. Haimovici H, et al: *Ann Surg* 164:990, 1966.
2. Haimovici H: *J Vasc Surg* 2:684, 1985.
3. Haimovici H: *Surgery* 101:515, 1987.

A Study of Estrogen and Progesterone Receptors in Spider Telangiectasias of the Lower Extremities

Sadick NS, Niedt GW (Cornell Univ, Ithaca, NY; Yeshiva Univ, Bronx)
J Dermatol Surg Oncol 16:620–623, 1990   21–5

Background.—Certain vascular tumors are associated with estrogen receptors, and vascular telangiectasias are associated with high levels of circulating estrogen. Estrogen and progesterone receptors were studied in patients with spider telangiectasias of the lower extremities.

Methods.—Thirteen women aged 22–50 had onset of lower extremity telangiectasias during pregnancy and/or oral contraceptive therapy. The diameters of the vessels ranged from .1–.6 mm. Frozen sections of biopsy material were cut and stained by the Golden-biotin-peroxidase method. Rat antibody to the human estrogen receptor and progesterone receptor was used, with diaminobenzidine as chromagen. All 13 women were assayed for antibody-to-estrogen receptors, and 8 were also assayed for antibody-to-human-progesterone receptors.

Results.—None of the women had positive estrogen receptor staining with the monoclonal antibody to human estrophilin. Nor did any have positive progesterone receptor staining with the monoclonal antibody to human progesterone.

Conclusions.—Apparently, telangiectasias of the legs with onset during pregnancy or oral contraceptive therapy do not arise from elevated levels of estrogen or progesterone receptors in the lesions. Because estrogen receptors seem to be absent in such lesions, the theory that estrogens mediate the formation of these vascular lesions is questionable.

▶ Because estrogen and progesterone clearly have profound effects on the venous system, it is disappointing that estrogen and progesterone receptors are not found in spider telangiectasias. This study shows that many aspects of venous pathophysiology remain to be elucidated.

A Comparison of Sclerosing Agents: Clinical and Histologic Effects of Intravascular Sodium Morrhuate, Ethanolamine Oleate, Hypertonic Saline (11.7%), and Sclerodex in the Dorsal Rabbit Ear Vein

Goldman MP (Univ of California, San Diego)
J Dermatol Surg Oncol 17:354–362, 1991   21–6

Background.—Sclerosing solutions (only sodium morrhuate, ethanolamine oleate, and sodium tetradecyl sulfate have been approved by the

US Food and Drug Administration) produce endothelial damage that eventuates in endofibrosis. The effects of various concentrations of sodium morrhuate, ethanolamine oleate, hypertonic saline 11.7%, and Sclerodex on the dorsal rabbit ear vein were assessed.

Methods.—The dorsal marginal ear vein was injected with Sclerodex; hypertonic saline 11.7%; 2.5%, 1%, and .5% ethanolamine oleate; or .25 mL of 2.5%, 1%, or .5% sodium morrhuate. The clinical appearance was graded and documented photographically just before injection and biopsy. Biopsies were done at 1 hour, 2 days, 10 days, and 45 days after injection.

Results.—The only vessel that had clinical and histologic evidence of endosclerosis with microangiopathic recanalization was the vessel injected with 2.5% sodium morrhuate. Partial clinical sclerosis and luminal recanalization was seen histologically with 2.5% ethanolamine oleate. All other solutions, except for .5% ethanolamine oleate, caused immediate clinical and histologic endothelial damage and thrombosis. However, they did not produce enough endothelial damage for endosclerosis to occur. Extravasated red blood cells occurred in vessels injected with 1% and 2.5% ethanolamine oleate and 1% and 2.5% sodium morrhuate at 1 hour and 2 days. They did not occur in vessels injected with sodium morrhuate .5%, ethanolamine oleate .5%, Sclerodex, or hypertonic saline 11.7%. There was no apparent hemosiderin discoloration or cutaneous necrosis.

Conclusions.—Because the extent of extravasation of red blood cells is related to the degree of endothelial destruction, it appears that more concentrated and stronger sclerosing solutions produce a higher incidence of postsclerotherapy hyperpigmentation. They also appear to produce a higher degree of perivascular and intravascular inflammation. Thus, at least as seen in this animal model, endothelial destruction sufficient to cause endofibrosis may also result in extravasation of red blood cells.

▶ Endothelial destruction is an essential element in obliteration of telangiectasias and varicose veins. If extravasation of red blood cells inevitably follows endothelial destruction, cutaneous pigmentation is to be expected. Unfortunately, such pigmentation is frequently permanent and is highly undesirable.

Sclerotherapy of Varicose and Telangiectatic Leg Veins: Minimal Sclerosant Concentrations of Hypertonic Saline and Its Relationship to Vessel Diameter

Sadick NS (Cornell Univ, New York)
J Dermatol Surg Oncol 17:65–70, 1991   21–7

Background.—As sclerotherapy has increased in popularity, the number of sclerosants that are available for this procedure has also increased. Side effects such as ulceration, pigmentation, and vascular neogenesis may be related in part to endothelial disruption, a function of sclerosant concentration. The effects of increasing concentrations of a sclerosant (hypertonic saline) with regard to vessel diameter, clinical efficacy, complications, and discomfort were tested in a double-blind, paired-comparison study.

Results.—Six hundred women with bilaterally symmetrical starburst telangiectasias or varicose veins were treated. Sodium chloride 11.7% was the lowest sclerosant concentration of saline that produced the most effective sclerosis of vessels measuring less than 8 mm in diameter; it also caused the fewest complications. With this concentration, 17.5% of the patients had cramping; 9%, thrombus formation; 5.5%, thrombophlebitis; 2.5%, postsclerosis telangiectatic mats; and 2%, postsclerotic pigmentation. None of the patients had extravasation necrosis.

Conclusion.—Although the 11.7% concentration of hypertonic saline appears to be the optimal sclerosant for vessels less than 8 mm in diameter, the optimal concentration of a particular agent may vary with the diameter of the vessels being treated.

▶ Hypertonic saline as a sclerosant agent would not be associated with anaphylactic reactions but is a highly caustic material that produces pain on injection. These studies by Sadick will be helpful in decreasing the deleterious effects of highly concentrated hypertonic saline.

Pulsed Dye Laser Treatment of Telangiectases With and Without Subtherapeutic Sclerotherapy: Clinical and Histologic Examination in the Rabbit Ear Vein Model

Goldman MP, Martin DE, Fitzpatrick RE, Ruiz-Esparza J (Univ of California, San Diego)
J Am Acad Dermatol 23:23–30, 1990   21–8

Introduction.—Sclerotherapy is most often used to treat telangiectases of the leg, but postsclerosis pigmentation and telangiectatic matting are frequent problems. Various forms of laser treatment have also been used but have produced adverse sequelae in excess of those seen with sclerotherapy. A subtherapeutic concentration of sclerosing solution was combined with use of a pulsed dye laser to specifically damage the endothelium of subcutaneous vessels.

Methods.—The 585-nm pulsed dye laser was used alone and combined with sclerotherapy in the rabbit ear vein model. A .25-mL volume of .25% polidocanol was injected immediately after laser treatment.

Results.—The laser by itself was effective at a level of 10 J/cm². When combined with injection of sclerosant, endosclerosis took place using laser energies of 8–10 J/cm². Sclerotherapy alone produced no evidence of endothelial damage. Combined treatment did produce endothelial damage as well as organizing thrombus formation. Endofibrosis or perivascular fibrosis was evident within 10 days. At 45 days there was evidence of recanalization in vessels treated with 8–9 J/cm², but not in those treated with 9.5–10 J/cm².

Discussion.—The pulsed dye laser enhances the efficacy of a sclerosing agent in this model. Telangiectatic matting may be reduced in laser-treated vessels because less perivascular inflammation develops.

▶ Usually, combined treatments cause enhanced side effects. This may not be true when laser energy is added to sclerotherapy, or it may be that hyperpigmentation will still occur because laser energy allows extravasation of red blood cells into the dermis of the skin.

Postsclerotherapy Hyperpigmentations: A One-Year Follow-Up
Georgiev M (Rome)
J Dermatol Surg Oncol 16:608–610, 1990   21–9

Introduction.—Early postsclerotherapy hyperpigmentation (PSH) usually fades and disappears in 1–3 years, but in some cases, unesthetic staining may persist.

Findings.—Of 100 patients with varicose veins who underwent sclerotherapy, 15 had some light brown pigmentation after 1–4 months of treatment. Pigmentation occurred following iodine/NA iodide injection in 53% of the patients and following polidocanol injection in 47%. Although other sclerosing agents may carry less risk of skin staining, they are too weak for use on larger veins. The mechanism of PSH is believed to be both hemosiderinic and melaninic (Fig 21–2). Topical medications with chelating agents did not prevent or cure PSH.

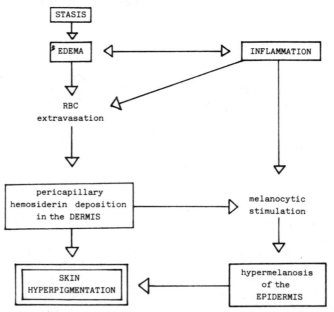

Fig 21–2.—Mechanism of skin hyperpigmentation; note the role of edema and inflammation. (Courtesy of Georgiev M: *J Dermatol Surg Oncol* 16:608–610, 1990.)

Results.—After 1 year, 1 patient still had some linear pigmentations and 4 others had barely visible pigmentation of no cosmetic significance. Only 1% of the patients (.66% of limbs treated) had cosmetically significant pigmentation after 1 year. Four other patients had resolved to barely visible pigmentation of no cosmetic significance.

Discussion.—Treatment of superficial veins produces the greatest risk of PSH. Controlling treatment factors such as concentration of the solution, paravenous injection, retention of blood and compression times minimizes visible signs of the inflammatory reaction. With proper sclerosing technique, the cosmetic risk of sclerotherapy is extremely low.

▶ Hyperpigmentation is an undesirable side effect of sclerotherapy of telangiectatic blemishes. Some of the hyperpigmentation is permanent, but, fortunately, most of it disappears over time.

Long Saphenous Vein Saving Surgery for Varicose Veins: A Long-Term Follow-Up

Hammarsten J, Pedersen P, Cederlund C-G, Campanello M (Hosp of Varberg, Sweden)

Eur J Vasc Surg 4:361–364, 1990   21–10

Background.—The autologous saphenous vein is the graft material of choice for infrainguinal arterial reconstructions. Hence, unnecessary removal of the long saphenous vein should be avoided. The long-term effects of long saphenous vein-saving surgery were compared with those of standard stripping in 42 patients with varicose veins.

Intervention.—Twenty-four patients were randomly assigned to standard stripping of the long saphenous vein and 18 to high ligation with division of the vein at the saphenofemoral junction. In both groups, local varicosities were avulsed. Perforators were ligated on the basis of physical examination and phlebography. The suitability of the preserved long saphenous vein as a conduit for revascularization was assessed with high-resolution, real-time ultrasonography. The mean follow-up period was 52 months.

Results.—Excellent or good results were achieved in 88% of the group that had stripping and 89% of those having high ligation. Recurrence rates were 11% in the patients who had stripping and 12% in the group having high ligation. Based on the criteria of Seeger et al., 14 of 18 (78%) of the preserved long saphenous veins were suitable for arterial conduits. The maximum diameters of the preserved veins at different levels of the limb ranged from 3 to 3.7 mm. In 2 patients the preserved vein could not be identified; in the other 2, the maximum diameter of the vein was less than 2.5 mm.

Conclusions.—Removal of the long saphenous vein is of no therapeutic value if sufficient perforators have not been ligated. Elective venous surgery for varicose veins can be performed with good results and preservation of the long saphenous vein for future arterial reconstructions in most patients.

▶ The saphenous vein can indeed be preserved for future use in arterial surgery. However, treatment of the varicose condition itself is dependent on detachment of all insufficient perforating veins from the saphenous vein segment. This was achieved in the Swedish study by careful use of phlebography. In North America, surgery for varicose veins is not as far advanced as in Sweden and, therefore, removal of the long saphenous vein for gross reflux is still justifiable and predictably will give the best long-term results.

22 Chronic Venous Insufficiency

▶ ↓ As treatment of chronic venous insufficiency is relatively unsatisfactory, this chapter will explore newer theories of etiology of the syndrome and newer attempts at treatment.

Venous Muscle Pump Function During Pregnancy: Assessment by Ambulatory Strain-Gauge Plethysmography
Struckmann JR, Meiland H, Bagi P, Juul-Jørgensen B (Gentofte Hosp, Copenhagen; Univ of Copenhagen)
Acta Obstet Gynecol Scand 69:209–215, 1990   22–1

Background.—Previous studies have suggested that compression by the growing uterus and a hormonally modulated increase in venous distensibility may both cause decreased circulation to the lower extremities in late pregnancy; 5% to 10% of pregnant women have such venous disorders in the lower extremities. Changes in the function of the venous muscle pump during pregnancy were studied.

Methods.—Ten primiparous and 14 multiparous women aged 20–37 years were examined at weeks 16, 30, and 38 of normal pregnancy and at 3 months after delivery. At each examination subjective claims of fullness, cramps, unrest, itching, swelling, and pain were registered, and objective clinical signs of edema, pigmentation, eczema, induration, varicosities, and incompetent perforating veins were noted. Blood samples were taken for radioimmunoassay study of levels of estradiol, estriol, and progesterone; ambulatory calf volume strain-gauge plethysmography was done to calculate venous return time (RT) and expelled volume (EV); and occlusion strain-gauge plethysmography was performed to measure total venous volume, maximal venous outflow, and arterial inflow.

Results.—Effectiveness of the venous muscle pump decreased in the last trimester, as indicated by a significant mean reduction in RT from 79.3 seconds at 16 weeks to 64 seconds at 38 weeks, and returned to the initial mean value of 81.5 seconds 3 months post partum. During pregnancy EV did not change significantly but it increased significantly post partum. In 17% of patients overall there was abnormal function of the venous muscle pump between 16 and 38 weeks of pregnancy. By week 38 of pregnancy, 66% of women had indications of vascular insufficiency, particularly swollen legs (Fig 22–1). A significant reduction in arterial inflow was found in late pregnancy.

Discussion.—Although RT decreased during pregnancy, this effect could not be correlated with levels of estradiol, estriol, or progesterone.

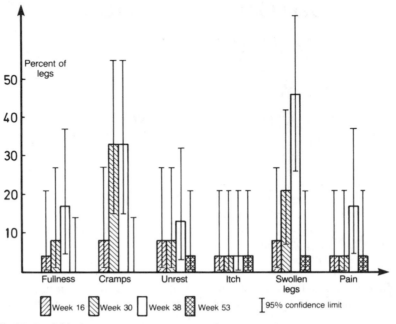

Fig 22–1.—Subjective symptoms in pregnancy weeks 16, 30, and 38, and 3 months postpartum (week 53). Proportion of patients with each quality is presented. *T* indicates 95% confidence limits. (Courtesy of Struckmann JR, Meiland H, Bagi P, et al: *Acta Obstet Gynecol Scand* 69:209–215, 1990.)

Thus it is likely that increased venous reflux is caused by mechanical obstruction of the inferior vena cava and iliac veins by the growing uterus or by increased venous distensibility caused by hormones other than those tested. The late pregnancy (38 weeks) decrease in arterial inflow could prolong venous refilling time and produce an underestimate of venous reflux at this time. Because venous hemodynamics normalize spontaneously after delivery, venous insufficiency during pregnancy should be handled conservatively; the use of compression stockings in the second and third trimesters may alleviate the problem.

▶ Because the hormones progesterone, estradiol, and estriol are clearly important to venous stasis, this study assumes relevance. Each of the hormones was found to peak at week 38 of pregnancy, coincident with the peaking of symptoms of fullness, swollen legs, and night cramps. Objective estimates of edema and development of pigmentation were made during this time. All of these are functions of venous distensibility and correlate clinically with maximal symptoms during the menstraul cycle that women express to the alert physician. That is, the symptoms of primary varicosities are maximal during the progesterone-dominated last 14 days of a menstrual cycle. They peak during the first 2 days of a menstrual period. Physiologic studies in the article reviewed in this abstract do not pinpoint the exact cause of these symptoms but do note the relationship.

Severity and Location of Venous Valvular Insufficiency: The Importance of Distal Valve Function

Rosfors S, Lamke L-O, Nordström E, Bygdeman S (St Göran's Hosp, Stockholm)
Acta Chir Scand 156:689–694, 1990   22–2

Introduction.—Chronic venous insufficiency results from loss of valvular function with venous reflux. In patients with severe chronic venous insufficiency, reflux is found more commonly in the deep than in the superficial veins. The regional distribution of venous reflux affects the results of different diagnostic tests in different ways. For example, plethysmography at foot or ankle level will not show reflux limited to the proximal veins. Venous calf pump function was evaluated with special reference to the distribution and severity of deep venous reflux at different levels.

Patients.—During a 2.5-year period, 98 patients aged 20–86 years were evaluated for venous insufficiency. All underwent ultrasonography, foot volumetry, and venous plethysmography; 32 patients also underwent phlebography and measurement of intravenous pressure. In 13 extremities there was known or strongly suspected earlier deep vein thrombosis. Surgery had been performed on the superficial venous system in 30 limbs.

Results.—There was a clear relationship between clinical stage of chronic venous insufficiency and location and number of segments with venous reflux. Clinically important deep venous insufficiency was found mainly in patients with reflux in the distal posterior tibial veins and was observed even if the patient had competent popliteal valves.

Conclusion.—The calf pump appears to be divided functionally into a series of venous pumps, with the distal valves in the lower leg being more important than the popliteal valves in the proximal part of the leg. Adequate assessment of venous calf pump function requires evaluation of venous valvular function at different levels.

▶ As the physiology of valvular reflux becomes more precisely defined, it becomes clear that a competent proximal valve (e.g., a popliteal or femoral) will not prevent totally the symptoms and findings of chronic venous insufficiency. Although the problem is confused by the finding of venous reflux in some asymptomatic limbs, these may be considered precursors of venous stasis. If this is true, then a clear relationship between number of segments refluxing and stage of chronic venous insufficiency is to be expected, a hypothesis that is proven by the article abstracted here.

Venous Hemodynamics in a Chronic Venous Valvular Insufficiency Model

Lalka SG, Unthank JL, Dalsing MC, Cikrit DF, Sawchuk AP (Richard L. Roudebush VA Med Ctr, Indianapolis; Indiana Univ, Indianapolis)
Arch Surg 125:1579–1583, 1990   22–3

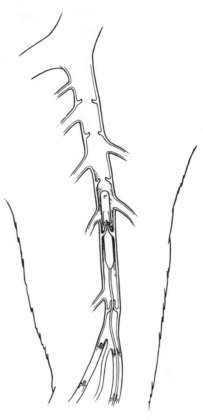

Fig 22–2.—Diagram of valve lysis procedure. Usually 5 to 8 valves are encountered in the iliac, femoral, and lateral saphenous veins. (Courtesy of Lalka SG, Unthank JL, Dalsing MC, et al: *Arch Surg* 125:1579–1583, 1990.)

Introduction.—Research into deep venous insufficiency is impeded by lack of laboratory models that allow the study of this problem and its surgical management. A large-animal model of long-term valve incompetence was developed for use in assessing various venous reconstructive techniques.

Method.—Thirteen adult dogs had unilateral hindlimb venous valve lysis. A valve cutter apparatus was pulled through the iliac, femoral, and lateral saphenous veins, where it usually encountered 5–8 valves (Fig 22–2). Bilateral venous pressure was measured before lysis, immediately after, and several times during a 14-week period with the dogs in the supine position, elevated 80 degrees semierect, and with their hindlimb venous system emptied.

Results.—Hemodynamic determinations disclosed shortened venous filling time, 90% venous refilling time, and elevated poststimulation venous pressure after valve lysis. All animals had hemodynamically documented venous valvular insufficiency at time of death. There was no external evidence of valvular insufficiency (e.g., ulcers, edema) during the 14-week period.

Conclusions.—This upright, large-animal model of venous valvular insufficiency facilitates the study of deep venous valve reconstructive surgery. The model was stable, reproducible, and hemodynamically monitored, successfully producing a verified venous valvular insufficiency model.

▶ This group from Indiana University is to be congratulated for creating an experimental model that allows study of venous pathophysiology. Other models of valve incompetence developed since 1965 have proven inadequate to the study of the important changes that occur when valvular insufficiency occurs in man.

Preliminary evaluation of the studies reveals that venous filling time, pressure, and venous recovery time were altered by the experimental valvular insufficiency. This situation is exactly what is found in physiologic studies in human venous stasis.

Fibrin- and Fibrinogen-Related Antigens in Patients With Venous Disease and Venous Ulceration
Falanga V, Kruskal J, Franks JJ (Univ of Miami; Vanderbilt Univ)
Arch Dermatol 127:75–78, 1991   22–4

Background.—Although several studies have implicated abnormalities in systemic fibrinolysis in the pathogenesis of venous ulcerations, little is known about the metabolism of fibrinogen and fibrin in patients with venous disease. An attempt was made to characterize the systemic fibrin abnormalities in patients with venous disease of the lower extremities.

Methods.—Using a technique that involves electrophoresis and densitometric analysis of captured fibrin-related antigens, the concentration and proportions of the individual fibrin and fibrinogen degradation products were measured in 18 patients and 15 healthy controls. Eleven patients had venous disease with ulcers and 7 patients had venous disease and lipodermatosclerosis but without ulceration.

Results.—In patients with venous disease with or without ulceration, the levels of total fibrin-related antigen and D-dimer, the terminal degradation product of cross-linked fibrin, were markedly elevated. In contrast, the levels of D-monomer, the terminal degradation fragment of fibrinogen and a measure of fibrinogenolytic activity, and non–cross-linked fibrin monomer were normal in all patients. In patients with ulceration, the levels of D-dimer were disproportionately higher than expected from the concentration of fibrin monomer. In individual patients, the levels of D-dimer were significantly elevated in 55% of those with venous disease with ulcers and in 43% with venous disease but no ulcers.

Conclusion.—Patients with venous disease have uniform evidence for enhanced fibrin formation, regardless of the presence of ulceration. Considering the previous finding of pericapillary deposition of fibrinogen/

fibrin products in skin taken from edges of venous ulcers, these observations suggest a pathogenic linkage of tissue-fibrin deposition and faulty fibrinolysis with the expression of venous disease and venous ulceration.

▶ In patients with venous disease, fibrinogen is important in 2 ways. The first is in formation of thrombi and the production of venous insufficiency characterized by the postphlebitic state. The second is the formation of pericapillary fibrin cuffs that interfere with oxygen transport in the areas of maximal venous stasis. The latter theory has not withstood the test of time. Attempts to enhance fibrinolysis by steroid administration have failed to find a place in treatment of the late effects of chronic venous insufficiency. On the other hand, the study abstracted here suggests that the thrombotic element remains in patients with venous stasis disesae. Elevated levels of total fibrin-related antigen and D-dimer in the serum suggest continuing thrombus formation and lysis in these patients.

Histological Study of White Blood Cells and Their Association With Lipodermatosclerosis and Venous Ulceration
Scott HJ, Coleridge Smith PD, Scurr JH (Middlesex Hosp, London)
Br J Surg 78:210–211, 1991   22–5

Background.—In patients with high venous pressure, "trapped" white blood cells may occlude the capillaries, which release superoxide radicals and proteolytic enzymes that damage the microcirculation. Conventional histologic techniques were used to quantify the white blood cell content of the skin in patients with venous disease, and the effect on white blood cell content of raising venous pressure in the limbs was assessed.

Methods.—The study sample comprised 19 patients with proven venous disease, all undergoing inpatient treatment for varicose veins. Eight of the patients had lipodermatosclerosis of the skin, and 6 had a history of ulceration. Patients were randomly assigned 2 groups, 1 studied after 30 minutes of lying supine and the other after sitting with the leg dependent to raise venous pressure. Punch biopsies of skin were taken, including an area of lipodermatosclerotic skin from affected patients, and then the groups were switched and another biopsy taken. White blood cells were counted by conventional histologic methods.

Results.—The median white blood cell count in uncomplicated varicose veins was 6.2/mm^2. In the lipodermatosclerotic samples the median count was 45 cells per mm^2, and in the samples from patients with a history of ulceration, median count was 217 cells per mm^2. Sitting with the limb dependent caused no significant alterations in these counts.

Conclusions.—Patients with venous disease have increased numbers of white blood cells in their skin, resulting in lipodermatosclerotic changes. The white blood cell count is particularly high in patients with a history of ulceration. It is unknown whether the increase in the white blood cell content of the skin causes or results from the skin changes.

▶ Now that the fibrin cuff theory of chronic venous insufficiency is in its waning phase, students of venous pathophysiology turn to the theory that centers on white blood cell trapping. This is represented by the article abstracted here. It is clear that limbs affected by chronic venous insufficiency retain many more white blood cells than normal limbs. Possible mechanisms of action include capillary occlusion and leukocyte activation, which causes release of superoxide radicals and proteolytic enzymes; this, in turn, damages the vascular endothelium. In the present histologic study, many more white blood cells were observed in the skin of patients with liposclerotic changes. Thus the indurative process is an obviously inflammatory condition. Let's hope that studies such as this will yield further information on the metabolic activity of white blood cells and the part played by their release of mediators of inflammation, such as cytokines, tumor necrosis factor, and interleukin-1.

Sequential Gradient Pneumatic Compression Enhances Venous Ulcer Healing: A Randomized Trial
Smith PC, Sarin S, Hasty J, Scurr JH (Univ College and Middlesex School of Medicine, London)
Surgery 108:871–875, 1990   22–6

Background.—Intermittent pneumatic compression (IPC) is an alternative to elastic compression for the management of venous ulcers. It is designed to promote venous blood flow and its use has enhanced systemic fibrinolytic activity.

Procedure.—A controlled study compared IPC with standard treatment, including débridement and the wearing of graduated compression stockings, in patients with venous ulcers present for at least 12 weeks. Patients with significant vascular disease were excluded. A sequential compression device (SCD) was applied over the compression stockings in study cases. The 21 study patients and 24 controls were clinically comparable. Both groups had had ulceration for 3½ to 4 years on average.

Results.—Ten patients treated with the SCD and 1 control patient had complete healing of all ulcers. Nearly half of all ulcers in the SCD group healed within 12 weeks, compared with 11% of those in control patients. Treatment was well tolerated. Many patients had attempted to use the device for a full 4 hours a day.

Conclusion.—It appears that sequential gradient pneumatic compression is an effective and safe approach to treating venous ulceration. Healing may reflect altered blood flow, changes in fibrinolysis, or white cell adhesion.

▶ This study is attractive for several reasons. The first is that the method of treatment advocated was added to best medical care, which included the wearing of heavy-weight elastic stockings. In addition, randomization was decided by a coin toss, which is eminently more understandable than a table of random numbers. Furthermore, the sequential compression avoided trapping of blood produced by uniform or 1-cell compression devices. It is entirely possible that sequential pneumatic compression enhances fibrinolytic activity, alters white blood cell adhesion, and improves oxygen transport by reduction of edema. Each of these concepts is an area for future fruitful research.

Reconstructive Surgery in Chronic Venous Obstruction of the Lower Limbs

Danza R, Navarro T, Baldizán J (Maciel Hosp, Montevideo, Uruguay)

J Cardiovasc Surg 32:98–103, 1991   22–7

Patients.—Forty-three operations to restore blood flow were carried out on 41 patients who had chronic venous insufficiency caused by venous trunk obstruction in the lower extremity. Indications for surgery included progressive limb edema, venous claudication while walking, and trophic lesions. Iliac vein obstruction was most frequent, followed by obstruction of the superficial femoral vein; 2 patients had obstruction at both levels.

Techniques.—Iliac vein obstruction was managed by autotransplantation of the great saphenous vein. Currently, the saphenous vein of the donor leg is excised and reanastomosed to the same vein. Isolated obstruction of the superficial femoral vein is bypassed using the great saphenous vein or an in situ saphenopopliteal bypass. For obstruction at both levels, free venovenous femorofemoral bypasses are done along with an in situ saphenopopliteal bypass. Three patients who had had the common femoral vein ligated in infancy and experienced postphlebitic syndrome underwent bypass from the superficial vein to the patent external iliac vein using the contralateral great saphenous vein.

Results.—Nearly 85% of patients had good to excellent results after free femorofemoral venous grafting of iliac vein obstruction. Good results generally were also obtained in patients with superficial femoral vein obstruction and iliac vein thrombosis associated with superficial femoral venous thrombosis. Femoroaxillary bypasses yielded good results in 3 patients with cavoiliac obstruction.

Discussion.—Only bypass operations and venous transplants have given consistently good results in direct venous surgery for chronic obstruction. Reconstruction with a polytetrafluoroethylene prosthesis remains experimental. Intraoperative and postoperative anticoagulation is essential.

▶ Each of the previous abstracts in this chapter was selected to elucidate the pathophysiology of chronic venous insufficiency and provide a rationale for conservative treatment. As surgeons, we are concerned with surgical reconstruction of veins in order to reduce disabilities of chronic venous insufficiency. In the article abstracted here, Danza et al. review their 20-year experience, during which time they concentrated on relief of the obstructive element of chronic venous insufficiency. Their work shows that autogenous tissue can be used for free femorofemoral venous grafts, the Palma procedure, and even in femoroiliac or femoroaxillary bypass. Unfortunately, methods of objective assessment of results were not used, nor was it possible to assess the long-term effects of bypass reconstructions. However, others have suggested that the results of distal reconstruction (e.g., saphenopopliteal grafting) are not good when followed over the long term.

Why Do So Few Surgeons Perform Reconstructive Venous Surgery? Reconstruction for Deep Venous Insufficiency in the 1990's
Eriksson I (Univ of Uppsala, Uppsala, Sweden)
Acta Chir Scand Suppl 555:187–191, 1990   22–8

Background.—Venous reconstruction overall has been far less successful than arterial surgery. High failure rates are ascribed to low pressure and flow in the venous system, low oxygen tension, and a tendency toward thrombogenicity. Adequate management of advanced chronic venous insufficiency requires precise and comprehensive anatomical and functional evaluation. It is especially important to define the degree of reflux, the chief feature of deep venous disease.

Outflow Obstruction.—Long-term patency can be achieved in bypass reconstruction for relief of outflow obstruction using grafts of autogenous venous tissue. Among synthetic prostheses, polytetrafluoroethylene is the only alternative. Bypass has a definite role in relieving sustained venous hypertension secondary to unilateral iliac vein obstruction. Femoral vein bypass surgery involving anastomosis of the saphenous vein on the affected side to the popliteal vein has given less encouraging results.

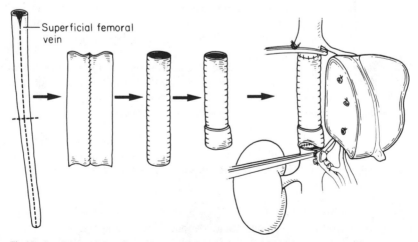

Fig 22–3.—Preparation and anastomosis of superficial vein graft for inferior vena caval replacement. (Courtesy of Schwartz ME, Schanzer H, Miller CM: *J Vasc Surg* 13:460–461, 1991.)

Deep Venous Reflux.—Several antireflux procedures have been used for repairing leaking deep venous valves directly. Valvuloplasty has been done most often on a valve in the superficial femoral vein; it is a reasonably durable procedure. Valve transposition is an alternative means of restoring competency to the deep venous system. Most transplants, however, have functioned for only a short time.

The Future.—An adequate tissue is needed for use in valve transplantation. Prospective studies should be done comparing conservative management with valve surgery. Single- and multi-level repairs also should be compared.

▶ As suggested by the previous abstract, reconstruction of the venous system for obstruction appears to be promising when the reconstructions are in proximal veins. When the reconstructions are at the superficial femoral or popliteal level, the results are less good. Valve reconstruction procedures, on the other hand, remain in the category of experimental surgery. They must be done, but they must be evaluated objectively so that progress can be made in this field of endeavor.

Use of the Superficial Femoral Vein as a Replacement for Large Veins
Schwartz ME, Schanzer H, Miller CM (Mount Sinai School of Medicine, New York)
J Vasc Surg 13:460–461, 1991   22–9

Background.—The need for reconstruction of large veins is infrequent, but current vascular techniques and grafts allow for safe and effective reconstruction. Synthetic grafts have provided high patency rates and a low incidence of thrombosis, especially compared with prosthetic grafts. The use of autogenous vein grafts, particularly the saphenous vein, has yielded the best patency rates, low rates of thrombogenesis, and good resistance to infection. The superficial femoral vein (SFV) has been proposed as an alternative to the saphenous vein in lower limb revascularization.

Case Report.—Woman, 34, underwent repair of the vena cava; the SFV was used with good results. Preparation of the graft was relatively simple and quick, and the diameter of the graft matched the vena cava well. Eversion of the graft at the lower end allowed for perfect tailoring of length (Fig 22–3).

Conclusion.—On the basis of graft patency at long-term follow-up in this case, and good results in using SFV for portal vein replacement in another patient, the SFV is recommended as the preferred graft for replacement of large veins.

▶ Transplantation of the SFV for use as an arterial conduit has produced remarkably little objectively measurable venous insufficiency. It is important in the case described here that normal venous physiology was objectively measured in the donor limb. Thus the SFV may be regarded as a possible tissue bank for autogenous replacement of large veins.

Subject Index

A

Abdomen
abscess, *Salmonella choleraesuis,* 117
vasculature, ultrasound of, duplex
Doppler, 207
Abscess
abdominal, *Salmonella choleraesuis,*
117
Acrocyanosis
in anorexia nervosa, 35
Aged
endarterectomy, carotid
over 75, 194
predicting complications, 194
stroke and carotid artery stenosis, 169
Amputation
of lower extremity, outcome, 154
Anastomosis
aortoprosthetic, end-to-side, CT of, 259
femoral noninfected anastomotic
aneurysm, 273
prosthetic anastomotic false aneurysm,
etiology, 274
vascular, with absorbable suture
material (in dog), 275
Anesthesia
epidural, and deep vein thrombosis after
knee arthroplasty, 334
epidural with general, in aortic surgery,
58
Aneurysm(s)
aortic
abdominal, atheromatous, hemoptysis
due to, 103
abdominal, disease, inflammation in,
112
abdominal, epidemiologic necrospy,
73
abdominal, family study results, 74
abdominal, immune-mediated
response in, 83
abdominal, inflammatory, 113
abdominal, inflammatory, cells in
parietal infiltrate of, 113
abdominal, inflammatory, as disease
entity, 115
abdominal, inflammatory, histological
analysis, 115
abdominal, infrarenal, surgery results,
97
abdominal, inheritance of, 75
abdominal, with perianeurysmal
fibrosis, 114
abdominal, repair, and coronary
artery disease, 61
abdominal, repair experience, 92

abdominal, repair, with myocardial
revascularization, 109
abdominal, resection, elective,
experience with, 94
abdominal, resection, long-term
survival, 96
abdominal, rupture, Harborview
experience, 100
abdominal, rupture, management, 99
abdominal, rupture, presenting as
colonic obstruction, 104
abdominal, rupture probability in
unrelated operative procedure, 98
abdominal, *Salmonella* infection in,
116
abdominal, small, CT of, 86
abdominal, surgical volume and
experience in, hospital type and
mortality, 93
abdominal, survival after operative
and nonoperative management, 84
abdominal, survival and size, 101
CT of, ultrafast, 90
diameter aortic diameter ratio in
rupture risk, 89
dissecting, elastic architecture
alterations in, 65
embolization in, distal, 91
mutation in gene for type III
procollagen in, 77
repair, arteriography for assessment,
87
repair, tube, aneurysmal change in
iliac arteries after, 107
rupture, 67
rupture, repair, perigraft pseudocyst
complicating, 110
surgery, kidney failure after, 111
arterial
in children, classification, 237
models of, 21
brachiocephalic, early recognition and
repair, 239
elastase-induced (in rat), 78
femoral artery, mycotic, antibiotics for,
238
femoral noninfected anstomotic, 273
form of aortoarteritis, 80
hepatic artery, diagnosis and treatment,
241
humeral circumplex artery, thrombus
from, 232
intestinal artery, surgery of, 242
popliteal
artery, follow-up and surgery results,
248
conservative management, 247

Author Index

A

Aabech, J., 49
Aarts, J.C.N.M., 52
Abbott, R.D., 1
Abbott, W.M., 187
Abdool-Carrim, A.T.O., 96
Abet, D., 312
AbuRahma, A.F., 94, 348, 352
Adams, D.H., 19
Admani, A.K., 169
Adu, D., 111
Adzick, N.S., 202
Agrifoglio, G., 273
Aguilar, J.L., 36
Agus, G.B., 273
Åkesson, H., 342
Alachkar, F., 192
Albat, B., 264
Albers, J.J., 5
Alberts, J., 311
Albrand, J.-J., 216
Alexander, J.B., 69
Alimi, Y., 216
Almgren, B., 114
Ameli, F.M., 50, 107
Amplatz, K., 4, 26
Amundsen, S., 93
Anderson, F.A., Jr., 332
Anderson, R.J., 191
Andria, G., 11
Andris, D.A., 351
Andros, G., 53
Anidjar, S., 78
Ansari, H., 312
Anthmyr, B.A., 336
Aota, M., 355
Archie, J.P., Jr., 172
Arias, J.D., 205
Arlart Von, I.P., 249
Armstrong, S., 33
Arnetz, B.B., 46
Arnold, W.P., 229
Artru, B., 219
Arvanitis, D.P., 293
Astara, C., 47
Athanasoulis, C.A., 57
Attar, S., 70
Azancot, M., 294

B

Baert, A.L., 223
Baethge, B.A., 326
Bagi, P., 365
Baird, R.N., 33
Bakal, C.W., 227
Baker, P.L., 338
Bakhos, M., 109
Baldizán, J., 372
Balfe, J.W., 221
Balslev, I.B., 118

Bandyk, D.F., 29
Barber, G.G., 101
Barnett, H.J.M., 179
Barr, H., 255
Barry, J., 60
Bartholomew, J.R., 317
Bartlett, S.T., 142
Bartoli, J.M., 135
Basil, A., 304
Bass, A., 86
Batellier, J., 209, 211
Bates, W.B., III, 110
Baudouin, C.J., 292
Baxter, B.T., 91
Beals, R.K., 290
Beaman, M., 111
Beckett, W.C., 291
Becquemin, J.P., 271
Bell, D.D., 87
Bell, W.H., III, 182
Belli, A.-M., 292
Benichou, H., 190
Benson, L.N., 288
Berg, P., 260
Bergentz, S.-E., 222
Bergeron, P., 190, 268
Bergmark, C., 138
Bergqvist, D., 114, 222, 330
Berisa, F., 111
Berland, L.L., 56
Bermann, M., 311
Bernhard, V.M., 193
Bernstein, E.F., 86, 197
Berry, R., 347
Bertuch, H., 228
Besancenot, J., 180
Beschu, D., 156
Beta, E., 18
Beven, E.G., 203
Bhanji, S., 35
Binaghi, F., 47
Birnbaum, E., 99
Bissett, J.K., 4
Bisson, B.D., 5
Black, I.W., 286
Blakeman, B., 109
Blanksma, C., 113
Blue, J.M., 241
Boland, J.P., 94, 352
Bonijoly, S., 341
Bonnefoi, B., 166
Bonneville, J.-F., 180
Bookstein, J.J., 256, 296
Boontje, A.H., 113
Bornstein, N.M., 176
Bosch, J., 311
Bouchier-Hayes, D., 106
Bour, P., 260
Bourseau, J.C., 97
Bouvard, J., 192
Bower, T.C., 147, 239
Bowyer, R.C., 247
Bradshaw, M.W., 269
Branchereau, A., 135, 262, 274

Brand, F.N., 1
Brand, R., 248
Brandjes, D.P.M., 323
Breitbart, G.B., 191
Brewster, D.C., 187
Brook, R.H., 194
Brophy, C.M., 112
Brown, G., 5
Brown, M.M., 184
Bryan, D.J., 233
Brzowski, B.K., 291
Buche, M., 344
Buchwald, H., 4
Buckner, N.K., 296
Büller, H.R., 323
Bunt, T.J., 59
Burch, J.M., 303
Burdick, J.F., 131
Burney, D.P., 241
Burrows, P.E., 288
Butler, P., 184
Bygdeman, S., 46, 367

C

Cahalane, S., 10
Callam, M.J., 266
Callejas, J.M., 325
Calligaro, K.D., 227
Cambria, R.P., 187
Camelot, G., 180
Cameron, J.L., 314
Camilleri, J.-P., 78
Camishion, R.C., 69
Campanello, M., 363
Campbell, D.R., 143
Campbell, G.S., 4
Campbell, J.J., 87
Campos, C.T., 4
Canzanello, V.O., 212
Capel, G.C., 238
Carbone, L., 11
Carboni, M.R., 47
Carney, W.I., Jr., 288
Carr, H.M.H., 246
Carrozzo, R., 11
Casals, A., 325
Case, W.G., 102
Cassel, W., 58
Castañeda-Zúñiga, W.R., 4, 26
Castelli, P.M., 273
Cattin, F., 180
Cavallaro, A., 155
Cavallino, R.P., 285
Cawthorn, S.J., 247
Cederlund, C.-G., 363
Celani, V.J., 151
Cenacchi, G., 113
Cernaianu, A.C., 69
Chaillou, P., 97
Chaing, F.L., 23

393